Principles and Practice of Gynecologic Laser Surgery

Principles and Practice of Gynecologic Laser Surgery

Joseph H. Bellina, M.D., Ph.D.

Director, Laser Research Foundation
New Orleans, Louisiana

and

Gaetano Bandieramonte, M.D.

National Cancer Institute of Milan
Milan, Italy

Plenum Medical Book Company • New York and London

Library of Congress Cataloging in Publication Data

Bellina, Joseph H.
  Principles and practice of gynecologic laser surgery.

  Includes bibliographical references and index.
  1. Lasers in surgery. 2. Gynecology, Operative. I. Bandieramonte, Gaetano, 1946–
II. Title. [DNLM: 1. Lasers — Therapeutic use. 2. Genitalia, Female — Surgery. WP 660
B444p]
RG104.B36   1984   618.1'059   84-3434

ISBN-13: 978-1-4612-9684-3   e-ISBN-13: 978-1-4613-2713-4
DOI: 10.1007/978-1-4613-2713-4

Dedicated to our children
Shawn and Todd
Viviana and John

Foreword

One of the first applications of lasers was for surgery on the retina of the eye. That, and the evident analogy to the old dreams of powerful heat rays, led many to predict that lasers would quickly be used for all kinds of cutting and welding, including surgical applications. It was soon apparent that laser surgery could be performed in ways that caused little bleeding. Nevertheless, other surgical applications have been slower to arrive.

One difficulty has been the enormous range of possibilities provided by the many different kinds of lasers. Infrared, visible, and ultraviolet light beams each interact very differently with human tissues. Light pulses of enormously great peak powers became available from lasers, but their effects differed in surprising ways from those obtained with continuous beams. That provided both opportunities (i.e., treating or removing a very thin surface layer without affecting the underlying tissue) and problems with undesired side effects. Moreover, techniques were needed to deliver a precisely controlled amount of energy just where it was desired. Lasers also had to be engineered and manufactured with the desired power levels and a high reliability.

Thus, it has required the combined efforts of surgeons, medical scientists, physicists, and engineers to overcome these difficulties and to make lasers the increasingly useful surgical tools that they have become. Dr. Bellina is one of the leading pioneers of gynecologic laser surgery. He is a founder of the Gynecologic Laser Society, which has very successfully brought together people of various disciplines to develop and understand the new tools and their possibilities.

Foreword

It is entirely possible that future progress in this field will be even more dramatic than anything envisioned now. Surely anything that can be done will rest on the foundation that Dr. Bellina and his colleagues have created, and on the cooperative efforts they have fostered. But the techniques that are available now are dramatically powerful, and deserve the widespread application that this book will help to make possible.

Arthur L. Schawlow
Nobel Laureate
Stanford University
Stanford, California

Preface

The past decade has witnessed the proliferation of several types of lasers, as well as applications for these instruments in medicine. This text will primarily address the molecular gas laser (and provide a brief overview of additional laser models), with particular attention being given to the carbon dioxide laser, as applied to gynecologic procedures.

It was in view of the recent explosive growth in the number of surgical procedures, which have embraced the advantages of the laser, and the untoward effects which can result from limited knowledge of the tool, that we were prompted to write this book. The laser must be approached with respect and caution, and one should be meticulously prepared before attempting to use it. It is with this approach that we have undertaken to prepare this tutorial. We have assumed that the reader knows little or nothing about lasers or their application to surgery and, thus, we have addressed such basic questions as *What is a laser? How and in what circumstances may it be used?* and *What are the advantages of using a laser over other modes of treatment?* In pursuit of answers to these questions, we have endeavored to begin by presenting the laser physics theory in a readily digestible form and to progress to the advanced theory, offering a menu to suit a variety of palates.

The major thrust of the research is the clinical investigation of the carbon dioxide laser and its effect on neoplasias, vulvar dystrophies, and other premalignant diseases of the external genital tract. Step-by-step, both verbally and graphically, the reader will be taken through the selection of laser surgery candidates; preoperative, operative, and postoperative treatment; and management of the patient. We will address the action, reaction, and interaction effects of laser-treated tissues. And, in like fashion, the reader will be guided through the technical aspects of preparing the surgical suite, selection of instruments, and ancillary personnel requirements. Safety and biological considerations are outlined and a review of federal and local regulations is included, as well as instructions for obtaining certification.

We hope the text will serve as a source of reference and a stimulus to advance laser surgery to the status of an exact technique in all branches of medicine. It was our intention to make this book readable, practical, and concise, while providing a comprehensive guide to surgical care of the gynecologic patient with this advanced, less traumatic, and most modern of surgical techniques.

Joseph H. Bellina
Gaetano Bandieramonte

Acknowledgments

We are indebted to numerous colleagues and friends for their help and contributions, and permanently indebted to the members of the Laser Research Foundation who have made it possible for us to produce this work. We are particularly indebted to Jeff Jackson and Linda Hoang for their help in preparing this manuscript, and to Alessandra Melchiorre for her devoted and loving attention to this book and the endless tasks associated with it. In addition, our thanks to Delia Malone for her artwork.

This work was supported in part by the National Research Council (Rome, Italy) and the National Oriented Project on Laser Medical Applications who supported a postdocotral fellowship for one of the authors (G.B.) at the Laser Research Foundation in New Orleans.

Special thanks go to Professor Emanuelli, Director of the Laser Center of Medical Applications at the National Cancer Institute of Milan, and to Professor V. Veronesi, Director of the National Cancer Institute of Milan, for their support in allowing laser gynecologic activity to be successfully realized at the Cancer Institute and in encouraging our collaboration by facilitating the necessary working meetings. Thanks also go to Drs. G. Fava and R. Marchesini of the Health Physics Service, National Cancer Institute, Milan, who provided the comprehensive glossary of physical terms and reviewed the section on physics.

Deep thanks to the colleagues and friends of the Outpatient Department of the National Cancer Institute of Milan, directed by Professor S. Di Pietro, who have patiently contributed to the collection of the study population data and collaborated on the definition of the indications for laser treatment and participated actively in discussions of the possibilities and limits of, as well as the selection of patients for, laser treatment.

Additionally, we would like to thank our assistant editors, Patricia Moorehead and Wanda Bolleter.

Last, but not least, we would like to thank our families, in particular Delia, for being understanding during the time that the manuscript was in preparation and allowing us to devote the amount of time we had. We truly appreciate the sacrifice that they have made.

J.H.B.
G.B.

Contents

Chapter 1

An Introduction to Lasers 1

1.1. General Information 1
1.2. Theoretical Background 3
1.3. Historical Data 6
1.4. Basic Physics of Generating Laser Energy 6
    1.4.1. Energy Levels in Atoms 8
    1.4.2. Generation of Light 10
    1.4.3. Emission and Absorption 10
        1.4.3.a. Spontaneous Emission 10
        1.4.3.b. Absorption 11
        1.4.3.c. Stimulated Emission 11
        1.4.3.d. Additional Characteristics 11
    1.4.4. The Laser 13
        1.4.4.a. Active Medium, Pumping 13
        1.4.4.b. Optical Cavity 14
        1.4.4.c. Loss and Gain Phenomenon 15
        1.4.4.d. Steady State 16
        1.4.4.e. Standing Waves 16
1.5. The Molecular Gas Laser (Carbon Dioxide Laser): Energy
Levels in Molecules 17
    1.5.1. Ground Level at Zero Energy Level 17
    1.5.2. Excited Level (V_1) or Symmetrical Stretch Mode 17
    1.5.3. Excited Level (V_2) or Bend Mode 18
    1.5.4. Excited Level (V_3) or Asymmetrical Stretch Mode . . . 18

Contents

1.5.5. Energy Transfer 19
1.6. The Liquid Laser 20
1.7. The Solid-State Laser 20
1.8. The Semiconductor Laser 21
1.9. General Characteristics of Lasers in Medicine 21
    1.9.1. The Ruby Laser 24
    1.9.2. The Argon Laser 24
    1.9.3. The Neodymium-YAG Laser 25
    1.9.4. The Carbon Dioxide Laser 25
    References 25

Chapter 2

Carbon Dioxide Laser Instrumentation 27

2.1. General Description 27
2.2. Biophysical Data 31
    2.2.1. Terminology of Laser Irradiation 31
    2.2.2. Absorption and Reflection 32
    2.2.3. Significance of Coefficients 34
    2.2.4. Power Density 36
    2.2.5. Transverse Electromagnetic Mode and Its Significance 40
    2.2.6. Laser Modes and Effects of Temperature on Mode
        Stability 41
    2.2.7. Biophysical Parameters of CO_2 Surgical Lasers and
        Dosimetry 44
    2.2.8. Clinical Conclusions 45
2.3. Current CO_2 Laser Models 46
    2.3.1. Introduction 46
    2.3.2. Troubleshooting the System 62
    2.3.3. Basic Office System 63
    2.3.4. Office Suite Operating Room Supplies 63
    2.3.5. Operating Suite System 66
    2.3.6. Recording System 67
    2.3.7. Ancillary Equipment 67
        2.3.7.a. Evacuation System 67
        2.3.7.b. Waveguides 70
2.4. Laser Safety 70
    2.4.1. General Information 70
    2.4.2. Hazards of Medical Lasers 71
        2.4.2.a. Injury by Primary Action of the Laser Beam 72
        2.4.2.b. Injury by Secondary Effects of the Laser
            Beam 72

2.4.2.c. Protecting the Patient's Eyes from Laser
Radiation 72
2.4.2.d. Damage to Skin and Underlying Tissues 74
2.4.2.e. Protecting Skin and Underlying Tissues 74
2.4.2.f. Toxic or Pathogenic Effect of Smoke or Vapor
from the Intended Target 75
2.4.3. Government Regulations for Laser Safety 76
2.4.3.a. Federal Regulations 76
2.4.3.b. Local Regulations 78
References 78

Chapter 3

Bioeffects **81**

3.1. Introduction 81
3.1.1. Experimental Studies 82
3.1.2. Clinical Studies............................ 82
3.1.2.a. Cytologic Analysis 82
3.1.2.b. Histologic Analysis..................... 83
3.1.2.c. Scanning Electron Microscope Analysis 84
3.1.2.d. Clinical Findings 87
3.1.3. Theoretical Analysis and Experimental Verification ... 88
3.1.3.a. Theoretical Analysis of Heat Transfer—
General 88
3.1.3.b. Theoretical Analysis—Closed-Form Solution . 90
3.1.3.c. Experimental Verification 91
3.1.3.d. Summary of Theoretical Findings 93
3.1.3.e. Conclusion 97
3.2. Plume Emission Analysis 97
3.3. Photoacoustic Properties 99
3.4. Photon–Tissue Interaction 102
3.4.1. Experimental Design 102
3.4.2. Results.................................. 103
3.4.3. Discussion 103
References 108

Chapter 4

Applications in Gynecology with Emphasis on the Cervix **111**

4.1. Introduction to Laser Surgery 111
4.2. Clinical Applications in Gynecology 115
4.3. General Considerations of Applications in Cervical
Intraepithelial Neoplasia.......................... 115

Contents

4.4. Cervical Applications 117
    4.4.1. Epidemiology 117
    4.4.2. Pathology 118
    4.4.3. Preoperative Analyses 125
    4.4.4. Patient Selection 127
4.5. Technical Approach to CIN Lesions 127
    4.5.1. Microsurgical Procedures 127
    4.5.2. Instruments, Equipment, and Patient Preparation for
            Cervical Microsurgery 128
    4.5.3. Anesthesia 130
4.6. Vaporization Procedure 130
4.7. Excisional Conization 135
    4.7.1. Technical Approach 136
    4.7.2. Pathologic Examination 140
    4.7.3. Combined Procedures 140
4.8. Postsurgical Care 141
4.9. Evaluation of Healing 142
4.10. Follow-up Examinations 143
4.11. Current Research on CIN 144
4.12. Complications 148
4.13. Laser Technique versus Conventional Methods 149
    4.13.1. Laser Vaporization versus Cryosurgery and Diathermy 149
    4.13.2. Laser Conization versus Cold Knife Conization and
             Hysterectomy 151
4.14. Other Indications for Laser Surgery 153
    4.14.1. Stenosis 154
    4.14.2. Lacerations 155
    4.14.3. Bicollis Configuration 155
    4.14.4. Adenosis and Cervical Changes Associated with
             Diethylstilbestrol Exposure in Utero 156
    4.14.5. Polyps 156
    4.14.6. Leiomyoma 156
    4.14.7. Cervicitis 157
    References 157

Chapter 5
Laser Surgery of the Vagina, Vulva, and Extragenital Areas 165

5.1. Introduction 165
5.2. Vaginal Applications 165
    5.2.1. Adenosis 165
    5.2.2. Dystrophy and Neoplasia 167

5.2.3. Postoperative Care and Follow-up 168
5.2.4. Reconstruction 169
    5.2.4.a. Longitudinal Vaginal Septum 169
    5.2.4.b. Transverse Vaginal Septum 169
    5.2.4.c. Gartner's Duct Cyst and Other Vaginal
        Inclusion Cysts 170
5.3. Vulvar Applications 170
    5.3.1. Introduction 170
    5.3.2. Preoperative Analysis 171
    5.3.3. Dystrophic and Neoplastic Lesions 172
    5.3.4. Premalignant Disease and Degenerative Dystrophia ... 172
    5.3.5. Carcinoma in Situ 173
    5.3.6. Primary or Secondary Invasive Neoplastic Lesions 173
    5.3.7. Procedure 174
    5.3.8. Tissue Reaction 174
    5.3.9. Postoperative Management 175
    5.3.10. Complications, Results, and Follow-up 177
5.4. Lower Genital Tract Multicentric Viral Lesions 178
    5.4.1. Condyloma Acuminatum Lesions 178
    5.4.2. Preoperative Analysis 178
    5.4.3. Sequence of Therapy 179
    5.4.4. Technique of Management 180
    5.4.5. Postoperative Management 180
    5.4.6. Complications and Results 181
    5.4.7. Herpes Simplex Virus Type 2 182
5.5. Other Sites 183
    5.5.1. Peritoneal Labial Fusion 183
    5.5.2. Hymenotomy 183
    5.5.3. Anal Lesions 184
    5.5.4. Periurethral Lesions and Skene's Ducts 184
    5.5.5. Bartholin's Gland Abscess and Cyst Management 184
    5.5.6. Other Cutaneous Lesions 184
    References 185

Chapter 6

Intra-abdominal Applications **187**

6.1. Introduction 187
6.2. Instrumentation 190
    6.2.1. Current Laser System for Microsurgery 191
    6.2.2. Laser Micromanipulator 191
    6.2.3. Omega Modification of Laser Micromanipulator 193

Contents

6.2.4. Laser Scalpel 195
6.2.5. Laser Accessory Instruments..................... 195
6.2.6. Laser Laparoscopy 195
6.2.7. Operating Room Modification..................... 196
6.2.8. Recording System: General 198
6.2.9. Recording System: Specialized Video–Cine
       Modification 199
6.3. Microsurgical Procedures 199
6.3.1. Adhesiolysis 200
6.3.2. Fimbrioplasty and Salpingostomy 201
6.3.3. Tubal Reanastomosis 202
6.3.4. Cornual Reimplantation 202
6.3.5. Ectopic Pregnancy: Linear Salpingostomy 203
6.3.6. Endometriosis 204
       6.3.6.a. Endometrial Implants 204
       6.3.6.b. Endometrioma: Ovarian Type 205
       6.3.6.c. Bowel Endometrioma..................... 205
6.3.7. Uterine Anomalies 206
       6.3.7.a. Septal Defects........................ 206
       6.3.7.b. Bicornuate Uterus 207
       6.3.7.c. Uterine Leiomyomata 207
6.3.8. Tubal Anomalies 208
       6.3.8.a. Intraluminal Polyps 208
       6.3.8.b. Bifid Fallopian Tubes................. 208
       6.3.8.c. Defective Fimbria Ovarica 209
6.3.9. Ovarian Procedures 209
       6.3.9.a. Cystectomy............................ 209
       6.3.9.b. Incisional and Excisional Approach 210
       6.3.9.c. Wedge Resection 210
6.3.10. Rectovaginal Repair........................... 210
6.4. Conclusion 211
     References 212

Appendixes

Appendix A. Zeiss Operating Microscope 215
       I. Optical Principles, Illumination Systems, and
          Support Systems 217
      II. Individual Parts, Handling, Assembling, Focus-
          ing, and Balancing 223
     III. Accessories 233

xviii

IV. Documentation 239
V. Maintenance and Cleaning 253
Appendix B. Patient Information: Laser Surgery 257
Appendix C. Discharge Instructions 259
Appendix D. Informed Consent 261
Appendix E. Laser Certification 263
Appendix F. Societies 267
Appendix G. Publications 269
Appendix H. Glossary of Laser Terminology 271

Index 281

Principles and Practice of Gynecologic Laser Surgery

1

An Introduction to Lasers

1.1. General Information

The tools of surgery did not undergo significant modifications until this century. As the scalpel, scissors, and saw belong to the earliest period of medicine, high-frequency bipolar cautery and cryosurgery are tools of modern medicine, but generally all lack precision of application. The impetus of precise tissue removal and the tendency toward conservative treatments have stimulated innovative surgeons to investigate new surgical modalities—hence, a rapid proliferation of new surgical instruments described as LASERS. *What is a laser? What role does the laser play in modern medicine? Will the laser be of benefit to my patient?* These questions are being asked each day in medicine in advertisements and courses, and, the public media cry out: *Why not use the laser?*

LASER is the acronym for light amplification (by) stimulated emission (of) radiation. A similar acronym is RADAR or radio detection and ranging. LASER is simply a name for a family of systems used in energy transfer.

Investigation into the use of the carbon dioxide laser as a totally new surgical mode has been underway since 1967. The CO_2 laser has been demonstrated to have unique capabilities for surgical procedures and excellent results have been observed. Since completion of the experimental research phase around 1972,[1-4] the use of the CO_2 laser beam has rapidly spread, and now it is routinely used in a number of disciplines, for a number of procedures, in a variety of institutions throughout the world. Moreover, surgically, it can be used for cautery and to vaporize or excise diseased tissue. The devel-

1

opment of surgical applications has to be considered rapid in relation to the short period of time in which instrumentation has been available. Now there are more than 20,000 clinically documented cases in which the laser was the primary mode of treatment.

To report briefly on the number of disciplines and the variety of procedures now embracing the versatility of the laser, a number of examples may be cited. In otorhinolaryngology, excellent results have been obtained in the treatment of laryngeal papillomas and in tumor tissue resections of the pharynx, oral cavity, nose, and sinuses[5-9]—including microsurgical procedures.[3] In thoracic surgery, the CO_2 laser has been used to perform thoracotomies and has provided a less traumatic and more efficient mode of treating benign tumors of the trachea and bronchi.[10] Benign and malignant dermatologic tumors,[11] hyperplastic scars, keloids, burns,[12-14] and tattoos have been successfully treated with the CO_2 laser. Additionally, several authors have reported on the advantages of using the laser in neurosurgical and microsurgical techniques.[15-16] and since 1974, others have described the surgical application of the CO_2 laser in intra-abdominal disease and in the lower genital tract.[17] In gynecologic surgery, the laser can be attached to a surgical arm and handpiece, or to an operative microscope or colposcope for microsurgery. and, properly used, it can destroy or excise an extremely small or extremely large area of tissue to any depth.

The cervix, vulva, and vagina appear to be useful models in demonstrating the expediency of the CO_2 laser in the treatment of patients with neoplastic disease in an easy but effective way, when compared to more conventional methods. Hysterectomy is now considered to be overtreatment for many neoplastic cervical lesions and the gynecological surgeon chooses not to sacrifice large areas of normal tissue in order to excise a focal area of disease. This accounts for the increasing use of cervical cryodestruction and diathermy under colposcopic direction. Consequently, it has been demonstrated that hysterectomy and even cone biopsy can be avoided in many cases and laser procedures can be performed on an outpatient basis with minimal discomfort.

Since the layers of damaged cells after laser treatment are often merely a few cells in width and depth, laser surgery represents the epitome of conservatism and has revolutionized the management of gynecologic disorders, including malignancies and premalignancies. It has the added benefit of the exclusive and precise removal of the diseased area, respecting and preserving the adjacent healthy tissue. Nevertheless, lack of familiarity with this instrument can create skepticism. A misunderstanding of the role and the practical principles of physics of the CO_2 laser not only can lead to disappointing results and deviation from the exact application of this newest surgical mode, but may also inhibit the recognition of its enormous potential in surgery and prohibit beneficial exploitation of this instrument. Thus, principles of physics pertinent to the application of the CO_2 laser will be summarized, in addition to the effects of tissue irradiation, in order to identify the advantages of using the laser in gynecologic procedures.

1.2. Theoretical Background

A young, brilliant scientist, whose name is synonomous with $E = mc^2$—Einstein—literally changed the course of history with his theoretical basis of laser action—stimulated emission of radiation—which he first proposed in 1917.[18] Early in his thinking, he noted that light and color were the result of wave properties and interaction with **photons.** The photon is the "other" property given to light when the wave theory fails. Interestingly, today, scientists are still discussing *What is light? . . . wave or particle?** It can be assmed that both can be correct under given circumstances. With this basic assumption in mind, we delve into the realm of physics.

First, we begin with a single atom with the electron cloud and nucleus in harmony at the resting state. This resting state of the electron cloud, or **ground zero,** is assigned a quantum number to indicate that the system (nucleus and electron) is resting or at the lowest energy level. Now consider what would happen if the electron orbit becomes disturbed and shifts away from the nucleus. In order to achieve this new suborbit, energy must be supplied to overcome the nuclear pull on the electron. This energy can be supplied by applying heat to stimulate the atom's electron cloud. This phenomenon is easily seen by heating an iron skillet. The resting *cold* (skillet) iron molecules are black and solid, but as you heat the skillet it becomes hotter until it is red in color. The electrons have gained energy from the fire so that they are no longer resting and *black* but now move at *red-hot speed.* Further heating or stimulation results in *white-hot* electrons where the electron energy has shifted to yield all visible wavelengths (i.e., white spectrum). This phenomenon represents the electron orbit shift during heating and cooling. As the skillet cools, the stimulated orbits return to a resting state and the black color returns. We have now seen quantum shifts and the effect they demonstrate by direct observations. The colors described were produced by

---

*Christian Huygens (1629–1695), physicist; proposed wave theory of light. Sir Isaac Newton (1642–1727), mathematician and physicist; proposed particle theory of light.

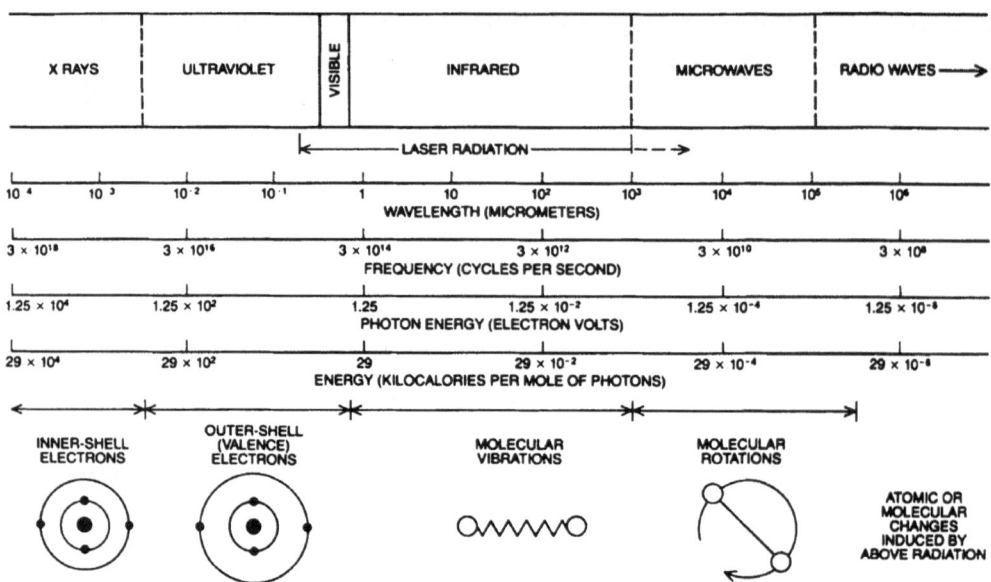

Figure 1.1. The electromagnetic spectrum spans from gamma rays into the long-range radio waves. The human eye can detect electromagnetic wavelengths from 390–780 nm.

the photons or symphony of wavelengths released in the heating and deexcitation processes.

With this background, let us take a step further. Each color we observed while heating the skillet (i.e., stimulating process) resulted in our retina detecting the colors (photon emissions) whose wavelengths were either red (600–650 nm) to white or a mixture of all color, including wavelengths of (400–780 nm in length). This means that color is related to wavelengths and changes in energy stages. Some colors are detectable, others are invisible. Our retina can detect between 390 and 780 nm in wavelength. However, other wavelengths exist, such as infrared or ultraviolet. How far can we take this model if we could see all the waves known to man? The electromagnetic spectrum ranges from γ rays to radiowaves (Fig. 1.1) and each wavelength has a particular property and each photon has a predictable color or effect. For example, X rays have one effect while radiowaves have another. The effect is a function of the wavelength and the energy stored in the photon. Again, we must consider each case separately.

Let us first discuss the X-ray photon. This photon has a wavelength that is extremely small (i.e., 1×10^{-4} μm). Compare this to the radiowave of 1×10^6 μm. Now remember that all light travels at the same speed; in the air the velocity is $\sim 3 \times 10^{10}$ cm/sec. In this model, you should envision a very small and a very large wave moving in space. As you travel on this wave in your mind's eye you come upon an atom with many clouds of electrons such as the iron atom. What will happen? Due to the extremely small wavelength, the X ray flies past the outer electron clouds of the atom until it approaches the small compact clouds around the nucleus and here it collides similarly to billiard balls. And, as with billiard balls, something has to give: a particle (an electron) is dislodged and sent into space. This altered state results in ionization, a phenomenon well known to radiotherapists. Now consider the large radiowave. As you travel on this wave, you approach millions of atoms per second. The wave gently distorts this sea of atoms and the result is music or sound. By carefully exploring the total electromagnetic spectrum you can go from X ray to radiowave and predict the properties based on wavelength and photon energy.

Now that this basic physics has been mastered, let us return to the stimulated atom. We understand that the stimulation effect is predictable; that is, X amount of heat to make red hot, Y amount of heat to make white hot. This predictable property (X or Y) is a **quantum** of energy. Each atom shift occurs in a predictable fashion and will reverse in a predictable fashion. The reversibility or release of stored energy (quantum) is a major premise in the making of a laser. Assume that if two stimulated atoms collide, each will release its quantity of energy simultaneously and in equal amounts. This simultaneous release of energy is known as **temporal** behavior—this denotes that all the photons (waves) are coherent or marching together like waves on the sea. This phenomenon was described by Einstein as stimulated emission of radiation. Remember, radiation relates to electromagnetic radiation (i.e., X ray to radiowave) and that it is a physical term to denote movement.

To complete the laser, it is necessary to amplify the light or waves. This is easily accomplished by placing mirrors in the path of the waves and adjusting the mirror surfaces to reflect the waves back and forth. This amplification causes the waves to be in time (temporal), equally spaced (spatial), and of the same wavelength (quantum). We now have **coherent** or laser light. How do we get the light past the mirrors? The easiest and most effective way is to simply make one of the mirrors 90% reflective. This means that 10% of the light will pass through the mirror and, thus, a laser is born. Finally, as all light behaves according to the natural laws of physics, it can be reflected or refracted in a predictable fashion. This means that electromagnetic waves produced by lasers can be focused, reflected by appropriate surfaces, and even put into wave guides or light pipes. Today there are solid, liquid, and gas lasers. Atoms, molecules, and solid state materials can be made to laser. The same properties of stimulating the atom, distorting the molecule, or creating stress in semiconductors can result in a predictable quantum change in energy, which, if properly harnessed, can be used to benefit mankind.

At this point, we wish to apologize to physics and engineering students for the oversimplification of the laser, but we must confess that this is the way we came to understand lasers. Now, let us return to advancing our understanding of light and its properties.

1.3. Historical Data

The concept and mathematical principles for lasers were set forth by Einstein. In 1954,[19] Gordon and colleagues, as well as Basov and Prokhorov,[20] set forth the physical principles of the MASER (microwave amplification by stimulated emission of radiation). This work revealed that wavelengths of various sizes could be made to act in accordance with Einstein's principles of stimulated emissions. In 1958 Schawlow and Townes extended the principle of the maser into the optical frequency range.[21] Maiman, in 1960,[22] created the first working ruby laser. This laser, a most complex system, was composed of a synthetic ruby made of an aluminum oxide crystal, into which a small amount of ionic chromium had been introduced as an impurity in the medium. The first gas laser, a helium–neon (HeNe) laser, was created by Bennett and co-workers in 1961.[23] In the same year, Johnson and Naussau developed the neodymium–yttrium–aluminum–garnet (Nd-YAG) laser. In 1964, C. K. N. Patel created the CO_2 laser for Bell Laboratories.[24] The CO_2 laser was designed for rapid communication, using the 10.6 μm wavelength as the carrier signal. In 1968, at the American Optical Laboratories, Bredmeier and Polanyi, in collaboration with Jako, began animal experimentation with the CO_2 laser.[25] The CO_2 system was modified to be used in conjunction with an operating microscope and the first description of this system in gynecologic surgery was described by Bellina.[17]

The extraordinary characteristics of laser stirred the imagination of researchers and raised the hope that lasers would offer help in the fight against cancer. As with all new modalities, success tempered with moderate disillusionment was the rule. With the advent of the carbon dioxide laser, again new hopes rose in he field of surgical ablation of neoplastic tissue (Table 1.1).

1.4. Basic Physics of Generating Laser Energy

To explain in full detail how a laser works, a great deal of advanced physics and mathematics is required; but for a qualitative picture, one needs

Table 1.1.   Historical Data

Year	Investigator(s)	Discovery
1667	Isaac Newton	Corpuscular light theory
1670	Christian Huygens	Wave theory
1917	Einstein	Stimulated emission
1953	Weber	Population inversion
1954	Gordon, Zeiger, Townes, Basov, and Prokhorov	Proposed principles of MASER
1958	Townes and Schawlow	Initially proposed principle of laser
1960	T. Maiman	Constructed the first pulsed ruby laser
1961	Bennett, Herriott, and Javan	First gas laser at the Bell Laboratories (He–Ne gas)
1961	Johnson and Naussau	Developed the neodymium-HAG (Nd-YAG) laser
1962	Bessis and Coll	First microscope coupled with the ruby laser for cellular microsurgery
1964	Patel	Investigated molecular gas laser for communication purposes using monatomic, diatomic, and other molecular media for a laser effect (Bell Laboratories, New Jersey)
1964–1966	Yahr and Strully	Application of ruby laser. First investigations of surgical properties of CO_2 laser. Ruby was later abandoned (heavy impact of this pulsed laser caused spreading of viable tumor cells in the tissue surrounding the tumors) because of the appearance of argon, CO_2, and Nd-YAG (American Optical)
1966		Appearance of argon laser and application in experimental ophthalmology
1968	Patel	Built the first CO_2 laser
1968	Polanyi, Jako, and Bredemeier	Micromanipulator adaptation for microsurgical use
1970		Appearance in the commercial market of argon as photocoagulator
1971		Hall defined the effects of CO_2 laser on tissues
1972	Jako	CO_2 laser began to be used in laryngeal surgery in humans (American Optical, Boston)
1973	Verschueren	CO_2 laser in tumor surgery
1974	J.H. Bellina	CO_2 laser in gynecologic surgery
1977		Proliferation of techniques in gynecology throughout the world
1980		CO_2 laser used in a number of medical centers around the world for surgical procedures

only to accept some of the results of the advanced theories, which can be simplified and in most cases easily visualized.

1.4.1. Energy Levels in Atoms

Light can be generated in atomic processes, which will be reviewed briefly; laser light is a consequence of these atomic processes.

The atom consists of a small, positively charged nucleus and of negatively charged electrons. The nature of the systems of nuclei and electrons cannot be described by the familiar Newtonian laws of classic mechanics, which apply to ordinary bodies and to the sun and planets. For the submicroscopic particles of atomic size, a new type of mechanics is used that is called **quantum mechanics**. The most important concept of quantum

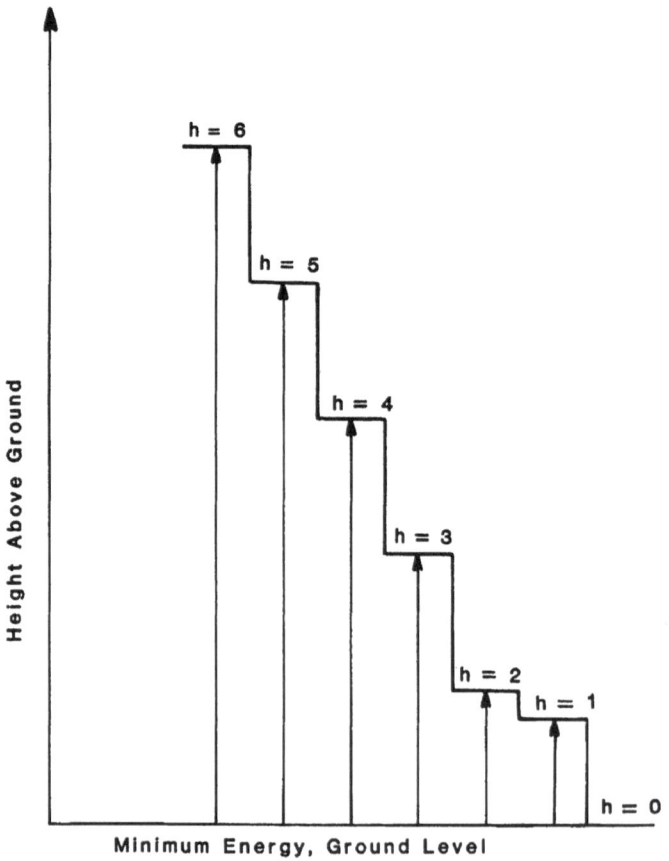

Figure 1.2. Potential energy staircase.

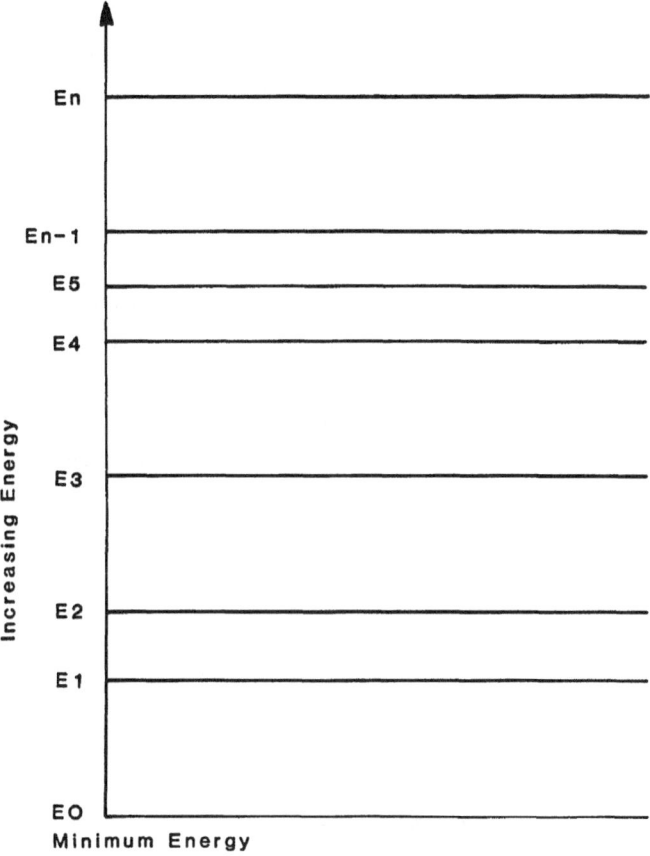

Figure 1.3. Energy level diagram.

mechanics is that the energy values of an atom are discrete; they cannot have any arbitrary value. These specific values or energy levels are characteristic for each atom. Atomic species differ from each other by the number of electrons and the charge of the nucleus. As the number of electrons increases, the structure of the energy levels becomes more and more complex, but the basic fact that the possible energies of atoms are discrete remains true in all cases.

One can visualize the concept of energy levels with the analogy of a ball on a staircase (Fig. 1.2). The (potential) energy of the ball on a step will have only the discrete values given by the heights of the steps above ground level; of course, these steps need not be equally spaced. Usually, one makes a diagram of the energy levels of an atom by drawing straightline segments one below the other, each segment denoting a possible energy level for the atom (Fig. 1.3). When the ball is on the ground-level step, it cannot go any lower. The atom is said to be at the ground level or in the ground state when it has

9

its lowest possible value of energy. When the atom is not at its ground level, it is said to be excited; in Fig. 1.2, levels $E_1 \ldots E_n$ correspond to excited levels of the atom, E_0 to the ground level. Ordinarily, atoms are in their ground state.

1.4.2. Generation of Light

The production of light by a quantum system (an atom) is intimately related to the energy levels of the system, because light which has frequencies only in the vicinity of certain characteristic values can be generated, and each of these characteristic frequencies, ν_{ab} for example, is connected to two energy levels of the atom by the simple relation first discovered by **Neils Bohr**:

$$\nu_{ab} = \frac{E_a - E_b}{h} \tag{1}$$

Here E_a and E_b are allowed energies of the atom. The h is called Planck's constant; the value is 6.63×10^{-34} J·sec.

1.4.3. Emission and Absorption

Under what circumstances will light be produced by an atom? How does light interact with the atom? Einstein answered these questions in the early part of this century. He deduced that there are three distinct processes possible:

a. Spontaneous emission
b. Absorption
c. Stimulated emission

1.4.3.a. Spontaneous Emission   Imagine that an atom is in one of its excited energy levels, E_a (see Fig. 1.4A). After a time, the atom has undergone a transition to one of its levels of lower energy, E_b and accompanying the energy loss $(E_a - E_b)$ suffered by the atom is the appearance of light of frequency ν_{ab}, as given in Eq. (1), (see Fig. 1.4B). This light contains an amount of energy equal to that given up by the atom; energy is conserved in the various atomic processes, just as in the more familiar Newtonian mechanics. Thus, the atom has undergone a spontaneous transition to a lower level and in so doing, has *spontaneously emitted light*.

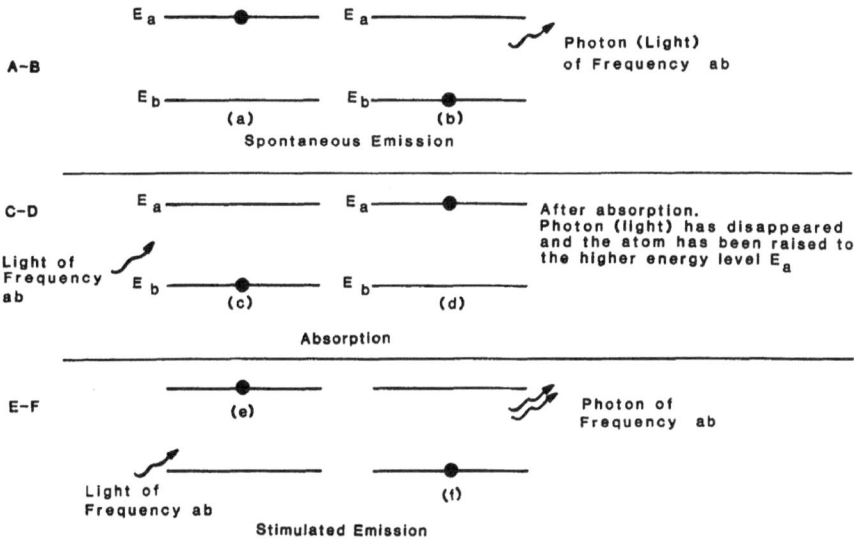

Figure 1.4. Interaction of light and atoms. (A,B) Spontaneous emission of photons; (C,D) absorption of a photon; (E,F) stimulated emission.

1.4.3.b. Absorption   Now imagine that the atom is initially in the level of lower energy E_b and is, in addition, being irradiated with light of the same frequence ν_{ab} (Fig. 1.4.). In time, the atom will remove the energy $(E_a - E_b)$ from the light and make a transition to the level of energy E_a (Fig. 1.4). The atom has been stimulated by the light irradiating it to undergo the transition to the higher energy level, thereby *absorbing* some of the light. Objects have color because some constituent colors of (usually) white light are absorbed, as just described. Then the light not absorbed, which we see, is no longer white.

1.4.3.c. Stimulated Emission   To understand the third process, imagine that the atom is in the upper energy level E_a. As we have just pointed out, sometime later on the atom can make a spontaneous transition to the lower level and emit light. We find that the introduction of light frequency ν_{ab} increases the likelihood of the transition to the lower level. The atom is *stimulated* to *emit* by the external light. The energy difference $(E_a - E_b)$ is delivered as light, which adds to the incident light. The process, called stimulated emission of light, is illustrated in Figure 1.4.

1.4.3.d. Additional Characteristics   At this point we need to mention certain other details of these three processes:
Spontaneous Emission   The light produced in spontaneous emission is emitted with equal probability in *all directions*. The frequency of sponta-

11

neously emitted light is not precisely ν_{ab} but is spread out over a narrow range centered at ν_{ab}.

Absorption   In the absorption process the light need not have a frequency of precisely ν_{ab}. However, the effectiveness of the light in stimulating the absorption diminishes rapidly as its frequency departs progressively from ν_{ab}.

Stimulated Emission   Light stimulating the atoms to emit also need not have a frequency of precisely ν_{ab}. However, in this process the *effectiveness* of the light in stimulating the emission diminishes rapidly as it departs progressively from ν_{ab}. Light from stimulated emission has the precise frequency and *direction* of the stimulating light; furthermore, it adds energy (constructively) to the stimulating light, thus increasing its intensity.

Stimulated Emission–Absorption Probability   For incident light of a given intensity, the chance or probability that an atom in the lower level will be stimulated to absorb in a certain time is equal to the chance that an atom in the upper level will be stimulated to emit in the same time.

Absorption and Amplification of Light   Moving a little closer to the laser by extending the phenomena discussed so far, we consider the case of a collection of identical atoms. We shall continue to refer to the same pair of excited energy levels, the upper one of energy E_a and the lower one of energy E_b; we consider two special cases.

All the atoms in the collection are in the lower level and light having a frequency close to ν_{ab} is propagating through the medium (a collection of solid, liquid, or gaseous atoms). Under these conditions, we know that atoms will be stimulated to *absorb* some light, and we expect that, as the light propagates, its intensity will *decrease* as its energy is being absorbed by the atoms.

Alternatively, let us start with all the atoms in the upper level: light will stimulate atoms to *emit* and the result will be an *increase* in intensity of the light as it propagates; the light has been *amplified*.

In general, whether the light intensity decreases or increases simply depends on the difference in the densities of atoms in the two levels. (This is just a consequence of the equal probability for absorption and stimulated emission stated above.) If the density of atoms in the lower level is greater than the density of atoms in the upper level, the medium will absorb the light of the right frequency. If, on the other hand, the density of atoms is greater in the upper level, the medium will amplify the light. If the densities of atoms in the two levels happen to be equal, the light will propagate unchanged in intensity as if there were no matter present at all. From these statements, we can predict that the ability of the medium to absorb or amplify the light will depend on the frequency of light. *The absorption of amplification properties* *of the medium will be greatest for light of frequency v_{ab} and will decrease rapidly as the frequency of the light deviates progressively from this value.*

Population Inversion   Usually, light absorption and light transmission are everyday phenomena, but this is not so in the instance of light gain or amplification because, under most circumstances, *there are far more atoms in the ground state than in any excited state. The higher the energy level, the fewer are the atoms in it.* To produce a laser, light gain is necessary. The major problem in designing a laser is in finding those rare cases of atomic systems (materials) in which it is possible, by some means, to accumulate more atoms in a higher level than in a lower one; this is called establishing a **population inversion.** Such an atomic system, whether it be gaseous, solid, or liquid, can have light gain and can produce a laser.

1.4.4. The Laser

1.4.4.a. Active Medium, Pumping   The laser has two basic components: an amplifying medium, as discussed previously, and an optical cavity (Fig. 1.5). Laser scientists call the amplifying medium an active medium (an active medium results, as stated earlier, when there is a greater density of

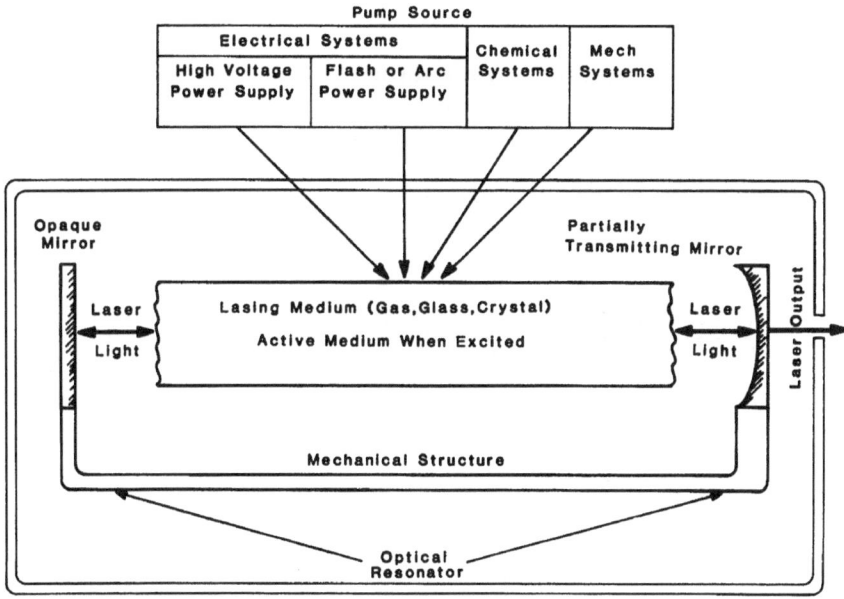

Figure 1.5. Laser optical cavity.

13

atoms in an upper excited level than in some lower level). This population inversion is characteristic of every active medium.

A source of energy is required to produce and maintain an active medium, because normally, each atom will be in its lowest energy level. The source of energy must not only raise atoms to excited levels, but it must also create a population inversion. This process is called **pumping** of the laser (Fig. 1.6). Many ingenious schemes have been proposed for doing this and many have been realized in practice. The pumping of the medium by the energy source must be continued if the population inversion is to be maintained, for if the pumping should be stopped, the atoms would rapidly return to their lowest energy level through the process of spontaneous emission.

1.4.4.b. Optical Cavity   The second basic component of every laser is a cavity in which the active medium is contained. Rather than discuss laser cavities in general, we shall discuss the role played in the laser process by the particular cavity used in the American Optical laser, which is formed by two mirrors carefully aligned in such a way as to have a common optical axis (Fig. 1.7). Plane mirrors or slightly curved mirrors can be used for the cavity.

If light strikes one mirror perpendicularly at its center, it will be reflected to strike the second mirror similarly and, again, be returned to the first mirror, continuing to infinity. Consider what happens when an active medium is placed between two such mirrors. Initially, light is emitted in all

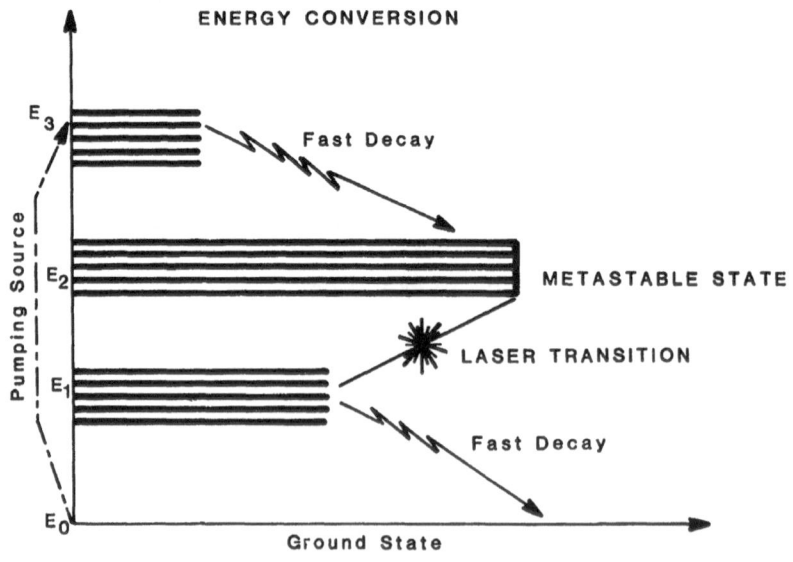

Figure 1.6. Population inversion is created by intense pumping to the highest energy state, followed by a fast decay to a metastable state (E_2).

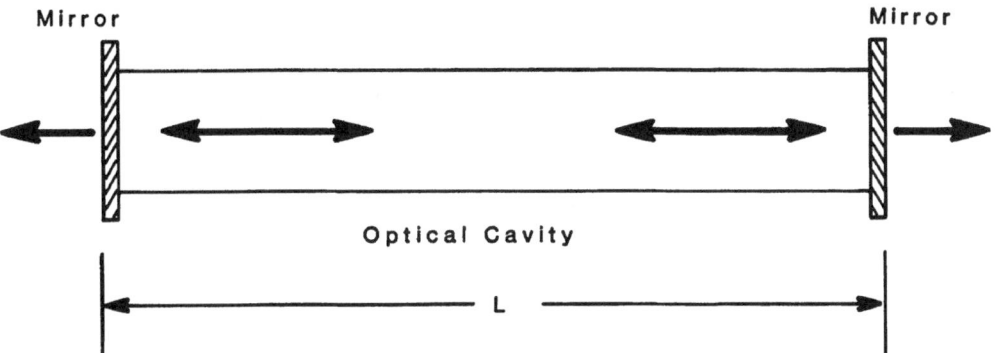

Figure 1.7. Optical cavity, simplified.

directions spontaneously by the atoms in the upper level of energy (E_a). The transitions which end up in the lower laser level of energy (E_b) produce light which has a frequency in the vicinity of ν_{ab}, and this particular light will be amplified as it moves through the active medium. The small fraction of light which is emitted spontaneously along the axis of the cavity (directed so that it is reflected back and forth between the two mirrors) will pass many times through the active medium. The light *stimulated* by this small initial amount of spontaneous emission always has the right frequency and the right direction to stimulate additional light and thus, the intensity of light increases with each traversal through the active medium. Thus, laser light is born.

1.4.4.c. Loss and Gain Phenomenon Let us go back a few steps now to consider in finer detail several aspects of the laser process. To begin with, not all of the light that strikes the mirrors is returned to the active medium. Some of it is transmitted or is scattered in some other direction. Indeed, in most lasers, it is the light transmitted through the mirrors that forms the useful output. But the fact that light is lost at the reflecting phase creates the condition on the active medium for the laser effect to occur. *The amount by which the light is amplified each time it makes a round trip in the cavity must be great enough to make up for the losses of light suffered at the two mirrors during the round trip.* Hence a minimum population inversion is required for lasering to occur. It should also be obvious, from what was stated previously about the frequency dependence of amplification, why the frequency or laser light is restricted to a narrow range about ν_{ab}. Remember that light having a frequency exactly equal to ν_{ab} is amplified best. When the frequency has deviated sufficiently from ν_{ab} so that the round trip amplification of the light no longer exceeds the round trip losses, then the laser effect will not be possible.

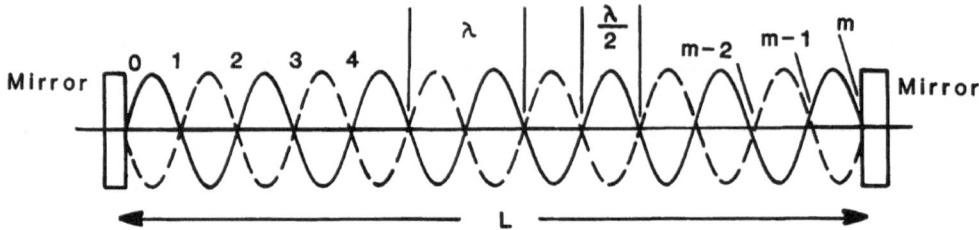

Figure 1.8. Standing wave inside optical cavity (L, length of optical cavity; m, number of waves; λ, wavelength).

1.4.4.d. Steady State   It is not clear, from the account of the laser process given so far, why a steady state should ever come about. What prevents the light in the cavity from continuing to grow in intensity indefinitely? As the laser output beam's intensity increases, the amplification of the medium is decreased due to depopulation of the higher energy excited state (E_a); however, continued pumping repopulates the state E_a. When the rate of pumping energy input is exactly equalled by the output of laser light (plus energy losses) a steady state condition is achieved. In the steady state, the round trip light amplification balances the round trip light losses (here including the laser output beam).

1.4.4.e. Standing Waves   One more important aspect of the laser process must be mentioned before we conclude the discussion of how a laser works. We have seen that the frequency of the laser light is limited to a narrow band centered about ν_{ab}, but within this band, the frequency is even further restricted. Consider light of a given frequency contained in an optical cavity between two mirrors. It consists of two waves traveling in opposite directions, resulting in a stationary wave pattern, or **standing wave.** When a mirror reflects an electromagnetic wave, a node (or zero of intensity) of the wave must be situated right at the surface of the mirror (Fig. 1.8). But in the laser cavity, we have two mirrors, and a node must be located at the surface of each. This condition puts a restriction on the possible wavelengths. If the mirrors are a distance L apart, then to get a node at each mirror only those wavelengths (λ) are allowed such that an integral number (m) of half-wavelengths is contained in L:

$$L = m \frac{\lambda}{2} \tag{2}$$

Wavelength and frequency are related to the speed of light (c):

$$\lambda \nu = c \tag{3}$$

By substituting c/ν for λ in Eq. (2) the possible frequencies can be obtained from Eq. (4):

$$\nu = \frac{mc}{2L} \tag{4}$$

We already know that the frequency must have a value in the vicinity of ν_{ab} which, in the case of red light, is about 5×10^{14} Hz. This means that, for a mirror spacing of 1 m, m is a fairly large integer: 3×10^6 in this case. An equivalent way of reaching this conclusion may be more enlightening. From the original definition of m, it is clear that $m + 1$ is the number of nodes between the mirrors, each separated by $\lambda/2$ from the next. In the case of red light, it is approximately equal to 6×10^{-5} cm; so for $L = 100$ cm, there are going to be many of these nodes—approximately 3 million of them. The answer is the same.[26]

1.5. The Molecular Gas Laser (Carbon Dioxide Laser): Energy Levels in Molecules

As with atoms, energy levels can be changed in molecules. With proper excitation, molecular gases can shift to higher energy levels. This energy is a shift in the rotational and vibrational configuration of the component atoms. The configurations that the linear carbon dioxide molecule can assume are depicted in Fig. 1.9.

1.5.1. Ground Level at Zero Energy Level

In this spatial arrangement, the molecule is at a resting or ground state. The CO_2 molecule has equispaced electron orbits at equispaced distances from the carbon electron orbits.

1.5.2. Excited Level (V_1) or Symmetrical Stretch Mode

In this arrangement, the atoms move in a symmetrical fashion. This level of energy is designated V_1.

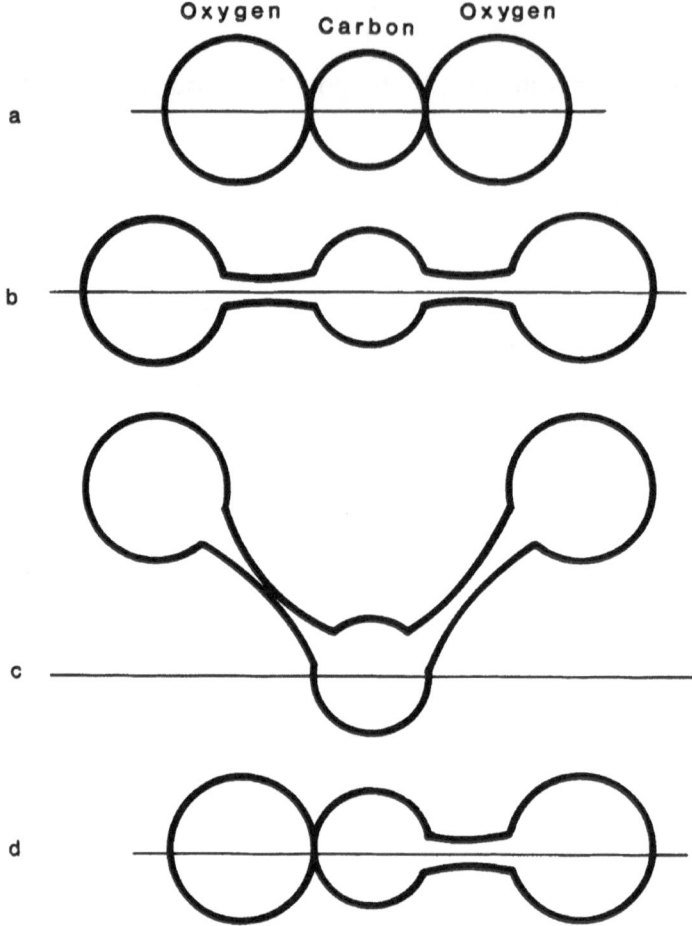

Figure 1.9. Vibrational energy transfer. (a) Ground level at 0 energy level; (b) excited level (V_1) or symmetrical stretch mode; (c) excited level (V_2) or bend mode; (d) excited level (V_2) or asymmetrical stretch mode.

1.5.3. Excited Level (V_2) or Bend Mode

In this arrangement, the interatomic axis is "bent" or distorted. This level of energy is designated V_2.

1.5.4. Excited Level (V_3) or Asymmetrical Stretch Mode

In this arrangement, the interatomic distances are asymmetrically placed and this level of energy is designated V_3.

1.5.5. Energy Transfer

In order to comprehend the photon emission in the various energy levels (V_1, V_2, V_3), an explanation of energy transfer is presented.

In quantum mechanics, the designators shown in Table 1.2 are used to quantitate the energy states.

From inspection, the CO_2 (001) vibrational energy state will decay to CO_2 (100) and CO_2 (020), releasing electromagnetic energy of wavelengths 10.6 μm and 9.6 μm.[27]

In the optical cavity, the addition of nitrogen gas (N_2), a diatomic molecule, allows the excited vibrational energy of the N_2 molecule to be transferred directly to CO_2. This transfer is a selective CO_2 excitation of CO_2 (000) to CO_2 (001). Thus, there is a high degree of efficiency in generating CO_2 (001). Furthermore, N_2 (0) is easily stimulated to N_2 (1) in one step. Remember, this molecule has only one degree of vibration, unlike CO_2, which has three.

$$CO_2\ (000) + N_2\ (1) \rightarrow CO_2\ (001) + N_2\ (0)$$

Now, we have two modes of stimulating a CO_2 (000) to CO_2 (001) level:

1. CO_2 (000) + electron + kinetic energy $\rightarrow$ CO_2 (001) by electrical discharge (low-efficiency energy transfer)
2. N_2 (0) + electron + kinetic energy $\rightarrow$ N_2 (0) then N_2 (1) + CO_2 (001) (high-efficiency energy transfer)

Finally, if the number of collisions per second of kinetic energy is increased, the population inversion of CO_2 (000) to CO_2 (001) would increase, thus achieving greater laser energy. It was found that pure CO_2 has approximately 100 collisions/sec; while N_2 (nitrogen under 1 ton of pressure) has 4000 collisions/sec. Thus, the increased number of collisions, with a high efficiency in N_2 transfer of energy to CO_2, completes the system; the final

Table 1.2. Basic Energy Levels

Configuration	Designator of energy[a]	Designator of spacial configuration	Relative energy
Asymmetrical mode	001	V_3	Highest
Bend mode	100	V_2	Higher
Symmetrical mode	020	V_1	Low
Ground state	000	V_0	Zero

[a]The designator CO_2 (001) is the highest energy level.

formula requires N_2, He, and CO_2 for an efficient CO_2 laser system.

The element helium is added to the above mixture because of its ability to transfer heat. In the decay process, heat is produced. This heat is efficiently transferred to the He atom and thence to the wall of the optical cavity. This is why the laser tube must be added. Water is usually used to conduct heat away from the optical cavity, however, air can be used. Remember that the laser's efficiency is dependent upon heat exchange, thus, each rise in external heat is equivalent to a loss in internal laser effect.

1.6. The Liquid Laser

Although not as common as the solid or gas laser, liquid lasers possess unique advantages for certain applications. Of the various types of liquid lasers, the dye laser is the most significant. The dye laser was discovered by Sorokin in 1965 at IBM Laboratories, and led to tunable outputs over a significant frequency range.[28] It differs from gas or solid lasers, which have a very narrow wavelength profile. Tunable lasers provide researchers with very narrow bands of highly coherent light. Such light is desirable in applications such as spectroscopy, cell sorting and counting devices, and isotope separation, as well as in the determination of molecular dissociation and energy of activation.

The active medium consits of organic dyes dissolved in solvent. When the dye is excited by external sources of a short wavelength, it emits radiation at longer wavelengths, or **fluoresces.** Dye lasers and fluorescence are now being used to investigate cancers. When the patient is premedicated with hematoporphyrins, the cancer will, when exposed to selective wavelengths, internally fluoresce, an oxidative process. This process causes cellular enzyme deactivation and death.[29]

In a similar and even more spectacular fashion, the krypton laser, using computer-accentuated imaging, can detect a 1 mm $\times$ 70 μm pulmonary carcinoma in situ.[30]

1.7. The Solid-State Laser

Solid-state lasers are made from crystalline or amorphous materials which incorporate unique ions whose physical properties allow an energy state transition. The ions, when excited by external pumping, change quantum states. Crystals, such as the ruby (Cr^{3+}: ion-activated aluminum oxide

Al$_2$O$_3$) or Nd-YAG laser (Nd^{3+}: ion-doped yttrium aluminum oxide Y$_2$Al$_5$O$_{12}$) can be used to create lasers. Mirrors at the poles of the crystal intensify (i.e., amplify) the laser effect.[28]

1.8. The Semiconductor Laser

Semiconductor lasers are the least expensive of all lasers available commercially because they can be mass-produced using the same techniques as for transistors. Because semiconductor lasers are efficient and of very small size (one could fit on your fingertip) they are well-suited as light sources for fiberoptic communications.

The name *conductor* implies the ability to carry a free charge or current. In semiconductors containing certain impurities, a stuation develops which allows for a shift of energy into the **band gaps** (spaces between the periodic crystal lattice structure of the atoms in a solid into which electrons can shift energy levels). There are two types of shifts: an n-type (negative) and a p-type (positive), and semiconductors can be of either type (Fig. 1.10). The shift of a semiconductor laser has a very narrow wavelength when compared to that of the LED (light-emitting diode) crystal (Fig. 1.11).

1.9. General Characteristics of Lasers in Medicine

Laser surgery must be approached in a responsible and conscientious manner, beginning with the education and training of the surgeon. It would be unthinkable to attempt to use a laser without a thorough working knowledge of the equipment and the biophysical properties of the wavelength chosen. To do so would be akin to being a Piper Cub pilot and thinking you were capable of confidently flying an X-15. Beware of the sales pitch: "This is so easy, all you have to do is press the red button, aim, and fire!" Hindsight can be very expensive, so in order to use a laser system properly in medicine, the following must characterize each application:

1. Delivery system promoting ease of application
2. Defined biophysical characteristics
3. Finite controls
4. Safety and fail-safe mechanisms
5. Proper physician training and education
6. System quality control

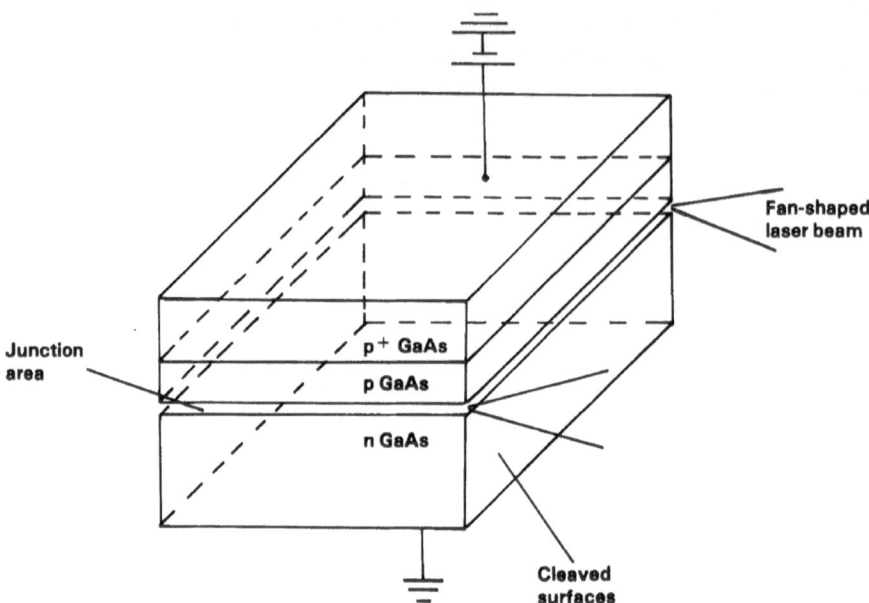

Figure 1.10. Model of semiconductor GaAs laser. (Reproduced with permission: Bellina JH: The carbon dioxide laser in gynecology, Part I, in Leventhal JM (ed): Current Problems in Obstetrics and Gynecology. Vol IV, Chicago, Year Book Medical Publishers, 1981, pp 1–34.)

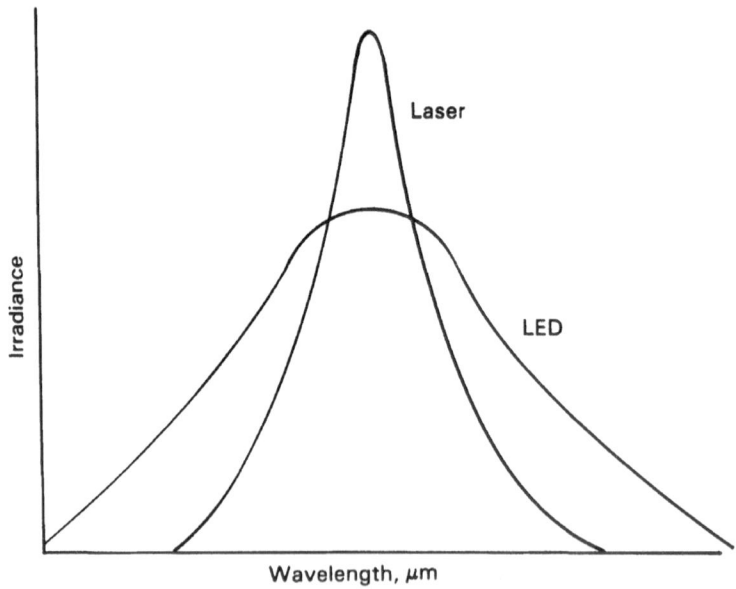

Figure 1.11. The laser wavelength is narrow in comparison to the light-emitting diode.

Table 1.3. Surgical Lasers in Use

Laser type	Wavelength (μm)	Power output (W)	Penetration depth (skin) (mm)	Main applications
CO_2	10.6	≤ 500	0.05	Cutting and vaporizing
Argon	0.488–0.514	≤ 20	0.2	Coagulation of retinal vessels and superficial skin lesions; neurosurgery
Nd-YAG	1.06	≤ 100	0.8–2.0	Coagulation of gastrointestinal tract bleeding tract bleeding
Ruby	0.6943	$> 10^6$		Ophthalmology; dark skin lesions
HeNe	0.633	0.8–2.0	—	Finder beam

Today, medicine is utilizing many laser systems, notably the ruby, argon, Nd-YAG, and CO_2 lasers (Table 1.3). Each system must have a delivery mechanism to direct the energy into precise areas for irradiation, and, even though manufacturers have improved the housing and delivery systems, much more work remains to be done (i.e., flexible, tunable systems and microprecision lasers).

Most of the laser models available today are more compact, with the chassis being mounted on wheels, making them easily transportable; thus, they are designed either for endoscopic surgery through an operating microscope or for surgery with an articulated arm. Also, a number of improvements have been incorporated which make lasers easier and less expensive to operate while allowing photographic and video documentation of surgical procedures.

The biophysical properties of the current wavelengths used in medicine are, in general, well defined, but additional work must be done in the areas of heat decay and transfer. The relationship of the transverse electromagnetic mode (TEM) to cutting or vaporizing versus injury and necrosis requires further research. Studies in acoustic properties of current medical frequencies are presented in this monograph (see Section 3.3).

The power output of lasers currently available in the United States is low and should be 100 to 300 W terminal output. Concepts in "core" type operating room lasers need to be expanded. Manufacturers have addressed the safety and fail-safe mechanisms, as defined by the Bureau of Radiological Health (see Section 2.4).

1.9.1. The Ruby Laser

The ruby laser (λ = 694 nm, visible, red) is a solid-state laser that was used early in ophthalmology for photocoagulation of retinal hemorrhages. Currently, it is being used extensively in the treatment of portwine stain lesions of the skin. This laser system is difficult to maintain but can result in exceptional cosmetic treatment of disfiguring lesions.

Ketchan used this laser in melanoma animal studies with poor therapeutic results.[31] However, the poor therapeutic outcome was the result of another property of pulsed lasers, the **photoacoustic phenomenon:** the shock wave (mechanical effect) resulting from the impact of very-high-energy pulsed photons on tumor cells. The ruby laser's usual power is between 10 and 100 mJ per pulse, and sufficient kinetic energy can be present to drive viable tumor cells deeper into tissues, which can result in rapid metastasis. The concept is similar to that of a small-caliber bullet fired from a high-powered rifle hitting bone—massive shattering occurs, usually causing loss of the limb and, occasionally, internal injuries from the shock wave effect. Compare this to the impact of a slow-moving bullet (i.e., a BB), in which tissue and bone damage is minimal. Thus "Q" switching or pulse lasers should not be used in tumor surgery unless a complete analysis of the photoacoustic profile is known. On the other hand, the carbon dioxide laser is a continuous-waveform laser which, like the BB, has a negligible to absent shock wave phenomenon. Ketchan's experiment demonstrates the absolute necessity for the surgeon to know all the properties of a laser system *before* surgery.

1.9.2. The Argon Laser

The argon laser (λ = 488–515 nm, visible blue–green) is an ion–gas laser. This sytem is currently in use in the fields of dermatology, urology, gastroenterology, otorhinolaryngology, and ophthalmology. Because of the wavelength property, fiber delivery systems are available which afford the surgeon a tremendous advantage. Argon's biophysical properties allow for photocoagulation of tissues and, under certain circumstances, tissue cutting. This laser is a continuous-waveform laser, unlike the pulsed ruby laser, but again the surgeon must have a thorough working knowledge of the wavelength properties before attempting to use this laser. The laser is from <1 to 20 W

1.9.3. The Neodymium-YAG Laser

The ND-YAG laser (λ = 1060 nm, invisible, near infrared) is also a solid-state laser. It is principally used in neurosurgery, urology, oncology, and gastroenterology. The best description of this laser and its properties was written by Hofstetter and Frank.[32] The laser output can vary from 1 to 100 W.

1.9.4. The Carbon Dioxide Laser

The carbon dioxide laser (λ = 10,600 nm, invisible, midinfrared) is a molecular gas laser (see Section 1.5). The remainder of this book will detail the biophysical effects of, animal experimentation with, and clinical results of the use of the carbon dioxide laser. This laser has a medical range of output from <1 to 300 W.

References

1. Mullins F, Jenning B, McClusky L: Liver resections with the cw carbon dioxide laser: some experimental observations. Am J Surg *34*:717–722, 1968.
2. Stellar S, Polanyi TG, Bredemeier HC: Experimental studies of the CO_2 laser as neurosurgical instrument. Med Biol Eng 8:549–558, 1970.
3. Jako GJ: Laser surgery of the vocal cords. An experimental study with CO_2 laser on dogs. Laryngoscope *82*:2204–2216, 1971.
4. Oosterhuis JW, Verschueren RC, Oldhoff J: Experimental surgery for the Cloudman S91 melanoma with CO_2 laser. Acta Chir Belg *74*:422–429, 1975.
5. Strong MS, Jako GJ, Polanyi TG, et al: Laser surgery in the aerodigestive tract. Am J Surg *126*:529–533, 1973.
6. Strong MS, Jako GJ: Laser surgey in the larynx. Am J Otol 81:791–798, 1972.
7. Jako GJ, Polanyi TG: Carbon dioxide laser surgery in otolaryngology, in Kaplan I (ed): Proceedings I International Congress on Laser Surgery. Jerusalem, Jerusalem Academic Press, 1976, pp 149–166.
8. Mihashi S, Hirano M: Surgical application of CO_2 laser in otolaryngology, in Kaplan I, Ascher PW (eds): Proceedings of the 3rd International Congress for Laser Surgery, Graz, OT-PAZ Tel-Aviv, Jerusalem, Academic Press, 1976, pp 293–308.
9. Wilpizeski CR: Otological applications of lasers, in Wolbarst ML (ed): Laser Applications in Medicine and Biology, Volume 3. New York, Plenum Press, 1977, p 289.
10. Christensen J: Use of the CO_2 laser in thoracic surgery, in Koebuez H (ed): Lasers in Medicine, Vol 1. Chichester, John Wiley and Sons, 1980, pp 39–45.

11. Goldman L, Naprstek Z, Johnson J: Laser surgery of a digital angiosarcoma. Cancer *39*:1738–1742, 1977.
12. Levine N, Ger R, Stellar S, Levenson SR: Use of a carbon dioxide laser for the debridement of third degree burns. Ann Surg *179*:246–252, 1974.
13. Fidler JP, Law E, MacMillan BG, et al: Comparison of CO_2 laser excision of burns with the thermal knives. Ann NY Acad Sci *267*:254–261, 1977.
14. Levine NS, Salisbury RE, Peterson HD, et al: Clinical evaluation of the carbon dioxide laser for burn wound excision. A comparison of the laser, scalpel and electrocautery. J Trauma *15*:800–807, 1975.
15. Stellar S, Cooper MD, Young J: Recent advance in neurosurgical treatment for the elderly. J Am Geriatric Soc *2*:848–860, 1970.
16. Goldman L: Laser surgery for skin cancer. NY State J Med *77*: 1897–1900, 1977.
17. Bellina JH: Gynecology and the laser. Contemporary Ob/Gyn *4*:24–34, 1974.
18. Einstein A: Zur quanten theorie der strahlung. Phys Zeit *68*:121, 1917.
19. Gordon JP, Zeiger HJ, Townes CH: Molecular microwave oscillator and new hyperfine structure in the microwave spectrum of NH_3. Phys Rev *95*:282, 1954.
20. Basov NG, Prokhorov AM: In Russia. Soviet Phys-JETP *27*:431, 1954.
21. Schawlow AL, Townes CH: Infrared and optical masers. Phys Rev *42*:1940, 1958.
22. Maiman T: Stimulated optical radiation in ruby masers. Nature *187*:493–494, 1960.
23. Bennett WR, Herriott DR, Javan A: Population inversion and continuous optical maser oscillation in a gas discharge containing a He-Ne mixture. Phys Rev Lett *6*:106–110, 1961.
24. Patel CKN: High power carbon dioxide laser. Sci Am *219*:733, 1968.
25. Polanyi TC, Bredemeier HC: Experimental carbon dioxide surgery of the vocal cords. Eye Ear Nose Throat Mon *52*:171–172, 1973.
26. Polanyi T, Tobias I: Principles and Properties of the Laser. Framington Center, Mass., American Optical Corporation Research Division, 1970.
27. Patel CKN: Vibrational energy transfer—an efficient means of selective excitation of molecules, in Kelley PL, Lax B, Tannenwald PE (eds): Physics of Quantum Electronics. New York, McGraw-Hill, 1966, pp 643–654.
28. O'Shea DC, Callen WR, Rhodes WT: Introduction to Lasers and Their Applications. Reading, Mass., Addision-Wesley, 1977, p 168.
29. Dougherty TJ, Kaufman JE, Goldford A, et al: Photoradiation therapy for the treatment of malignant tumors. Cancer Res *8*:2628–2635, 1978.
30. Doiron, DR, Profio E, Vincent RG, et al: Fluorescence bronchoscopy for detection of lung cancer. Chest *76*:27–32, 1979.
31. Ketcham AD, Hoye RD, Riggle GC: A surgeon's appraisal of the laser. Surg Clin North Am *47*:1249–1263, 1967.
32. Hofstetter A, Frank F: The Neodymium-YAG Laser in Urology. Basel, Switzerland, Roche Scientific Service, 1980.

2

Carbon Dioxide Laser Instrumentation

2.1. General Description

The CO_2 laser's energy is supplied by passing an electrical current (DC) through a mixture of helium, nitrogen, and carbon dioxide (this is in contrast to the ruby laser, which is excited by powerful flash lamps) that is contained in a cylinder with reflective mirrors at the end known as an optical cavity. The mirrors are aligned in such a manner as to have a common optical axis, whereby if a photon strikes one mirror it will be reflected to the second mirror and return in a similar fashion. Each pass through the optical cavity may result in photon absorption and yield stimulated emissions. In a short time, a population inversion and a laser effect are achieved. If a small optical opening is created in one mirror (i.e., a semitransparent mirror) a stream of photons that has the unique properties of being parallel and of the same frequency will exit. The energy density in the beam cross section is extremely high, and if this energy is passed through a lens system of appropriate material, an even greater cross-sectional density of energy can be achieved at the focal point. Using a system of gimbaled mirrors outside the optical cavity and on appropriate lens, the carbon dioxide laser has been harnessed for precision surgery (Fig. 2.1).

One of the carbon dioxide surgical laser systems used in our studies (American Optical Corporation) has been described in detail by Polanyi and colleagues.[1] To date, models of other water-cooled CO_2 lasers are of a similar

Stereo Operating Microscope
Microscope Objective
Laser Beam
Focusing
Lens (L)
Endoscope
Steerable Mirror (M)
Focusing Lens (L2)
Aiming Light
Fiber Optic
Aiming Light Source

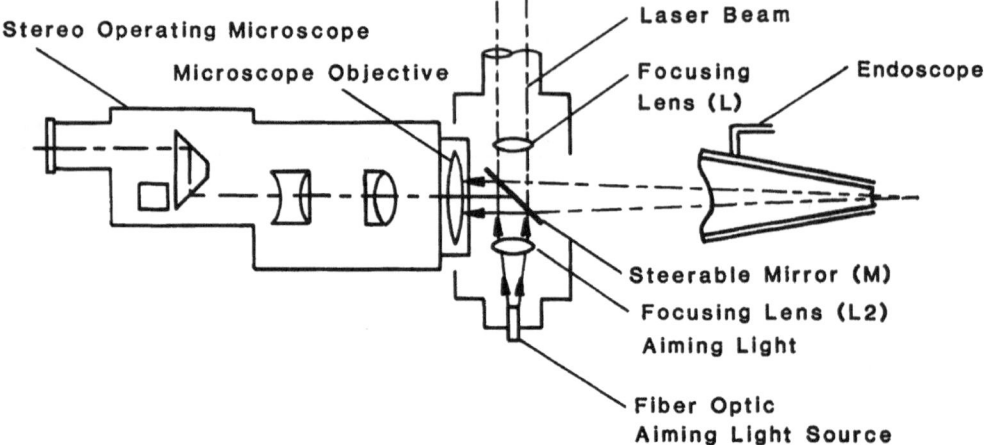

Figure 2.1. Internal structures of the colposcope and micromanipulator (side view).

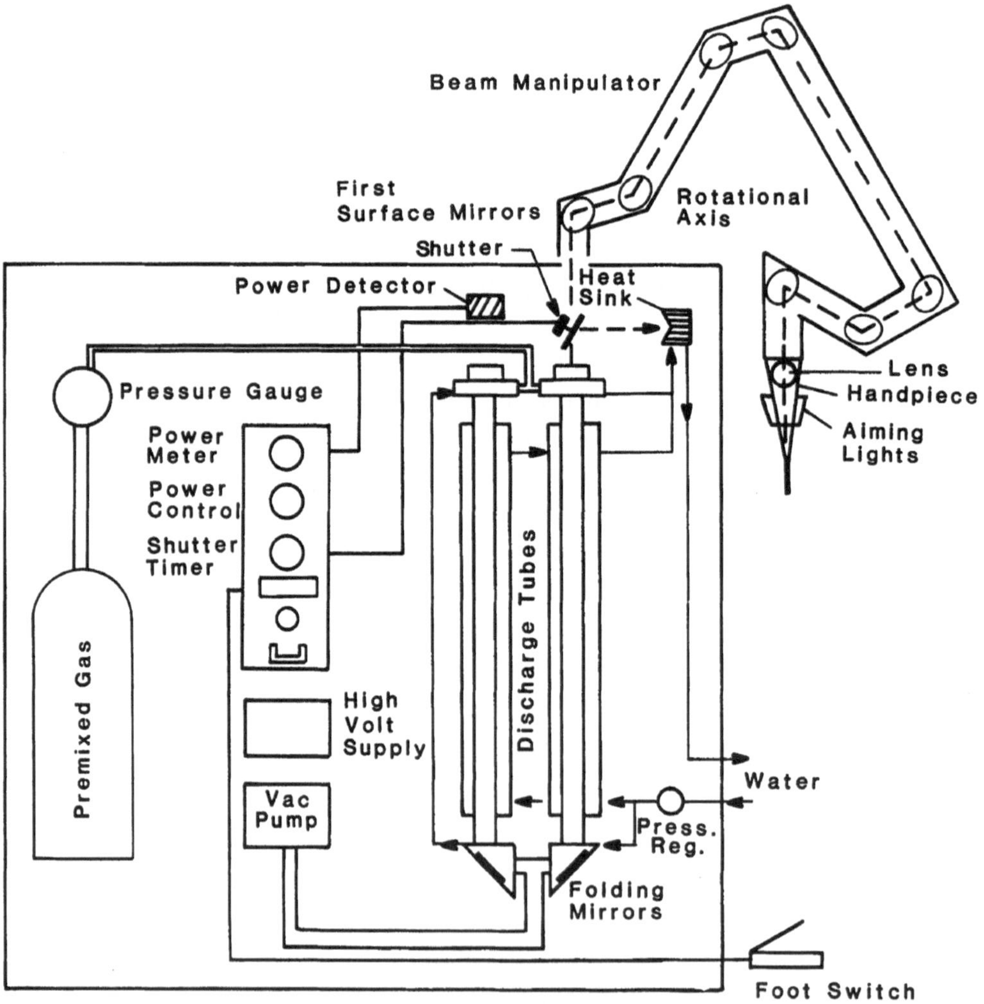

Beam Manipulator
First
Surface Mirrors
Rotational
Axis
Shutter
Heat
Sink
Power Detector
Pressure Gauge
Lens
Handpiece
Aiming
Lights
Power
Meter
Power
Control
Shutter
Timer
Discharge Tubes
Premixed Gas
High
Volt
Supply
Water
Vac
Pump
Press.
Reg.
Folding
Mirrors
Foot Switch

Figure 2.2. Anatomy of a surgical CO_2 laser system.

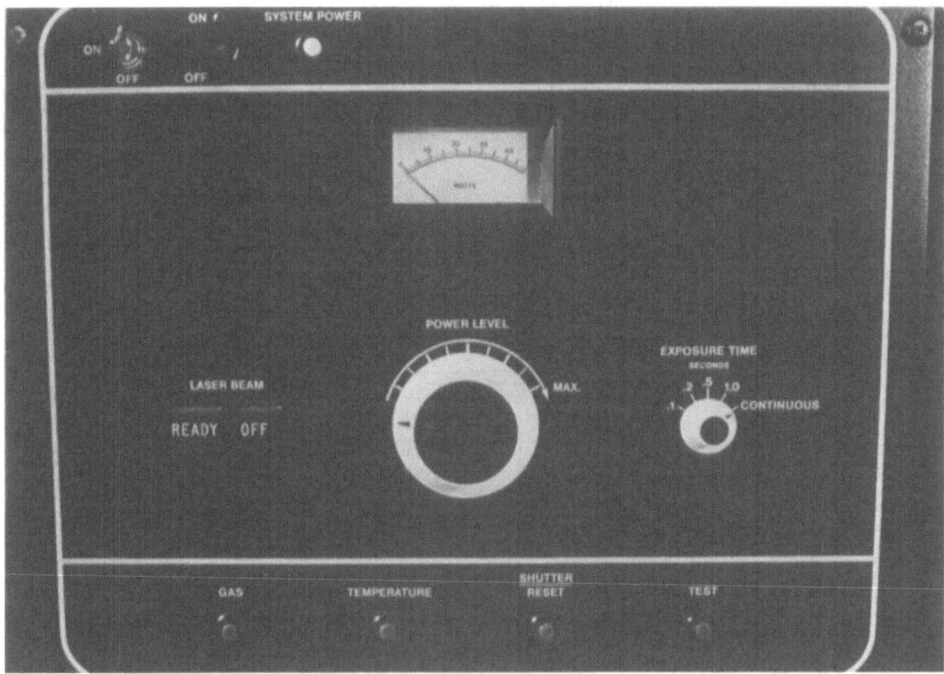

Figure 2.3. Control panel of a surgical system.

mechanical design. A standard electronic cabinet contains the gas supply for the laser, vacuum pump, power pack, operating controls, and safety interlocks. The water cooling system is self-contained; only a connection for the electric power source is needed. The laser beam is issued from the optical cavity and is directed into a beam-manipulating arm that contains several mirrors in rotating joints with a focusing lens at the beam exit. This arrangement allows the surgeon to apply the focused laser beam, which may be directed to any point within a large area, from any direction (Fig. 2.2).

When not in use the beam is deflected into a heat sink by a reflecting shutter. This shutter is opened by a foot switch to allow the laser beam to reach the target, which is pinpointed by a luminous spot or helium neon laser (i.e., the target beam). Either continuous exposure or time exposure can be used, and the power can be varied from zero to its maximum, about 25 W, by adjusting a knob on the control panel (Fig. 2.3).

For microsurgery, the colposcope or operating microscope is attached to both the manipulator and a special gimbaled mirror. The narrow laser beam entering from above strikes a gimbal-mounted mirror which is located between the optical axes of the stero microscope. The mirror is positioned at 45° to the primary incident laser beam and deflects the energy along the

29

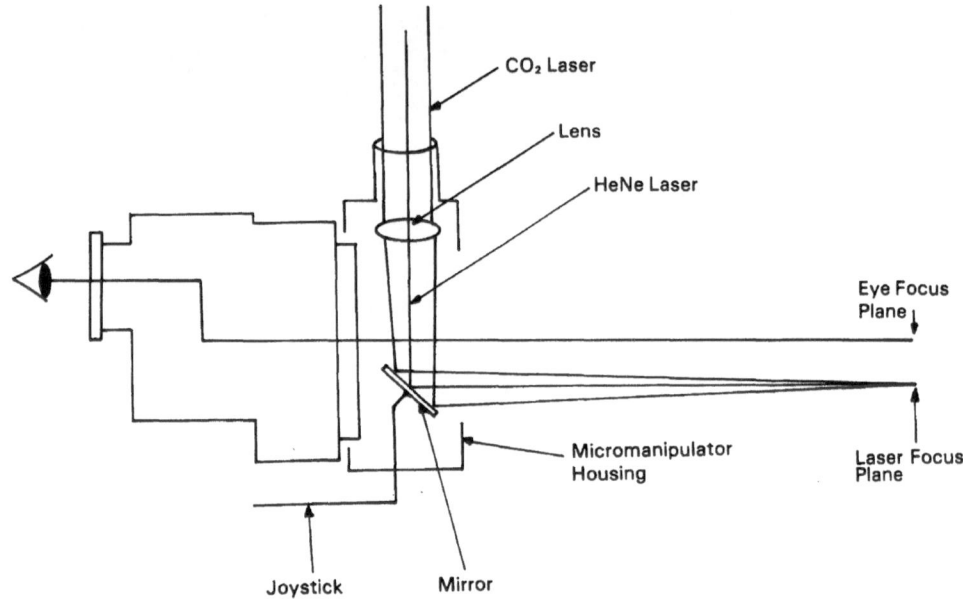

Figure 2.4. Micromanipulator with internal focusing lens. (Reproduced with permission: Bellina JH: The carbon dioxide laser in gynecology, Part I, in Leventhal JM (ed): Current Problems in Obstetrics and Gynecology. Vol. 4, Chicago, Year Book Medical Publishers, 1981, pp 1–34.)

viewing axis of the microscope. Apertures in the mirror permit normal viewing with the microscope. A lens located in the primary incident laser beam focuses the energy to a spot at a distance equal to the working distance of the microscope objective. By appropriate lens selection (i.e., germanium, gallium arsenide, or zinc selenide) this distance can be varied from 10 to 50 cm or more (Fig. 2.4). The gimbal-mounted mirror permits steering of the beam to any location within $\pm 3°$ of the central axis of the microscope. The diameter of the working area is, therefore, about one tenth of the working distance. To move the mirror about the gimbal axis, a joystick type of control is provided in a convenient location a few inches to the right or middle of the microscope. The mechanical linkage between the joystick and the gimbal is arranged to make the motion of the beam directly proportional to the same joystick movement with a demagnification of seven to one. The sensitivity and naturalness of this adjustment allow the surgeon to position the beam with confidence and precision at any preselected location.

One additional feature is necessary to predict with accuracy, prior to exposure, where the focused energy will make contact with the work site. A marker system projects a visible image of a light source into the focal plane of the microscope eyepiece. If the marker light from a beam splitter attached to and located in the same plane as the metal mirror which directs the laser beam is reflected, the image of the visible marker appears on the work surface and moves in a one-to-one relationship with the impact point of the laser beam. A similar arrangement, but using a helium–neon laser, is coupled to the other laser systems. The markers coincide with the CO_2 laser impact point.

2.2. Biophysical Data

2.2.1. Terminology of Laser Irradiation

In order to converse with the physicist, the physician must speak the same language. Table 2.1 shows a simple but precise outline of the physical parameters one must understand.

The term **power** (P) is related to the watts or heat output produced by the system. This measurement is taken using a power meter. Most, if not all, laser systems have a power meter built into the system. A rheostat controls the voltage input and/or the gas flow to the optical cavity and allows the surgeon to vary the laser output power (Fig. 2.3).

Energy (E) is a term related to the time of exposure to power. Energy is the product of power (W) and time (sec). The time-related nature of energy is illustrated in Table 2.2, while different combinations of power and time that will create the same quantity of energy are given in Table 2.3.

Since energy is time- and power-dependent, tissue injury is not directly related to energy but rather to time and power interdependently. In particular, time is of maximum importance and power of less importance. The reader must fully understand this concept, as the remainder of this text will expand upon this basic concept. The following is a simple example of this

Table 2.1.   Variables Used in Laser Terminology

Term	Symbol	Unit
Power	P	W (watt)
Time	t	sec (second)
Energy	$E = P \times t$	$W \cdot sec = J$ (joule)
Area	A	cm^2
Power density	$I = P/A$	W/cm^2
Energy density	$L = E/A$	$W \cdot sec/cm^2 = J/cm^2$

Table 2.2. Relationship of Constant Power and Time to Energy

Power (W)	Time (sec)	Energy (W·sec or J)
20	1	20
20	0.5	10
20	2	40

Table 2.3. Relationship of Variable Power and Time to Energy

Power (W)	Time (sec)	Energy (W·sec or J)
20	1	20
40	0.5	20
10	2	20

principle. A hot skillet is touched by your finger for a moment. Assume the skillet has 40 W of power and your touch is for 0.5 sec or 20 J of energy exposure. The burn on your finger is scant and well defined (i.e., small blister). The extent of injury is related to the short time of heat transfer. Now assume you put a soldering iron on your finger and then plug it in. As the tip begins to heat from ambient temperatures, the energy is transfered gradually until 20 J have been transferred. During the heating, you must keep your finger in place until it receives a total of 20 J. During each second of contact the amount of tissue heating and energy transfer is resulting in a large burn. Thus, by the time 20 J have been received the burn could be two to three times as great as that from the 0.5-sec contact at 40 W.

2.2.2. Absorption and Reflection

Since human tissue is 70–90 % water, the absorption of the carbon dioxide in tissue can be related to the water content of the tissue. From Fig. 2.5, one can evaluate the absorption of various wavelengths in aqueous media.[2] Argon (λ = 0.488–0.515 μm) requires approximately 1000 mm of water, while CO_2 (λ = 10.6 μm) requires approximately 0.01–0.1 mm of water to reduce the incident energy to 90% of its original energy. This stopping or absorbing of energy is related to the absorption coefficient. This property follows the Beer–Lambert law:

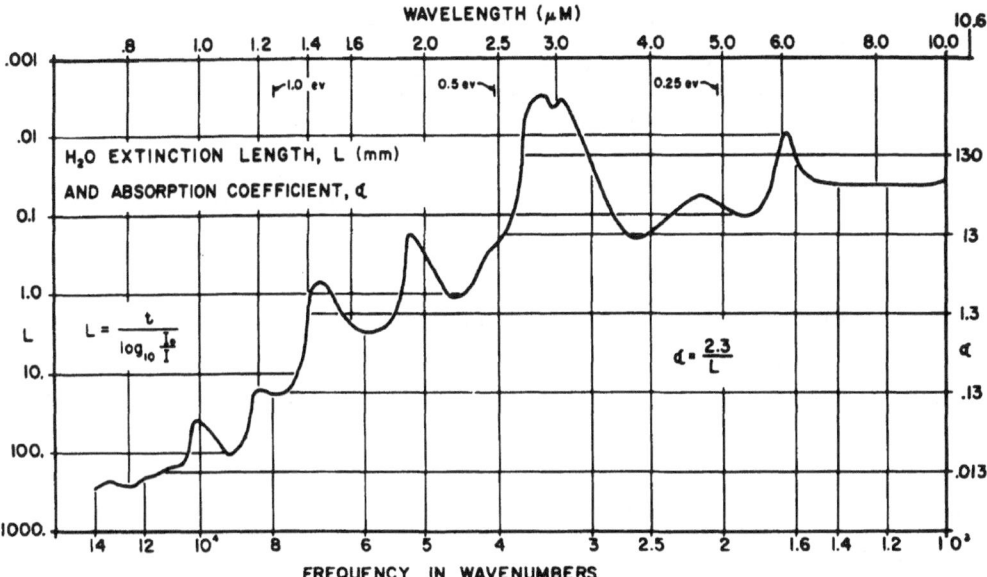

Figure 2.5. Absorption coefficient and extinction lengths of wavelengths from <0.8 to 10.6 μm. (Adapted from Bayly JT et al: Infrared Physics 3:211, 1963.)

$$I = I_0 e^{-(a+b)x}$$

where I is the intensity at depth, I_0 is the incident intensity, a is the absorption coefficient, b is the reflectance coefficient, x is the depth, and e is the base of the natural logarithm (2.71828).

Applying this law with the coefficients given in Table 2.4 to tissue at depth x, one can appreciate the effects of the different lasers. The extinction length (L) of the radiation in water is related to the wavelength and expresses the thickness of water that absorbs 90% of the incident radiation (Table 2.5). For comparison, a 300-mm layer of water is required to absorb 90% of the radiation of the argon laser, while only 60 mm of water absorbs 90% of the

Table 2.4. Absorption and Scattering Coefficients for Water at Different Wavelengths

Laser	Absorption (cm^{-1})	Reflectance (cm^{-1})
CO_2	200	0
Nd-YAG	0.23	21
Argon	0.03	>3

33

Table 2.5. Properties of Lasers

Laser	Wavelength, λ (μm)	Extinction length, L (mm)
Nd-YAG	1.06	60
CO_2	10.6	0.03
Argon	0.488–0.515	230

radiation from the Nd-YAG laser. In contrast, only 0.02 mm of water is required for the carbon dioxide laser beam. Because human tissue is composed of 70–90% water, precise control of the depth of destruction is possible.

2.2.3. Significance of Coefficients

1. CO_2 laser energy is totally absorbed within a depth of 90 μm. The energy remains where the beam strikes the tissue, because lateral scattering or reflectance is negligible. This property makes the CO_2 laser eminently suitable for precise surgical removal of tissue, since typical lesions are less than 2 mm in diameter. However, it makes the CO_2 laser poorly suited for coagulating deep or broad areas of tissue (Fig. 2.6).
2. The energy of the beam of a Nd-YAG laser is totally absorbed within a 30-mm depth in water, whereas in tissues it is totally absorbed within a few millimeters. A significant part of the energy is scattered laterally.* These facts make it well suited to deep coagulation of tissue, as in gastrointestinal bleeding, but poorly suited to precise local excision of tissue (Fig. 2.6).
3. The energy of the beam of an argon laser is totally absorbed within a depth of 230 mm, whereas about 100 times as much energy is scattered laterally as is directly absorbed. Hemoglobin absorbs at the argon laser's wavelength, thus in vascular tissue the argon laser will be absorbed in the first few millimeters. The argon laser is well suited to either retinal coagulation or coagulation at any site, but its color-sensitive absorption in living tissue and inherently deep penetration, combined with significant lateral scattering, make it poorly suited to precise surgical procedures (Fig. 2.6).

---

*Reflectance = 21 cm^{-1}, so the irradiated volume is greater than the definable geometrical one.

The unique properties of the CO_2 laser allow for precise vaporization of surface epithelium with a limited zone of injury. The argon and Nd-YAG can penetrate beyond the target surface; however, the forward scattering effect can, and occasionally does, result in additional injury to adjacent organs. But the CO_2 laser effect is precise and can be easily limited to the irradiated surface, because the scattering effect seen in argon and Nd-YAG lasers is not a characteristic of the CO_2 lasers. However, one must consider reflected energy: if the irradiated surface is reflective to the 10.6-μm wavelength, the ray can be deflected. Since polished surfaces, regardless of color, will reflect the CO_2 laser, nonreflective instruments or instruments of absorptive materials must be substituted for the usual highly polished stainless steel instruments. Nonflammable plastics, dulled metallic surfaces, or wet surfaces also absorb or fail to deflect the 10.6-μm wavelength. Glass contact lenses or plastic goggles will protect the eyes from accidentally reflected beams (see Section 2.4).

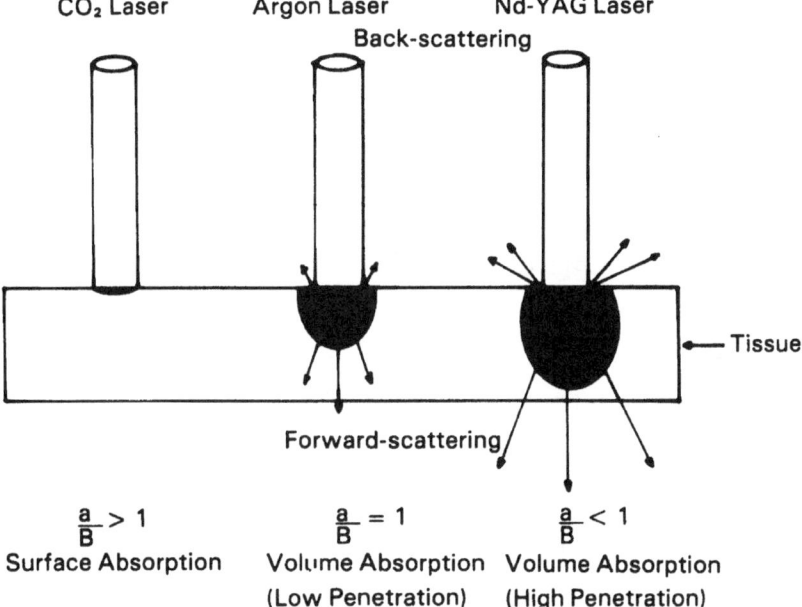

Figure 2.6. CO_2 laser vs. argon laser vs. Nd-YAG. Note the absence of reflection with CO_2 and the large amount of forward scatter with argon and Nd-YAG lasers. (Reproduced with permission: Bellina JH: The carbon dioxide laser in gynecology, Part I, in Leventhal JM (ed): Current Problems in Obstetrics and Gynecology. Vol. 4, 1981, pp 1–34.)

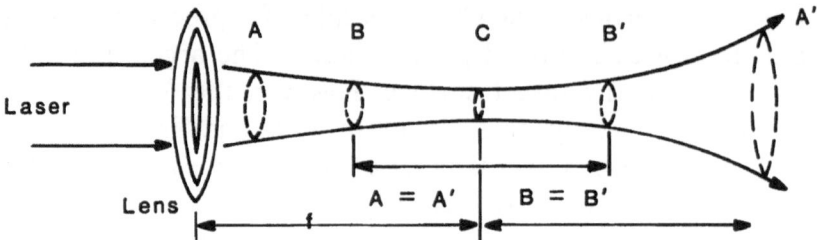

Figure 2.7. CO_2 beam diameter varies with focal length. Power densities are equal if beam diameters are equal.

2.2.4. Power Density

When the operating temperature has stabilized, most practical lasers will operate in a combination of lower-order transverse modes (the average net profile of power density across the beam will have low values near the edge of the beam, but comparatively higher values near the center), provided the mirror positions and other parameters have been properly adjusted. Because it is hopeless to attempt an analytical description of all the possible theoretical modes and combinations thereof, we shall consider only the most fundamental transverse mode, the **transverse electromagnetic mode** (TEM_{00}). For this mode, the variation of power density across any diameter of the beam is as shown in Fig. 2.7. In a gaussian (TEM_{00}) laser beam, the power density (PD) at any point can be calculated by the following formula:

$$PD = PD_0 \frac{W_0}{W} e^{2-2(r^2/w^2)} K$$

where PD_0 is the power density of the diameter of the beam axis at the waist, W is the radius at which the E field falls to $1/e$ of its value at the center (the so-called half-width of the beam), W_0 is the half-width of the diameter of the beam at the waist, r is the radius to the point at which PD is measured, e is the base of the natural logarithm (2.71828), and K is a phase constant dependent primarily on the axial location of the cross section relative to the diameter of the waist of the beam, and in the radius of curvature of the phasefront of the beam.

The most important parameters of a surgical laser, operating at a given wavelength, are **power density,** which is expressed as watts/cm^2 [or, in simple algebra, PD = (watts $\times$ 100)/(spot size in mm)^2] and **time exposure,** or the amount of time a given spot is exposed to the laser beam. However, since the time exposure depends on the speed of incision, power density is the single most important factor when choosing a machine of lesser power. Later, we shall see that the range of power density employed determines whether a laser will coagulate, vaporize, or cut into living tissue.

How can power density be measured? Unfortunately, because the focal spots of most lasers used in surgery are less than 2 mm in diameter, actual measurement of the point-to-point power density of a real surgical laser is very difficult. However, **total power** of the beam and **average power density** are relatively easy to measure. Except in the case of a stationary beam, where peak power density determines the maximum depth of ablation, it is more useful to know average power density, which determines both the central depth and the rate of mass removal from the furrow made by a moving beam. Average power density can be determined rather easily by measuring the effective spot diameter and the total power of the beam if we assume a gaussian distribution (TEM_{00} mode). Even if this is not valid for all lasers, it is a plausible assumption for well-adjusted lasers at stable operating temperatures, depending on lasing cavity and defective optical components. The beam's spot diameter at a given wavelength and power output is a function of the focal length of the lens of the beam divergence and of the diameter of the beam before the focusing lens. The depth of the focus is determined by the square of the focal length; the longer the focal distance of the lens, the larger the spot size (i.e., for a 400-mm length spot size $= 0.8$ mm, where as for a 50-mm length spot size $= 0.1$ mm). Furthermore, for constant power output, the smaller the spot size produced by the laser beam, the higher the power density per unit area. Thus power density is a function of both spot size and power, and it varies inversely with the square of the focal length of the lens. The relationship of power density, wattage, and spot size is illustrated in Figure 2.8. Therefore, the higher the power density capability of the CO_2 laser, the greater its versatility of application in performing operations. Moreover, since the focused beam's spot has an unequal cross-sectional distribution of energy (produced by the different mirror alignment and geometric patterns within the laser resonator cavity) the power density describes only the *average* power density, while the "shape" of the beam is determied by the TEM_{00}. Other power-density profiles will, of course, yield different average values with a given total power and spot diameter, but stable modes of well-adjusted lasers will not produce drastically different average power densities than that of TEM_{00}, even though, for a given total power and spot size, they must cause higher peak power densities (Fig. 2.9).

The above discussion and formula are difficult to integrate into a gynecologist's daily working practice. Thus, the exponential formula was condensed. Recall the simple algebraic expression PD $= $ (watts $\times$ 100)/(spot size in mm)^2. The calculation of power density is straightforward, and the

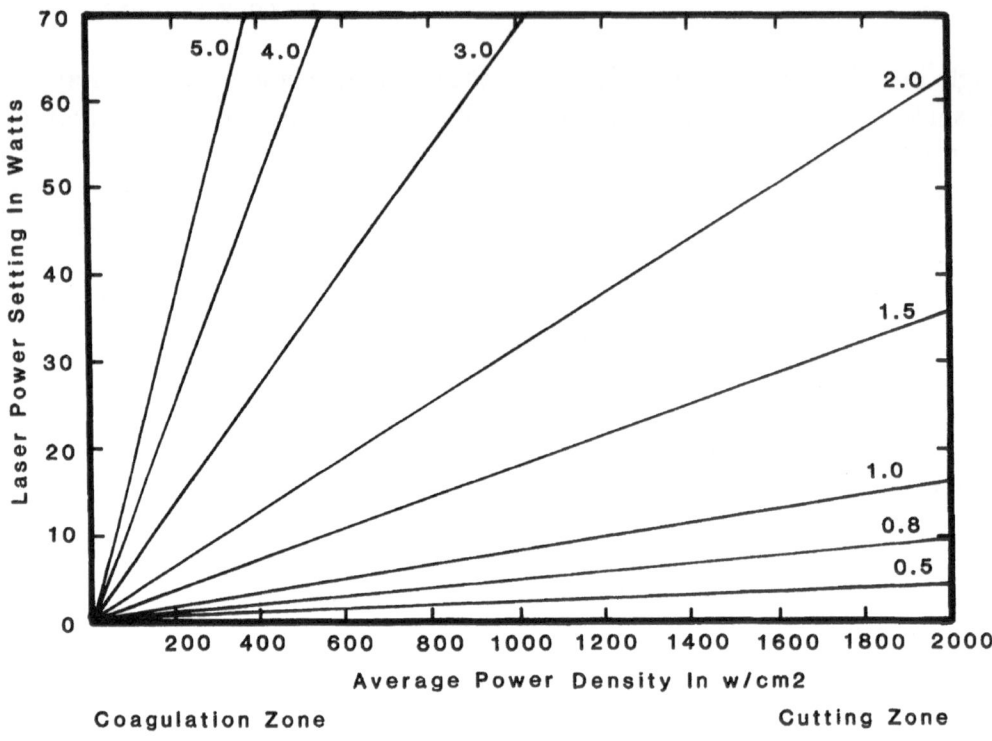

Figure 2.8. Chart showing the interrelationships of spot size, laser power setting, and average power density.

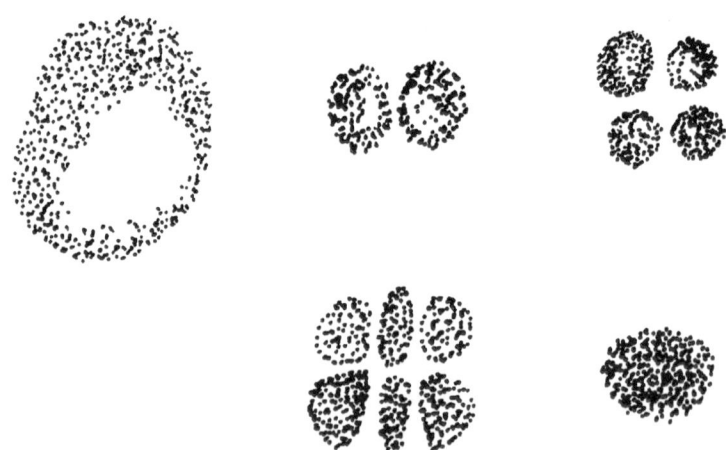

Figure 2.9. Variation in laser beam characteristic with respect to the shift in TEM. (Reproduced with permission: Bellina JH, Dorsey JH: Physics and bioeffects of gynecologic surgical lasers, in Bellina JH (ed): Gynecologic Laser Surgery, Proceedings of International Congress on Gynecologic Laser Surgery and Related Works, New Orleans, LA, Jan 1980. Plenum Press, New York, 1981.)

surgeon need only know the wattage of the laser, read from the inline power meter, and the diameter of the focal spot of the laser. The focal spot diameter can be easily measured by means of a millimeter ruler. The laser can be focused on any surface where an imprint can be measured. From this spot diameter in millimeters (SD) and the inline power meter on the laser instrument (W), the average power density (PD) to the tissue surface in watts/ cm^2 can be calculated as follows:

$$PD = \frac{\text{watts} \times 100}{SD^2}$$

where SD is the focused spot size diameter of the laser in millimeters.

Although πr^2 is the formula for calculating surface area, it has been found that the surface area does not need to be used to compensate for gaussian or average power distribution. The diameter of the spot size will give an excellent approximation when substituted in the formula. (The average power densities may also be determined from the chart in Fig. 2.10.)

Power is measured in watts, and energy is measured in joules. Energy equals power times duration of exposure. It follows then that power, energy, and tissue destruction are all directly proportional. The time of exposure is controlled by a shutter activated by a foot pedal. The great number of variations in combining power settings and duration of exposure allows the surgeon great flexibility in the application of laser energy. Different settings are appropriate for different surgical situations and produce different effects. A power density chart, showing the most utilized CO_2 combinations, is shown in Fig. 2.8.

If it is assumed that tissue reacts to laser impact as does water (due to its high water content) then, theoretically, when CO_2 laser energy is applied to this tissue, a cylindrical section with a diameter equal to the focal spot diameter of the laser beam would be vaporized. The depth of tissue destruction is precisely controlled by varying the power density of the beam and the duration of time for which the beam is applied. This assumes that all of this energy is used to vaporize tissue and that laser energy is evenly distributed over the area of the focal spot. In reality, however, some energy is reflected by the target tissue, and the energy distribution within the laser beam, which does vary due to a number of factors such as the shape and reflectivity of the mirrors and changes in temperature within the laser tube, causes expansion and contraction of its various elements. In small commercially available surgical lasers it would be difficult to eliminate these variations without tremendous expense. Fortunately the surgeon is usually not hampered by these deviations from the ideal, but recognizing the characteristics of the beam will allow for its optimum use.

P_0 = Total Power required in a gaussian laser beam to achieve specific values of average power density

P_{aw} = Average power density in the laser beam within the effective diameter, $2w$, in W/cm^2

2w = Effective diameter of laser spot in millimeters	10	50	100	200	300	400	500	600	700	800	900	1,000	1,500	2,000
0.1	0.001	0.005	0.009	0.018	0.027	0.036	0.045	0.055	0.064	0.073	0.082	0.091	0.136	0.182
0.2	0.004	0.018	0.036	0.073	0.109	0.146	0.182	0.218	0.255	0.291	0.327	0.364	0.546	0.728
0.3	0.008	0.041	0.082	0.164	0.246	0.327	0.409	0.491	0.573	0.655	0.737	0.819	1.228	1.637
0.4	0.015	0.073	0.146	0.289	0.437	0.582	0.728	0.873	1.019	1.164	1.310	1.455	2.183	2.911
0.5	0.023	0.114	0.227	0.455	0.682	0.910	1.137	1.364	1.592	1.819	2.047	2.274	3.411	4.548
0.6	0.033	0.164	0.327	0.655	0.982	1.310	1.637	1.965	2.292	2.620	2.947	3.274	4.912	6.549
0.7	0.045	0.223	0.446	0.891	1.337	1.783	2.228	2.674	3.120	3.565	4.011	4.457	6.685	8.914
0.8	0.058	0.291	0.582	1.164	1.764	2.328	2.911	3.493	4.075	4.657	5.239	5.821	8.732	11.642
0.9	0.074	0.368	0.737	1.473	2.210	2.947	3.684	4.420	5.157	5.894	6.631	7.367	11.051	14.735
1.0	0.091	0.455	0.910	1.819	2.727	3.638	4.548	5.457	6.367	7.276	8.186	9.096	13.643	18.191
1.1	0.110	0.550	1.101	2.201	3.302	4.402	5.503	6.603	7.704	8.805	9.905	11.006	16.509	22.011
1.2	0.131	0.655	1.310	2.620	3.929	5.239	6.549	7.859	9.168	10.478	11.788	13.098	19.647	26.195
1.3	0.154	0.769	1.537	3.074	4.611	6.149	7.688	9.223	10.760	12.297	13.834	15.372	23.057	30.743
1.4	0.178	0.891	1.783	3.565	5.348	7.131	8.914	10.696	12.479	14.262	16.045	17.827	26.741	35.655
1.5	0.205	1.023	2.041	4.093	6.140	8.186	10.233	12.297	14.326	16.372	18.419	20.465	30.698	40.930
1.6	0.233	1.164	2.328	4.657	6.985	9.314	11.642	13.971	16.299	18.628	20.956	23.285	34.927	46.569
1.7	0.263	1.314	2.629	5.257	7.886	10.515	13.143	15.772	18.400	21.029	23.658	26.286	39.429	52.573
1.8	0.295	1.473	2.947	5.894	8.841	11.788	14.735	17.682	20.629	23.576	26.523	29.470	44.205	58.940
1.9	0.328	1.642	3.284	6.567	9.851	13.134	16.418	19.702	22.985	26.268	29.552	32.835	49.253	65.670
2.0	0.364	1.819	3.638	7.276	10.915	14.553	18.191	21.829	25.468	29.106	32.744	36.382	54.574	72.765
2.1	0.401	2.006	4.011	8.022	12.033	16.045	20.056	24.067	28.078	32.089	36.100	40.112	60.167	80.223
2.2	0.440	2.201	4.402	8.805	13.207	17.609	22.011	26.414	30.816	35.218	39.620	44.023	66.034	88.045
2.3	0.481	2.406	4.812	9.623	14.435	19.246	24.058	28.869	33.681	38.492	43.304	48.116	72.174	96.232
2.4	0.524	2.620	5.239	10.478	15.717	20.956	26.195	31.434	36.673	41.913	47.152	52.391	78.586	104.781
2.5	0.568	2.842	5.685	11.370	17.054	22.739	28.424	34.109	39.793	45.478	51.163	56.848	85.271	113.695
2.6	0.615	3.074	6.149	12.297	18.446	24.595	30.743	36.892	43.040	49.189	55.338	61.486	92.229	122.973
2.7	0.663	3.315	6.631	13.261	19.892	26.523	33.153	39.748	46.415	53.046	59.676	66.307	99.460	132.614
2.8	0.713	3.565	7.131	14.262	21.393	28.524	35.655	42.786	49.917	57.049	64.179	71.310	106.964	142.619
2.9	0.765	3.825	7.649	15.299	22.948	30.598	38.247	45.896	53.546	61.192	68.845	76.494	114.741	152.988
3.0	0.819	4.093	8.186	16.372	24.558	32.744	40.930	49.116	57.302	65.488	73.674	81.860	122.791	163.721

Figure 2.10. Interrelationships of spot size, laser power setting, and average power density. $P_0 = 0.0090956 \times (p_{aw} \text{ in W/cm}^2) \times (2w \text{ in mm})^2$, where P_0 is the total power of the beam in watts. $p_c = 254.65 P_0/(2w \text{ in mm})^2 = 2.3162 p_{aw}$, where p_c is the power density at the center.

2.2.5. Transverse Electromagnetic Mode and Its Significance

The fluctuations in cross-sectional energy distribution can readily be demonstrated if one examines the imprint made by short bursts of laser energy on a tongue depressor. Some areas within the focal spot are obviously more scorched or burned than others. Often, energy density is higher at the center of the beam than at the periphery. Cross-sectional energy distribution in the laser beam is referred to as transverse electromagnetic mode (TEM). Usually the energy is most intense in the beam center, decreasing in intensity toward the periphery of the beam. This is best described in two dimensions by the gaussian distribution (Fig. 2.11). Other TEMs can occur in surgical lasers, as demonstrated in Fig. 2.12, and it is necessary for the surgeon to recognize the variations of energy distribution of his instrument in order to understand the anatomic configurations and pathology of the resulting laser lesions.[3]

2.2.6. Laser Modes and Effects of Temperature on Mode Stability

The term **mode** refers essentially to the geometric patterns of coherent radiation both inside the laser resonator, where reflections and amplification occur, and outside the laser, where the beam of radiation is used for some

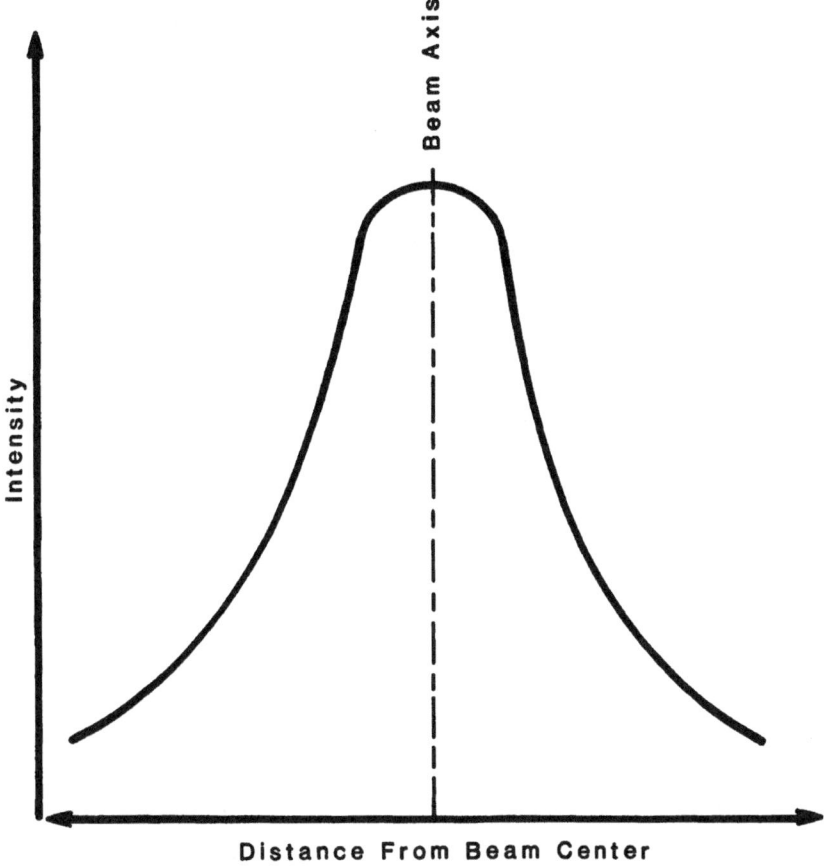

Figure 2.11. Two-dimensional intensity profile of the laser beam. The distribution is gaussian and beam intensity diminishes in a reciprocal exponential function as distance from the beam axis increases.

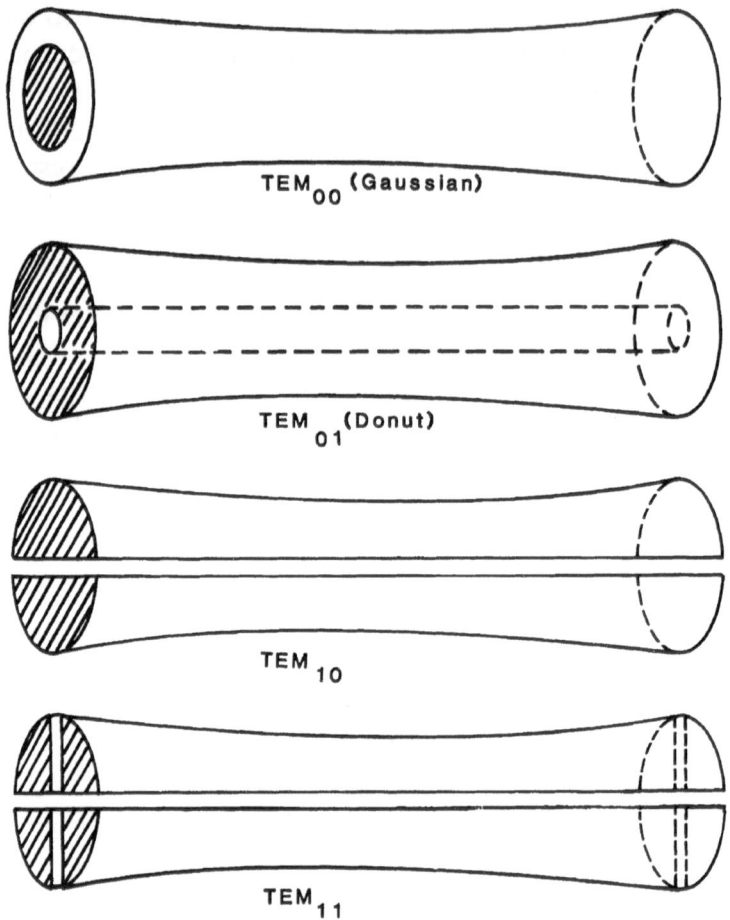

Figure 2.12. Different energy profiles of various laser instruments as demonstrated by their impact craters.

external purpose (Fig. 2.12). By **geometric patterns,** we mean not only the gross three-dimensional direction of the resonator, but also the density or distribution of the rays over any cross-section perpendicular to the axis of the resonator. Modes may be divided into longitudinal and transverse. Longitudinal modes relate to the number of half-wavelengths which can exist between the mirrors and the amplification and losses associated with each of these wave patterns. The longitudinal mode(s) of a laser determine the predominant wavelength(s) at which it will operate. The transverse modes of a laser determine the radial distribution of power across the laser beam. Each possible mode of a laser has an amplification factor and a loss factor associated with it. Each mode draws its power from the total inverted population of excited atoms or molecules available as the result of the "pumping" of these potential emitters of coherent radiation. In an ideal resonator, each of the possible modes is independent of all the others, but in real lasers, there is coupling between modes. Those modes which have high amplification and low loss will predominate. The resonator is often designed to accentuate certain modes and suppress the others, particularly those axial modes which generate wavelengths from the most desirable beam of the laser. Most practical lasers, or multimode lasers, will operate simultaneously in only a few axial modes and in several transverse modes. Each of the separate modes will augment the total output power of the laser, provided that there is a sufficient population of excited atoms so that power flowing into one mode does not deplete that flowing into the other modes.

For many physical and medical purposes, it is desirable to have only one *axial* mode, so that all of the output power of the laser can be concentrated at *one wavelength,* and to have only one *transverse* mode, so as to achieve a *smooth variation of radiant-power density* over the cross section of the beam. The former condition is relatively easy to achieve, but the latter is rather difficult.

The purpose for which the laser is to be used will determine the selection of the TEM. Fidler[4] has demonstrated that less power is required with a single-mode beam than with a multimode beam to achieve the same power density. This is due to the greater possibility of obtaining a smaller spot size because of easier focusing. Actually when a surgeon deals with a sophisticated biophysical instrument, he must recognize the concepts concerning all parameters of surgical lasers. Their energy delivery systems must be completely understood.

Energy distribution in the section of the beam does vary considerably from manufacturer to manufacturer and from CO_2 laser unit to CO_2 laser unit; in fact, some units are less stable than others and vary from minute to minute, primarily in temperature. This mode variation may not be significant when we consider that we define the working area or focus spot size as 2 mm; but in general, as the spot size diminishes, the TEM biological effect becomes more pronounced. When only total quantity of energy in watts is known, the physician can easily read the inline meter power output and obtain the watts being delivered by the source.

The transverse mode of the laser is most readily measured in practice by the profile of power density (power per unit area) across the beam. It is intuitively evident that this will be affected by the shape of the mirrors (i.e., plane, spherical, etc.) and by the variation of reflectivity across the surface of each mirror. In all real lasers of high output power (>5 W or so), heat is generated by the pumping system, and the temperature of the resonator will change from point to point and from time to time. Changes of temperature cause expansion and/or contraction of the laser tube or rod, the mirrors, and the supporting structures. These small thermal movements, in turn, cause shifting of the transverse modes of the laser. Only by very elaborate structural schemes, which are often prohibitively expensive and bulky, can these thermal shifts be minimized. Therefore, the surgeon must be aware that they exist, and modify his technique to accommodate them. One simple way to minimize thermal mode-shifts is to operate the laser at the desired power level for a period of 30–60 min before surgery to allow all parts of the laser to reach stable temperatures. Furthermore, one must remember that the transverse electromagnetic modes of a *real* laser cannot always be described by the the theoretical modes designated as TEM_{mn}, where m and n are integers.

2.2.7. Biophysical Parameters of CO_2 Surgical Lasers and Dosimetry

Wavelength = λ = 10.6 μm (far infrared).
Power output = 0–100 (maximum obtainable 300 W–9 kW) continuously adjustable or pulsed. Class IV = high-power system.
Beam spot size = 0.1- to 2-mm diameter (function of the focal length and the mode).
Divergence = angle by which the laser deviates from parallelism.
Exposure time = intermittent emission (duration less than 0.25 sec) or continuous wave (cw) emission (duration more than 0.25 sec) function of speed of incision.
Power density = $\dfrac{\text{Power output}}{d^2}$ = 0–2000 W/cm^2 (maximum, 10^6 W/cm^2).
TEM = gaussian (00) or multimode.
Focal length $\geq$ 50–500 mm.
Absorption coefficient = a = 200/cm in water (Beer–Lambert law:
$$I = I_0 e^{-ax})$$
Helium–neon: Guide light (finder beam) = 632.8-mm wavelength (or other guide light). Power 0.8 → 2 mW; spot size~1 mm.

2.2.8. Clinical Conclusions

The conclusions to be drawn from the foregoing analysis are as follows:

1. The total mass ablated by a laser beam which strikes a target body in one fixed place is directly proportional to the total power of the beam, and to the length in time of application, and inversely proportional to the energy per unit mass needed to preheat and vaporize the material, starting from its initial temperature.

2. The total mass ablated by a moving laser beam depends upon the same factors as for a stationary beam, but will be somewhat less, even if the total beam power and length in time of application are the same as for the stationary beam, since it depends on cutting speed.

3. The depth of ablation produced by a stationary beam is directly proportional to the maximum power density multiplied by the length in time of application, and inversely proportional to the energy per unit volume needed to reheat and vaporize the material, starting from its initial temperature.

4. The depth of ablation produced by a moving laser beam is directly proportional to the average power density of the beam diameter multiplied by the effective diameter of the beam, and inversely proportional to the velocity at which the beam sweeps across the surface, as well as to the energy per unit volume needed to heat and vaporize the material.

5. To avoid furrowing the crater when an area of surface must be ablated, it is essential that the beam be swept across the area in at least two directions, whose lines are mutually perpendicular. This is especially important in dealing with dysplastic tissue with oncogenic potential, because the small islands of unvaporized tissue formed by the ridges between adjacent parallel grooves can contain viable cells.

6. To insure destruction of all viable tissue in a dysplastic lesion, the margin (periphery) and the depth of the ablated volume must be greater than those of the lesion itself, insofar as this can be achieved without unacceptable destruction of adjacent healthy tissue.

7. The best procedure is to use the highest average power density that the surgeon can control without causing undesirable damage to proximal healthy tissue.

8. When the laser is used for coagulation, rather than vaporization, the average power density should not be more than $150 \, \text{W/cm}^2$. This can be achieved by adjusting the focus to increase the spot size or reducing the total beam power, or both.

2.3. Current CO$_2$ Laser Models

2.3.1. Introduction

The following companies offer equipment for gynecologic surgery that is presently on the United States market:

Cavitron Lasersonics
88 Hamilton Avenue
Stamford, Connecticut 06906

Merrimack Laboratories
34 Tower Street
P.O. Box 357
Hudson, Massachusetts 06149

Metricon, Ltd.
1931 Old Middlefield Way
Mountain View, California 94043

Advanced Biomedical Instruments
4 Plympton Street
Woburn, Massachusetts

Coherent
3270 West Bayshore Road
P.O. Box 10321
Palo Alto, California 94303

Advanced Surgical Technologies
Sharplan CO$_2$ Lasers
27 Wells Road
Monroe, Connecticut 06468

Valfivre Laser Surgical Systems
Via Panciatichi 70
50127 Florence, Italy

American Optical Corporation
P.O. Box 123
Buffalo, New York 14240

Biophysics Medical S.A.
10, Rue Des Barres
75004 Paris, France

Nippon Infrared Industries
4-8-8 Roppongi Minato-Ku
Tokyo 106, Japan

Cooper Medical Devices
600 McCormick Street
San Leandro, California 94577

Xanar, Inc.
2860 S. Circle Drive, Ste. 2203
Colorado Springs, Colorado 80906

Each system has its own peculiarities, but in general, the following discussion will be sufficient to understand the generalities of each machine (Figs. 2.13–2.20).

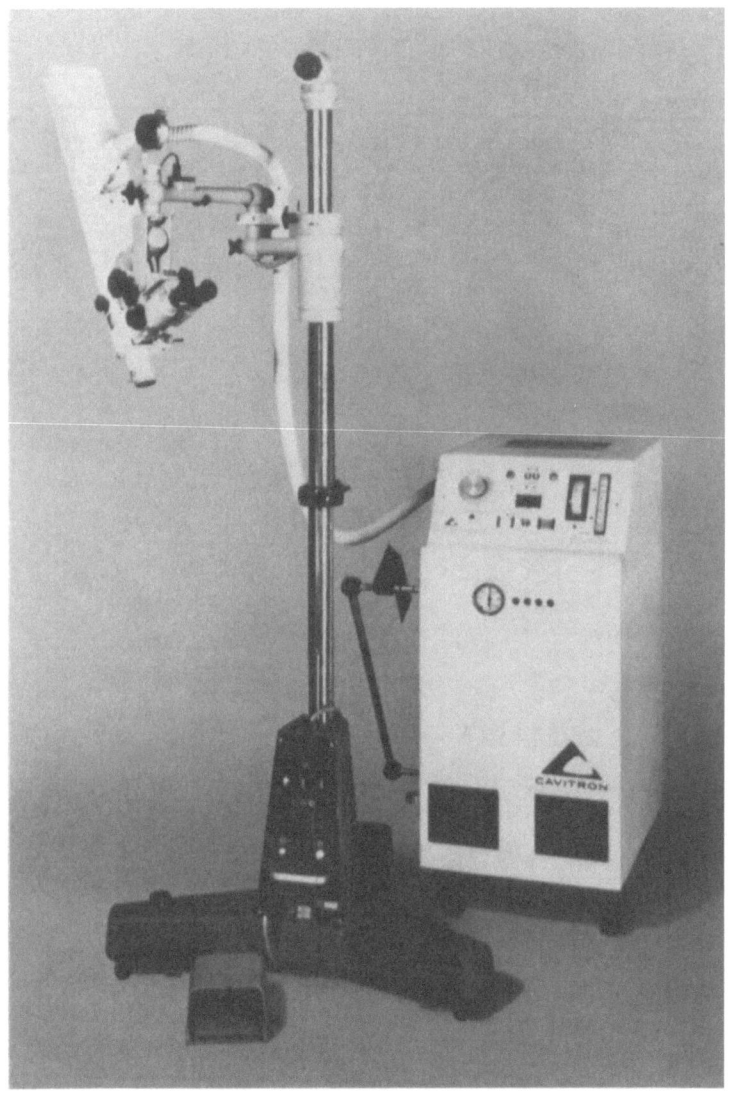

Figure 2.13. Cavitron Model 300 laser.

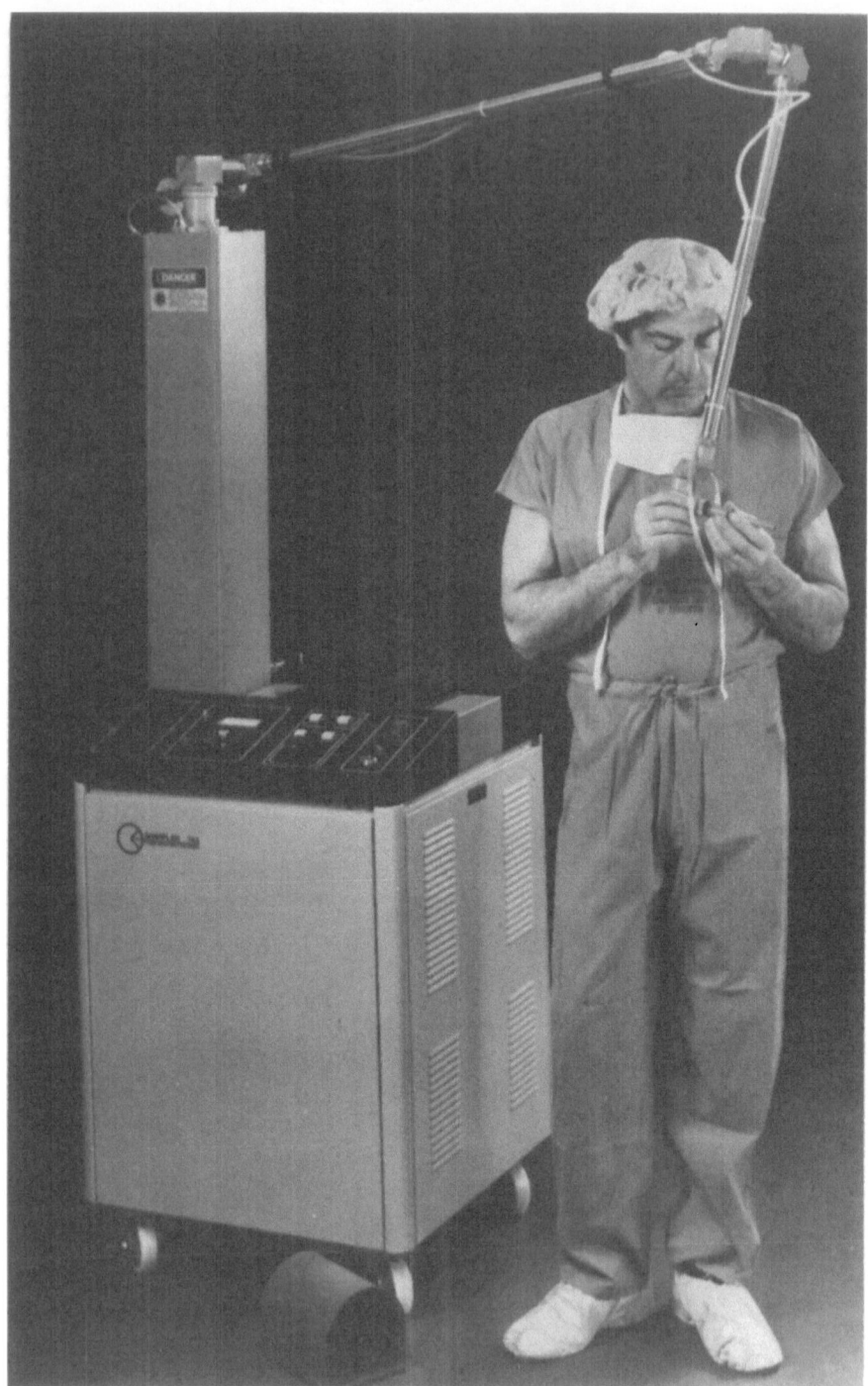

Figure 2.14. Advanced Surgical Technologies—Sharplan Model 733 laser.

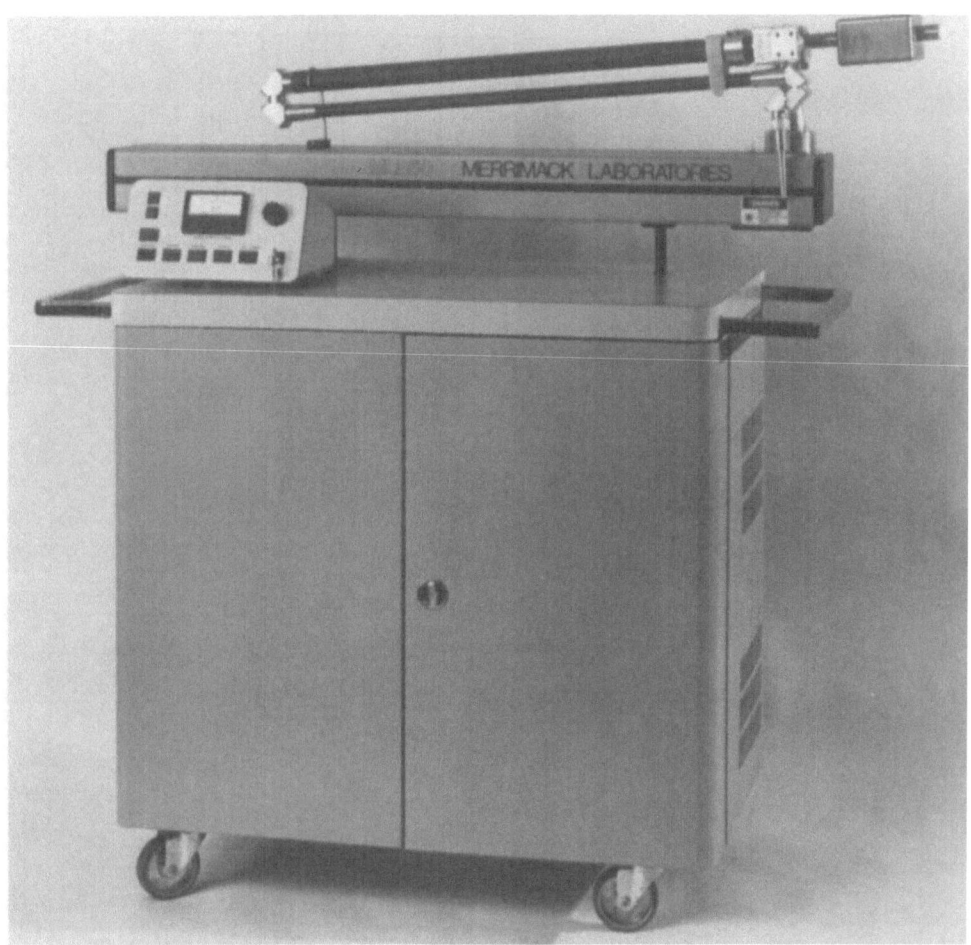

Figure 2.15. Merrimack laser.

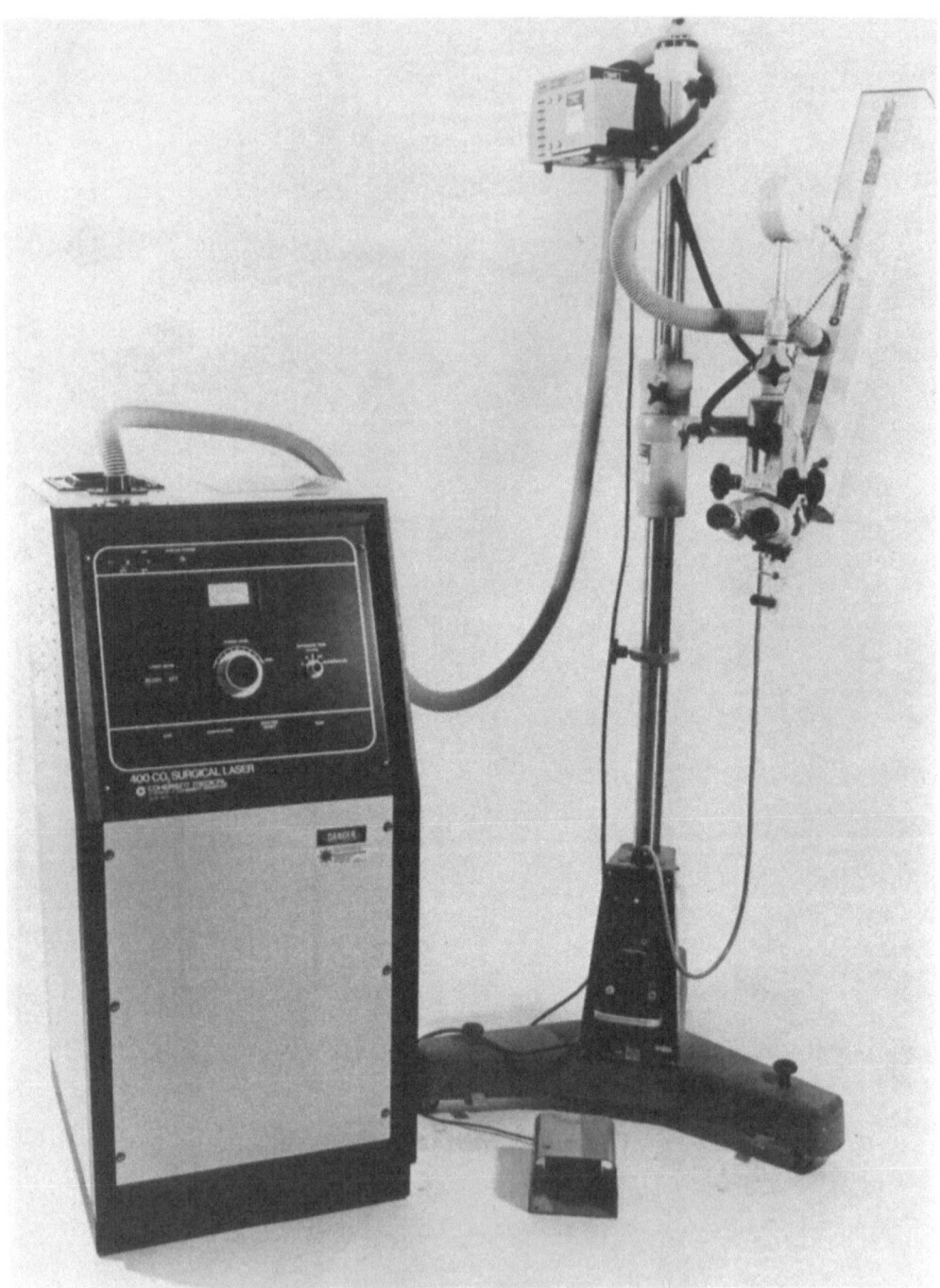

Figure 2.16. Coherent Model 400 laser.

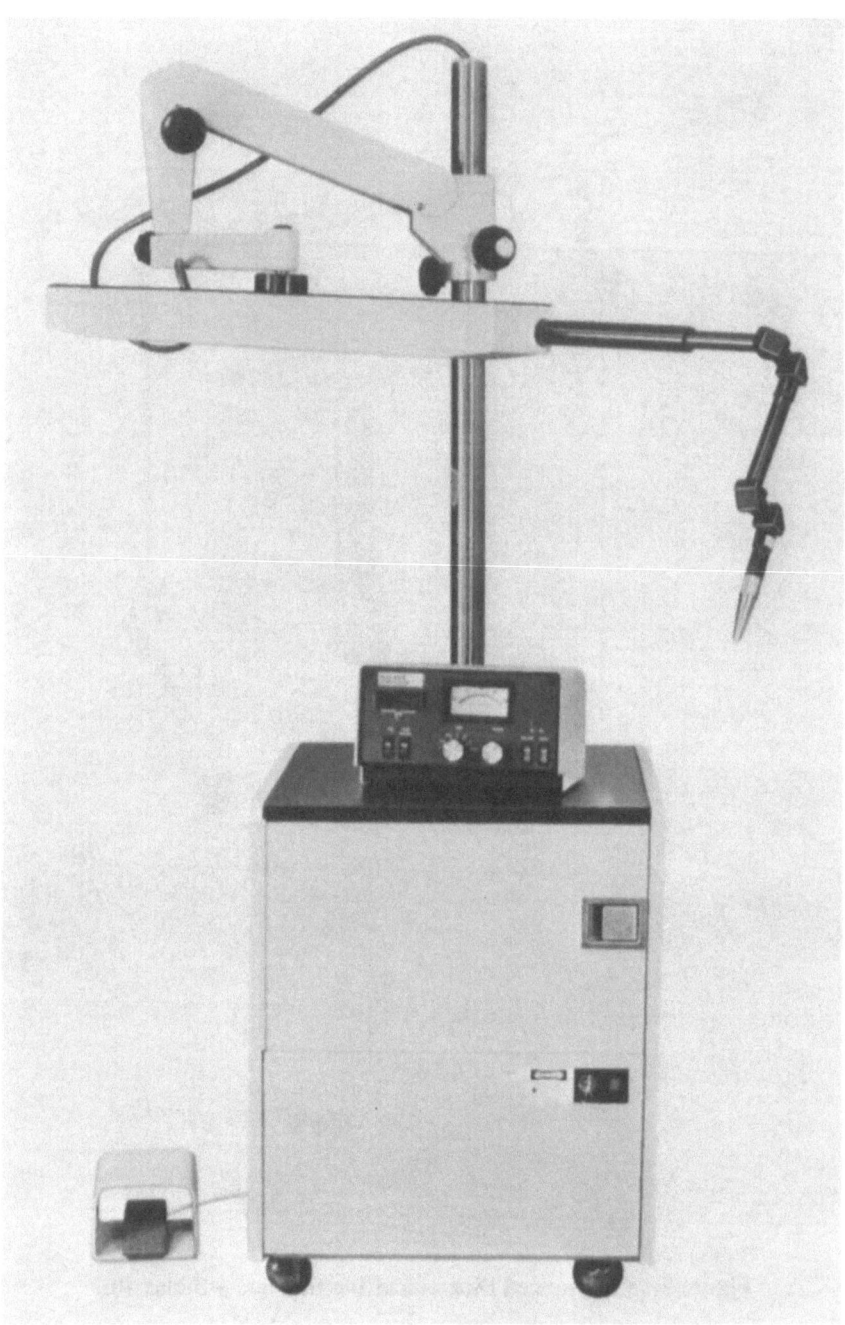

Figure 2.17. Xanar Model 370 laser.

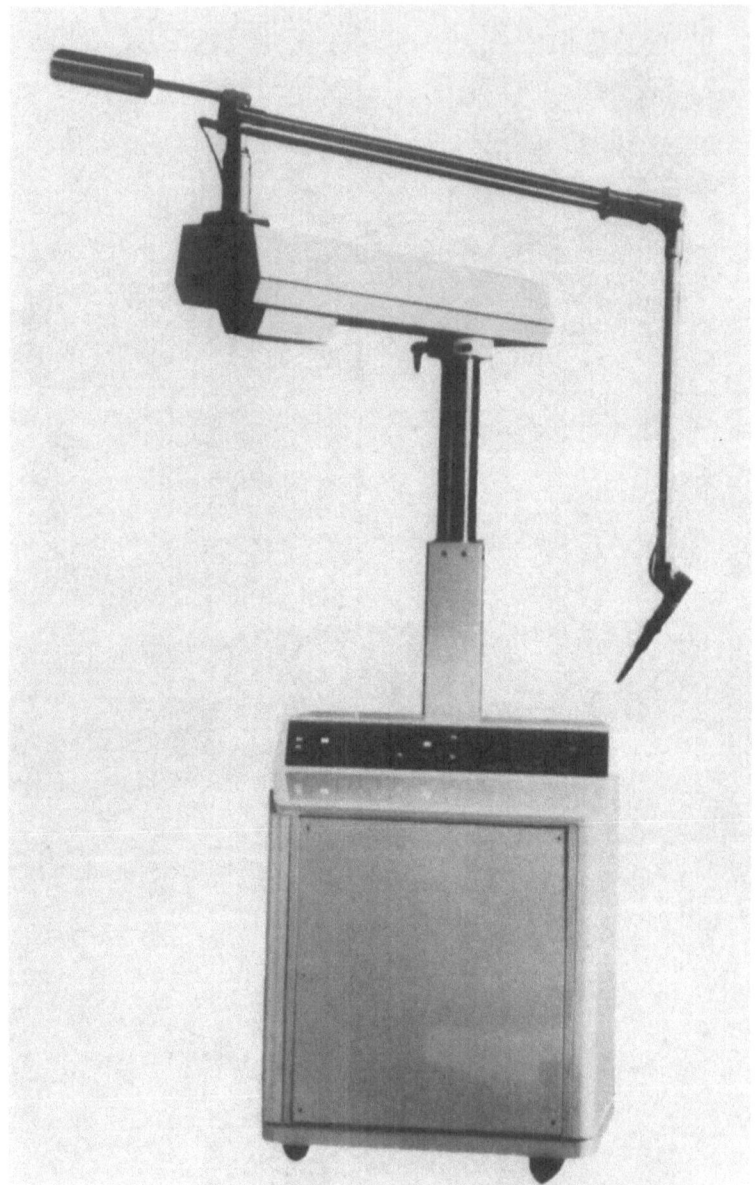

Figure 2.18. Advanced Biomedical Instruments—Biolas 40.

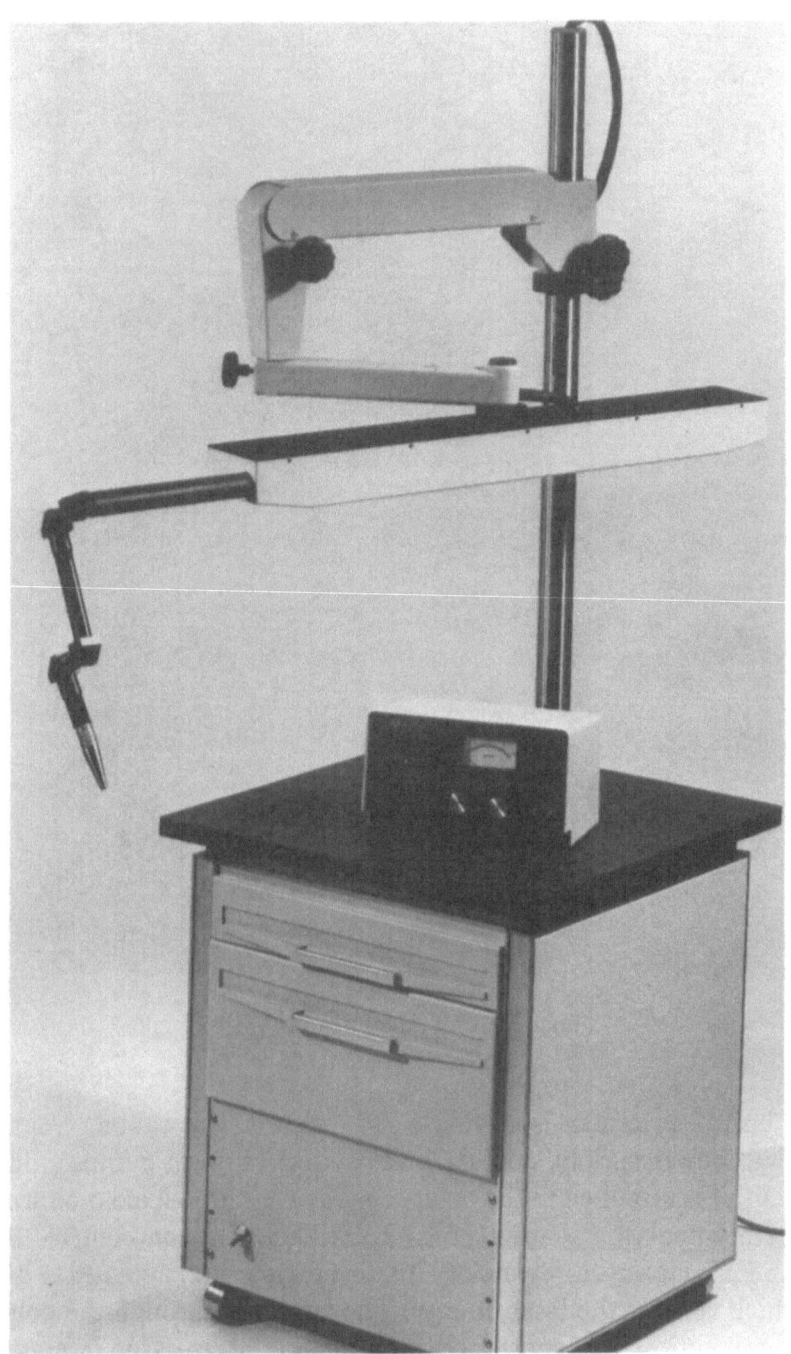

Figure 2.19. Valfivre Model LSS50.

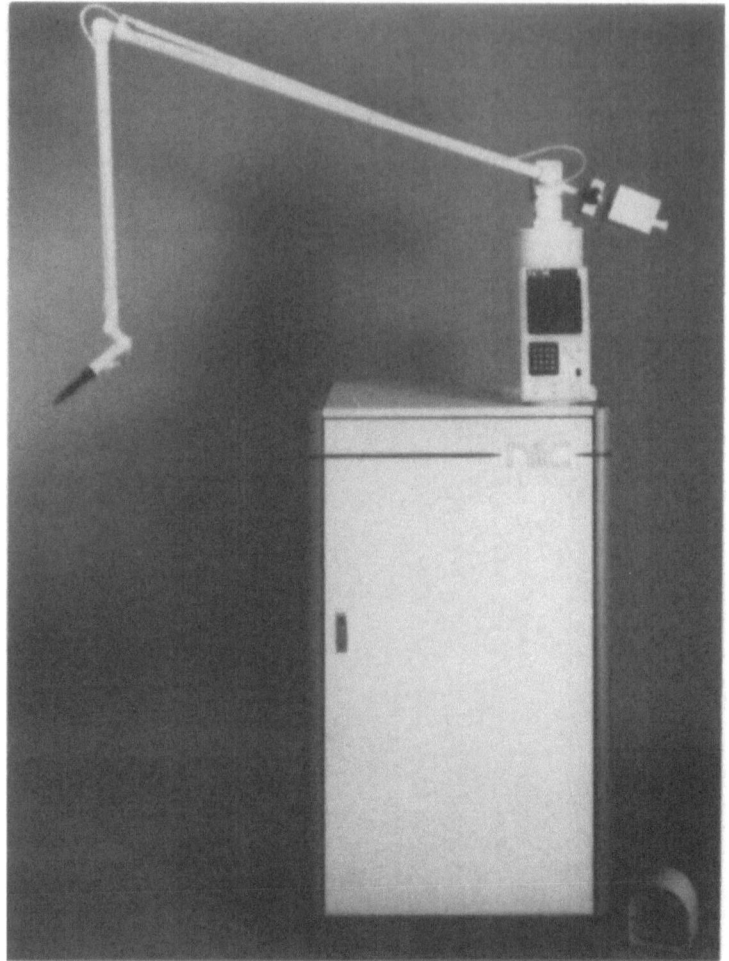

Figure 2.20. NIIC laser 130YZ.

The basic equipment is composed of an electrical cabinet housing, the high-voltage power supply, cooling pumps, and vacuum pumps (Fig. 2.21). The laser head is attached to the colopsocope by either a fixed mounting (Fig. 2.22) or a manipulator adaptor (Fig. 2.23). The surgeon controls the laser beam by manipulating a joystick. This lever system articulates a gimbaled mirror which reflects the laser energy. The surgeon, through the colposcope, under magnification, can constantly monitor the laser–tissue interaction.

In order to begin the activation sequence, the paramedical personnel should perform the following steps:

1. Open the access door in the rear or side of the electrical cabinets (Fig. 2.24) where a large bottle of premixed gas is stored (make sure

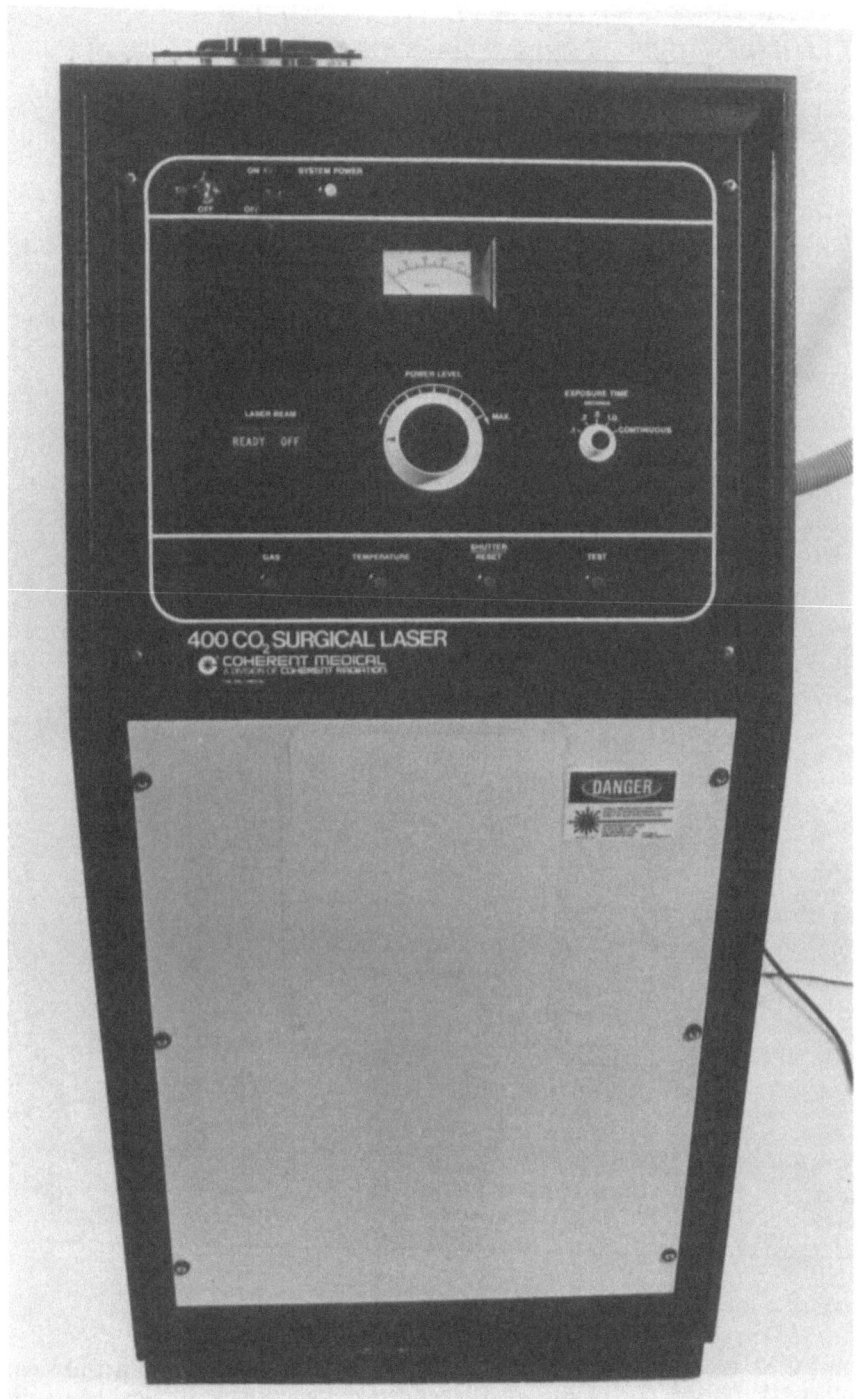

Figure 2.21. Basic laser electrical housing.

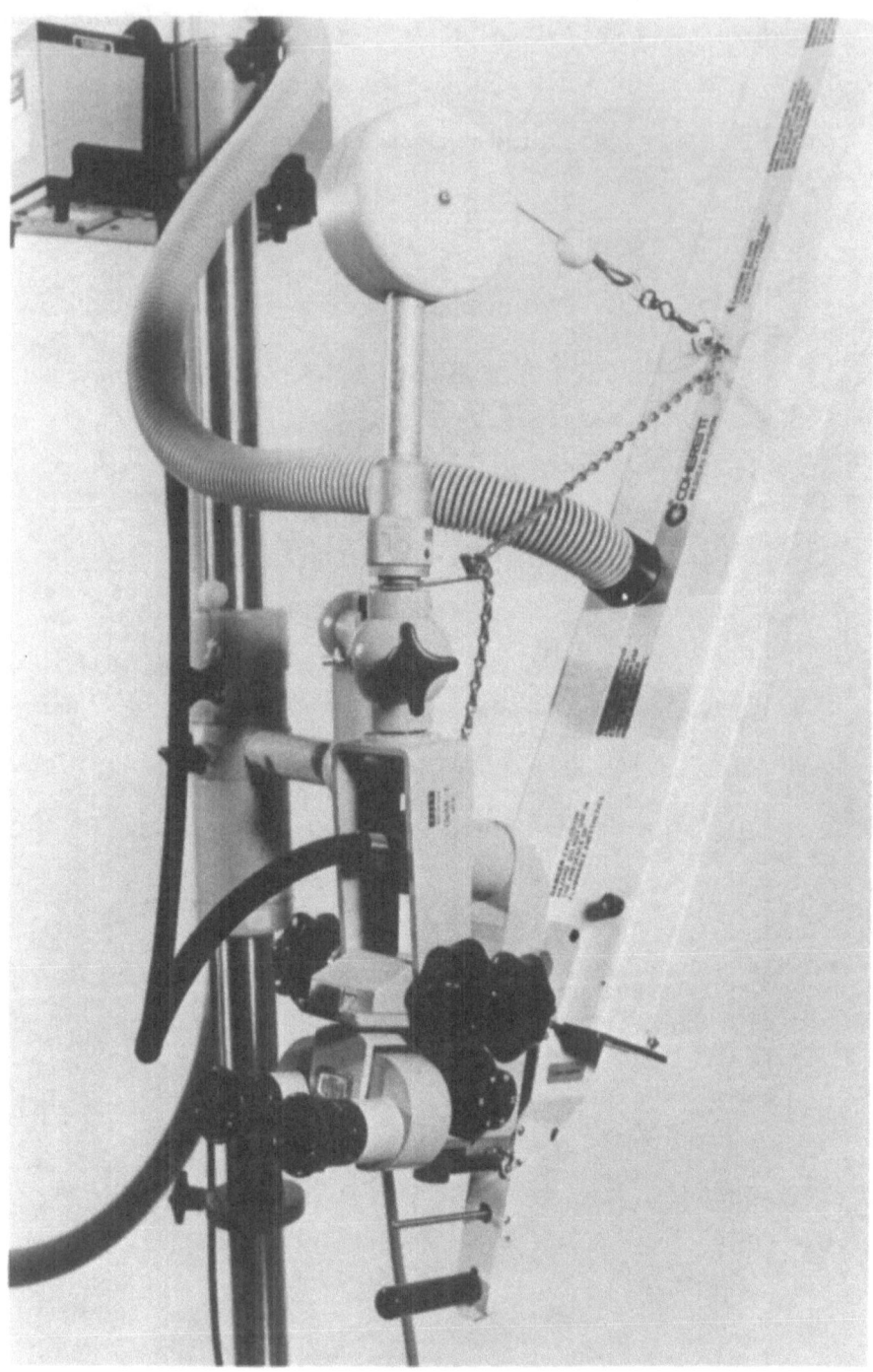

Figure 2.22. Laser head is attached to colposcope. (Reproduced with permission: Bellina JH, Dorsey JH: Physics and bioeffects of gynecologic surgical lasers, in Bellina JH (ed): Gynecologic Laser Surgery, Proceedings of International Congress on Gynecologic Laser Surgery and Related Works, New Orleans, LA, January 1980. Plenum Press, New York, 1981.)

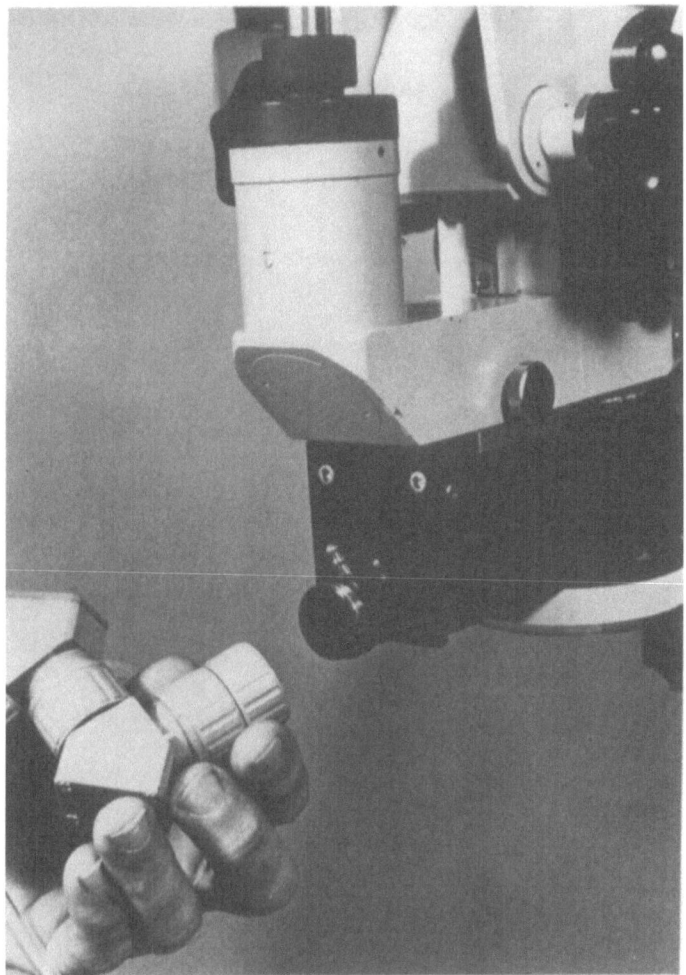

Figure 2.23. Laser head is attached to micromanipulator.

the proper gas mixture ratio is present, because each manufacturer uses a slightly different proportion of N_2, CO_2, and He).

2. Check the radiator water; if it is low, add distilled water. The cooling system needs periodic flushing and the engineer or paramedical personnel must be familiar with the manufacturer's manual.

3. If safety circuits are present, they must be placed in the *on* position.

4. The gas tank control valves must be opened. Usually there is a main control valve indicating inner tank pressure and a second valve indicating outflow in liters/min (Fig. 2.25). The flow rate gauge can be controlled by a second needle valve handle. It should be turned until

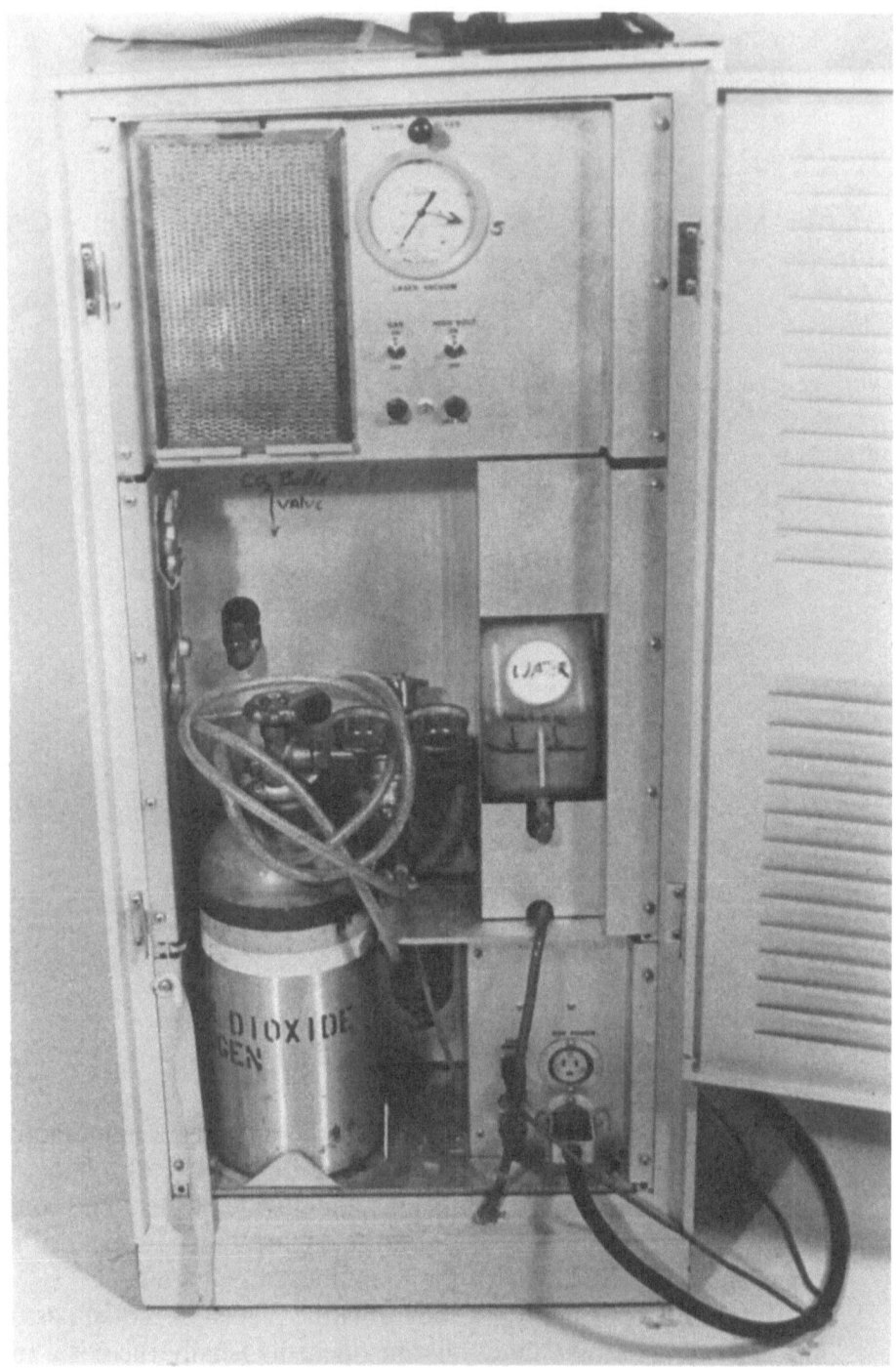

Figure 2.24. Access door to laser cabinet.

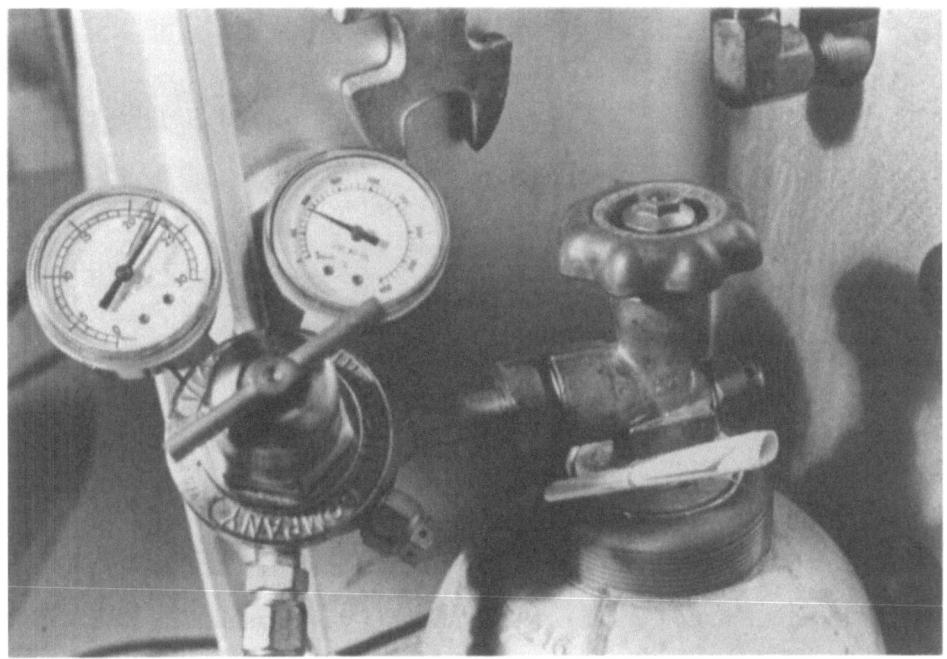

Figure 2.25. Gas pressure gauge and flow rate gauge.

the flow rate or pressure is proper, because each manufacturer may have a different setting. Consult your manual.

In order to activate the laser system electrically, the following general rules apply (there are slight variations from manufacturer to manufacturer). The control panel contains a keyed lock for maximum safety (Fig. 2.26) and the key should be kept in a safe place. Once activated, the electrical circuits can be turned on by the manual switch. Usually a *power on* light will indicate the system is activated. Next the *laser switch* is pushed to charge the optical cavity. A red light or warning signal indicates that the system is activated. The power in the system can now be controlled by turning the power level knob. The laser power is recorded on the power meter on the instrument panel. Finally, the time interval can be chosen.

The mode, continuous or pulsed, and the repetition rate are selected. Power output is expressed in watts (J/sec). Pulsed repetition rate (pps) and single pulse duration (sec) are specified when the output beam is emitted in the pulsed mode. The laser usually has a manual safety shutter (Fig. 2.27). When it is closed, the HeNe laser pointer cannot be seen. This safety feature allows the surgeon to stop the laser manually should an electrical circuit fail. To date, we know of no shutter failure; the shutter mechanism is one of the

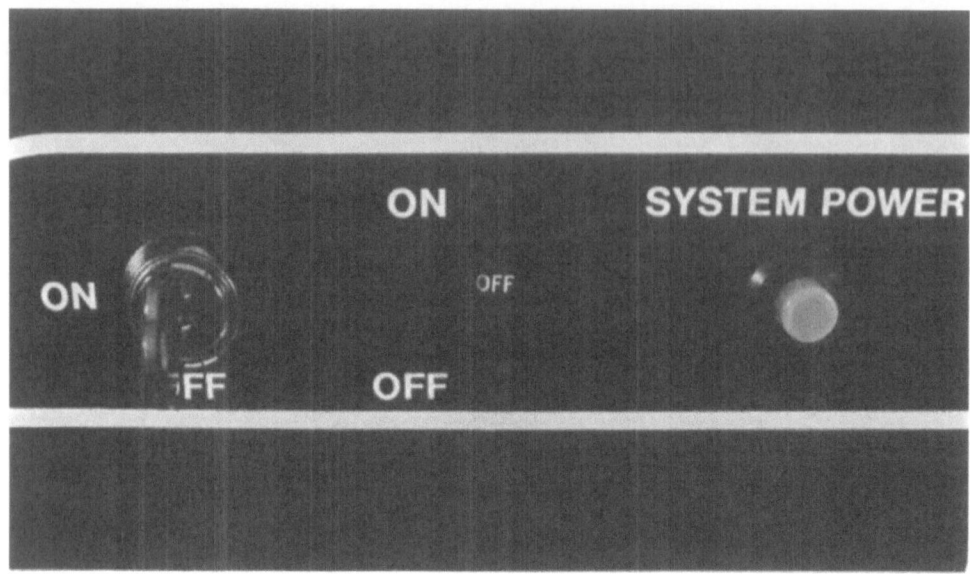

Chapter 3

Figure 2.26. Control panel with keyed lock for maximum safety.

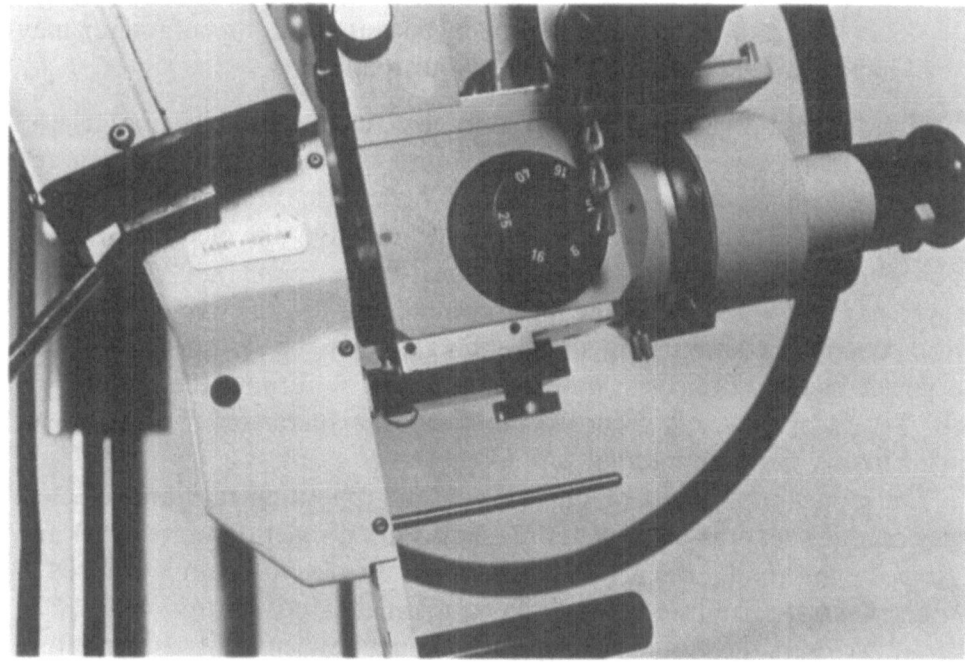

Figure 2.27. Manual safety shutter noted above laser aperture sign.

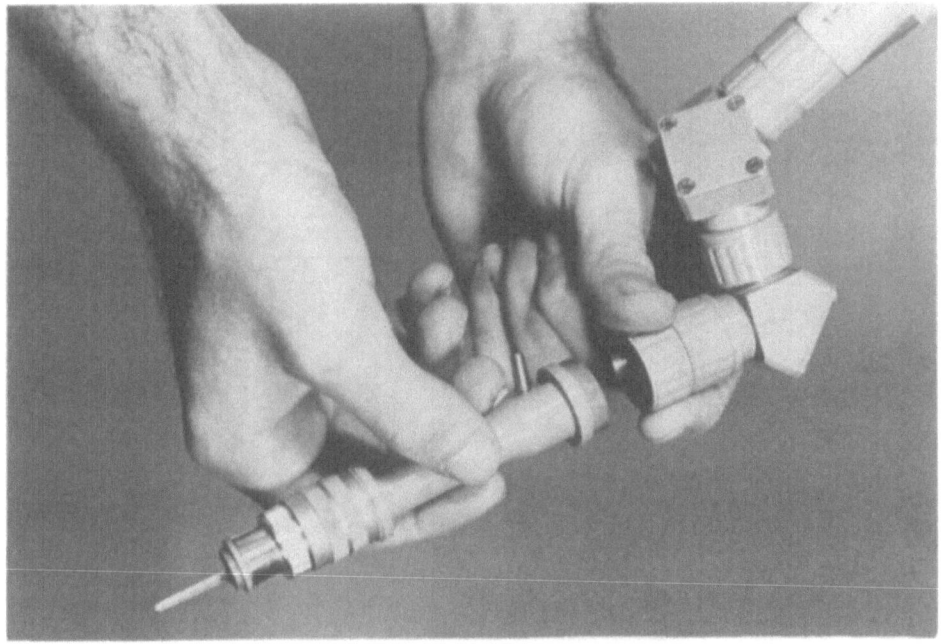

Figure 2.28. Laser hand assembly.

most tested systems in manufacturing. Once the manual safety shutter is opened, the laser can be activated by the foot pedal.

The laser head can be used with a free-hand piece scalpel or with an operating microscope (colposcope). The free-hand arrangement, available on most of the laser instruments, allows the surgeon to apply the focused laser beam to any point in a large area, and to remove tissue lesions selectively, since the laser beam is directed through the internal mirror system of a multiarticulated surgical arm. For microsurgery the colposcope or operating microscope is directly attached to the laser head and manipulator[1] by a simple snap lock connector.

Should the surgeon be using the laser hand scalpel (Fig. 2.28), then the appropriate lens must be chosen. Usually the manufacturer supplies a 125-mm and 50-mm focal length lens system. Each system has an extension rod to indicate the focal point. The entire hand assembly can be wet-sterilized. Do not autoclave the lens. The ethylene oxide will reduce the specialized lens coating and the focusing efficiency will be diminished. Finally, remember to attach the nitrogen lens jet wash tubing (Fig. 2.29). The lens is very expensive and should be handled accordingly. The jet wash protects the lens from spattering debris which could damage it. If it becomes necessary to clean the

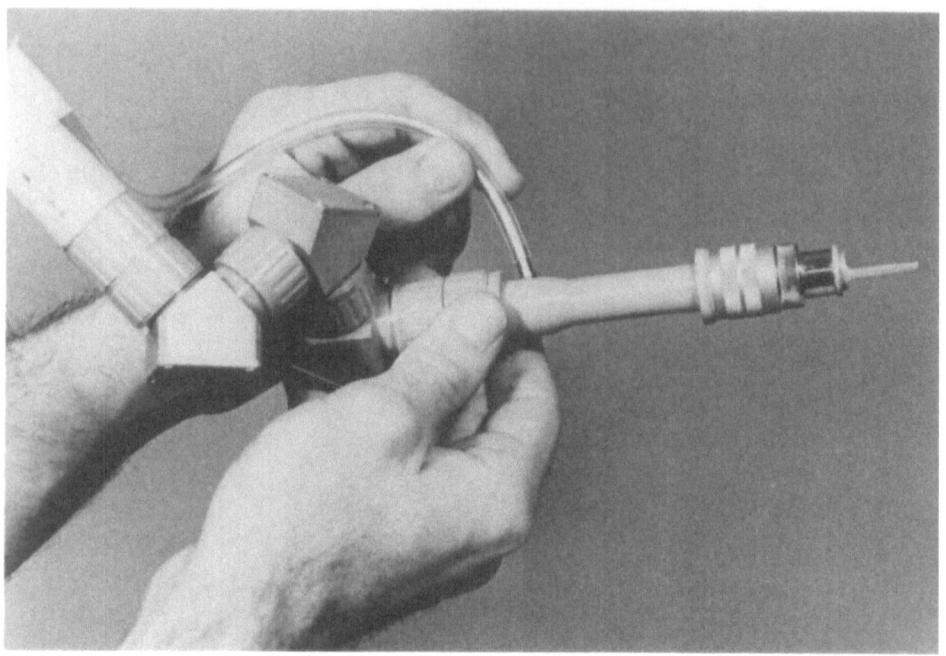

Figure 2.29. Nitrogen jet tubing attached to hand piece. (Reproduced with permission: Bellina JH, Dorsey JH: Physics and bioeffects of gynecologic surgical lasers, in Bellina JH (ed): Gynecologic Laser Surgery, Proceedings of International Congress on Gynecologic Laser Surgery and Related Works, New Orleans, LA, Jan 1980. Plenum Press, New York, 1981.)

lens by means other than the jet wash, consult the manufacturer, who will usually recommend absolute ethyl alcohol or acetone. Do not scrape the lens or wash it in detergent! The mirrored surface of the articulating arms or the micromanipulator is cleaned in a similar fashion. *When in doubt, call the manufacturer.*

2.3.2. Troubleshooting the System

Because lasers can be temperamental, you should have a thorough working knowledge of what can go wrong with the system and what you can do to rectify it.

First, the system should be checked prior to the anesthetization of the patient. Check the gas supply. If the intertank pressure is <500 psi, have a reserve bottle on hand. Check the water; if it is low, fill with distilled water.

Turn the laser on. Adjust the power supply to check your power output. Turn to the lowest setting and to the highest setting. If the laser output does not fluctuate properly, cancel the surgery. This problem cannot be easily corrected; you need the service representative.

Test fire the laser on a tongue blade. Did the laser impact coincide with the HeNe pointer? If not, an adjustment must be made by the company. Look carefully at the laser impact. Is the char equally distributed? If not, turn off the laser and check the mirror surfaces and the lens. If either is dirty, clean with the appropriate solvents. Remember to allow time for the volatile solvents to evaporate as the laser can ignite these materials.

During the surgery, if the temperature light is activated, there are problems in the radiator system. A trick to help "get you off the table" is to add ice cubes to the water reservoir, but as soon as the surgery is finished, call the company.

Occasionally, the shutter will "override" and a "reset" button or switch must be depressed to recycle the system.

2.3.3. Basic Office System

In establishing an office-based system, the physician must do the following:

1. Select a large room, preferably 12 × 12 ft or greater (Fig. 2.30), which has a window or easy access to the outside for plume exhaust.
2. Purchase or make an adequate suction system (Fig. 2.31).
3. Purchase or acquire a table that can be put in the Trendelenburg position and completely elevated.
4. Acquire the correct nonflammable or dulled speculum (Fig. 2.32).
5. Test the entire system.
6. Set up a system of recording data.

2.3.4. Office Suite Operating Room Supplies

The office set-up should contain Mayo stand and a tray with the following items (Fig. 2.33):

1. Bivalved speculum (nonflammable or dulled)
2. Biopsy forceps
3. Acetic acid solution (3%)

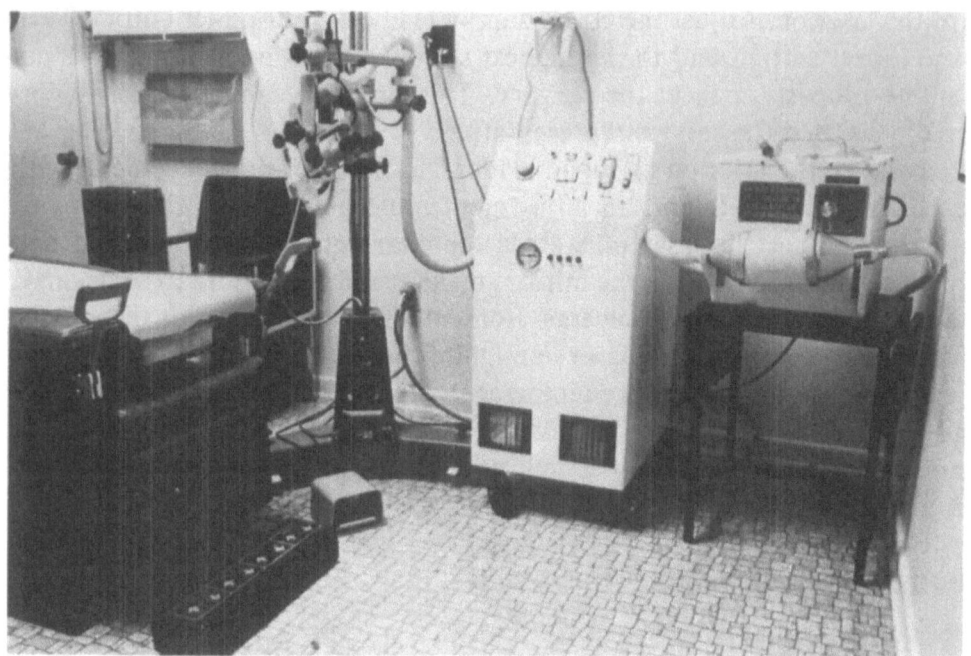

Figure 2.30. Properly equipped examination room.

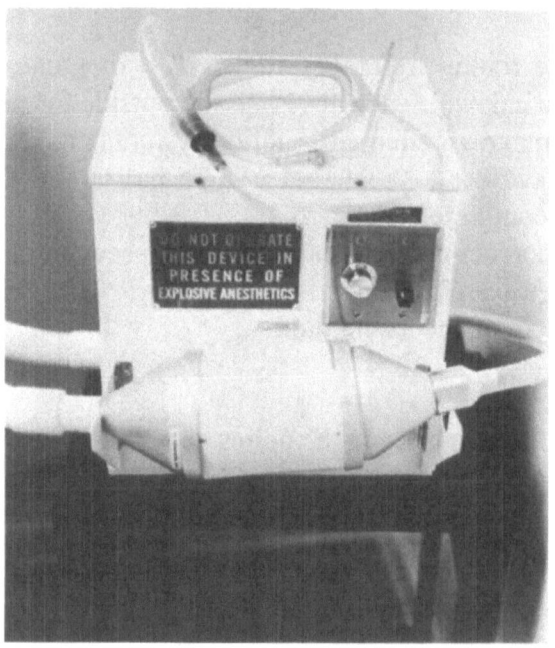

Figure 2.31. Adequate suction system must be available (Biovac® instrument).

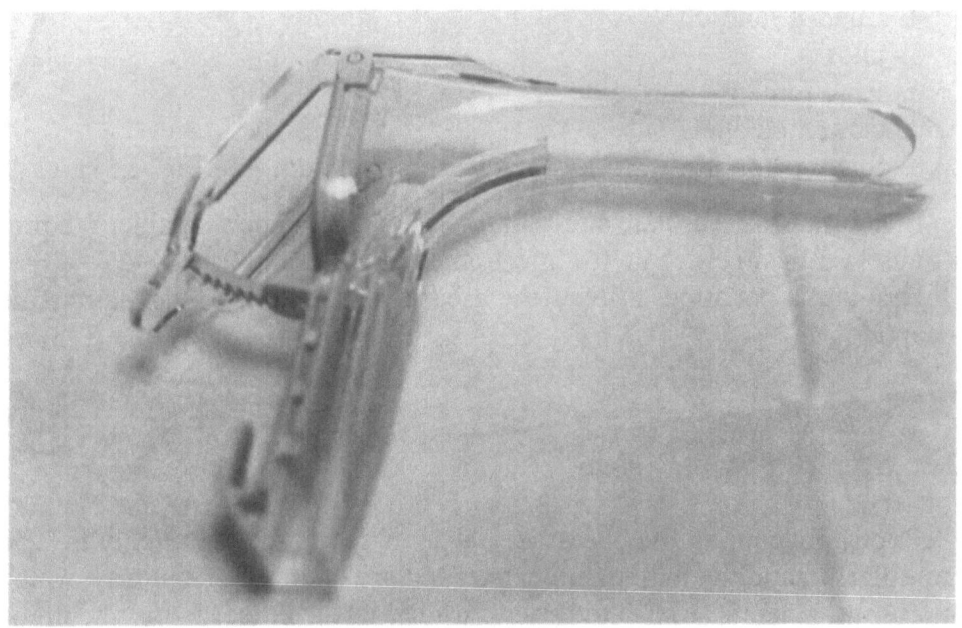

Figure 2.32. Nonflammable speculum.

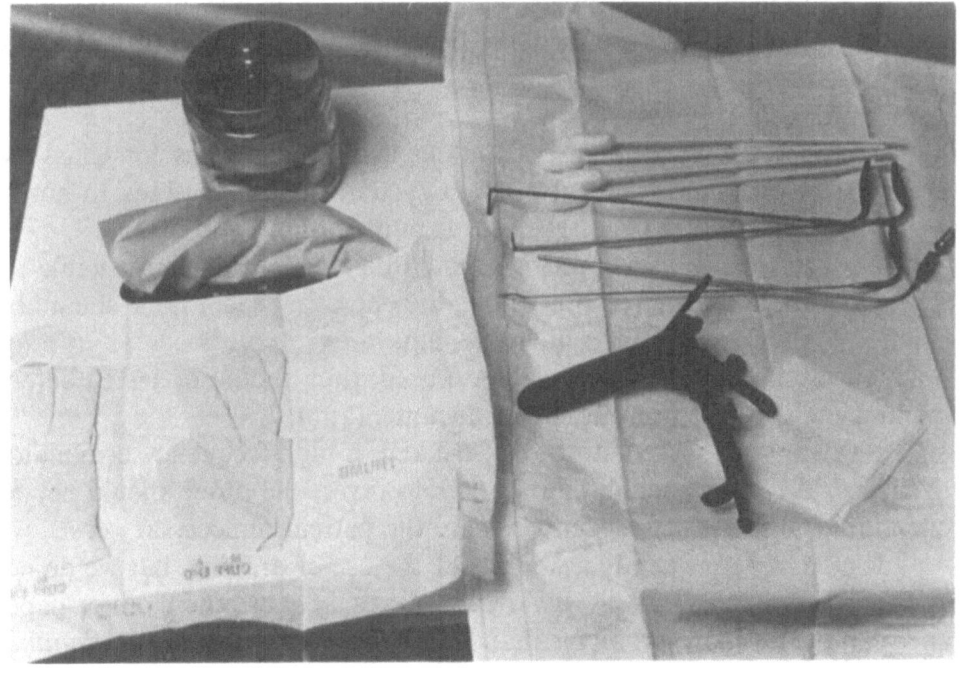

Figure 2.33. Properly equipped office laser tray.

4. Lugol's solution
5. Gloves
6. Ring forceps
7. Cotton pledgets
8. Suction apparatus, if not attached to speculum (see Fig. 2.31)

In addition, appropriate anesthetic solution should be available. We prefer to use a 30-gauge needle for injection of small lesions.

Draping is not used; instead the area is cleaned with a nonflammable antiseptic.

2.3.5. Operating Suite System

Prior to beginning the operation, the staff should be thoroughly trained in equipment handling and maintenance, and the operating room tray, which contains instruments similar to those provided in the office set-up, should be appropriately placed on a Mayo stand.

A periodic inspection of the laser system must be performed by the biomedical department, because a log must be kept of maintenance and it must be available for federal inspectors.

The maintenance department should install an in-line fiberglass filter system to prevent the wall suction from becoming clogged with vapor tars. A simple and very effective system is to put a fiberglass filter in the plastic canister used to trap fluids.

The proper size of Bureau of Radiological Health signs for Class IV lasers must be installed. (We also use a system of lighted signs to notify entering personnel that a Class IV laser is in operation.)

Glasses (or plastic eye covering) should be worn, or made available to, all operating room personnel. If possible, the operating room table should be positioned to face away from a door opening.

If television or recording devices are used, they should be tested before beginning each case to prevent loss of documentation.

If a vulvar procedure is to be undertaken, a high-frequency coagulator with disposable probe should be at hand. However, the probe should not be opened unless it is in fact needed, to spare the patient unnecessary cost.

Questions are frequently asked about the use of draping, but we do not drape for vaginal, cervical, or vulvar procedures, because the cloth or paper drapes can create more problems than they solve, and *they may be flammable*. The areas to be irradiated should first be cleaned with nonflammable solution.

2.3.6. Recording System

The Zeiss system operating microscope can be fitted with a beam splitter to create 35-mm still photographs, video tapes, and 16-mm motion picture documentation. In our operating room system, we have chosen to use the 50/ 50 beam splitter fitted to both a 35-mm automatic camera and a video recorder. The 35-mm camera should be motor driven and fitted with an electronically controlled shutter. A data bank should be used to record patient information. Cameras, such as described, are available through all camera stores. The film should be tungsten ASA 160 pushed two *f*-steps. The cost of the video system is not critical. Remember, order the correct adaptors from Zeiss. Zeiss can supply the necessary equipment, including cameras, if desired, and, even though it is slightly more expensive, you are assured of a properly integrated system (Fig. 2.34).

2.3.7. Ancillary Equipment

Figure 2.35 shows the current ancillary equipment for laser surgery in gynecology. The modified Graves bivalved speculum contains dual suction tubes and a dual fiberoptic light bundle and was designed for cervical and vaginal work. The suction tubes allow the surgeon to manipulate the speculum while having constant suction. The added fiberoptic light bundles are used for photographic illumination. The instrument to the right is a special detachable suction which clips on to a speculum rim, and has the advantage of being attachable to any speculum.

2.3.7.a. Evacuation System   Currently, the only available commercial evacuation system is produced by Biovac. This is a complete system. The inline charcoal tank absorbs the odor generated in tissue vaporization.

Another evacuation system can be homemade using a standard vacuum pump and an inline fiberglass filter. This filter prevents the pump mechanism from clogging. The fumes are then piped through a window (Fig. 2.36).

Still another system, for rooms without windows, is to pipe the exhaust into the water sink drain. By adjusting the cold water tap, a flow rate can be achieved that will wash the fumes into the drain. This type of apparatus is similar to those used in chemistry laboratories. It is inexpensive, simple, and never clogs (Fig. 2.37).

Whichever system you use, it is very important to exhaust or trap the fumes, as the effect of long-term exposure is not yet known. Besides, the odor can become quite irritating to you and to your patients.

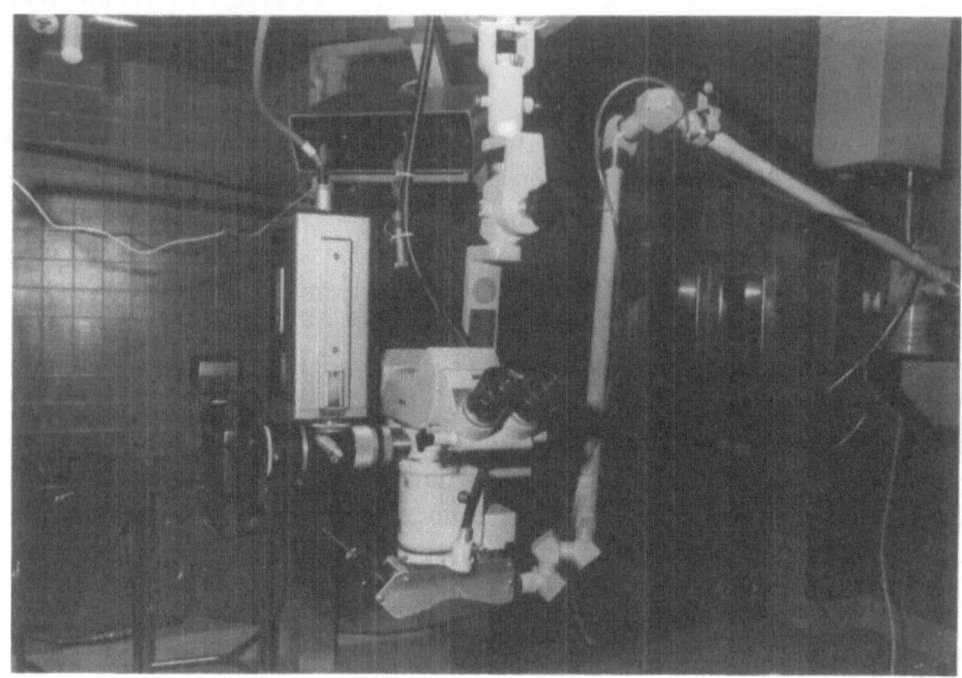

Figure 2.34. Operating microscope with complete photographic instrumentation including 35-mm still photography and video recording system by Zeiss.

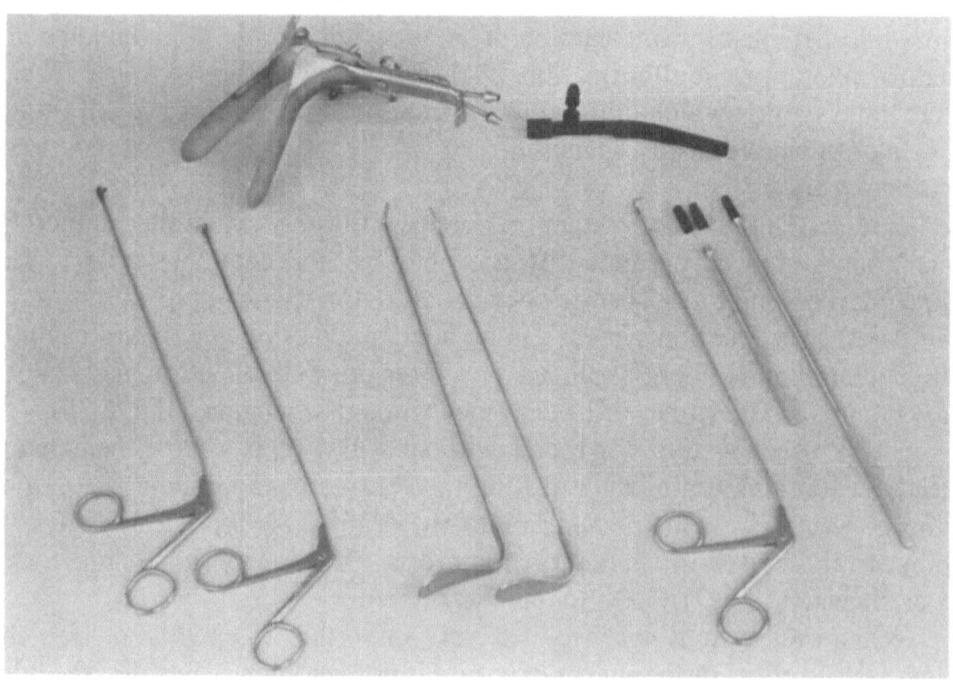

Figure 2.35. Ancillary equipment by Narco Pilling Company.

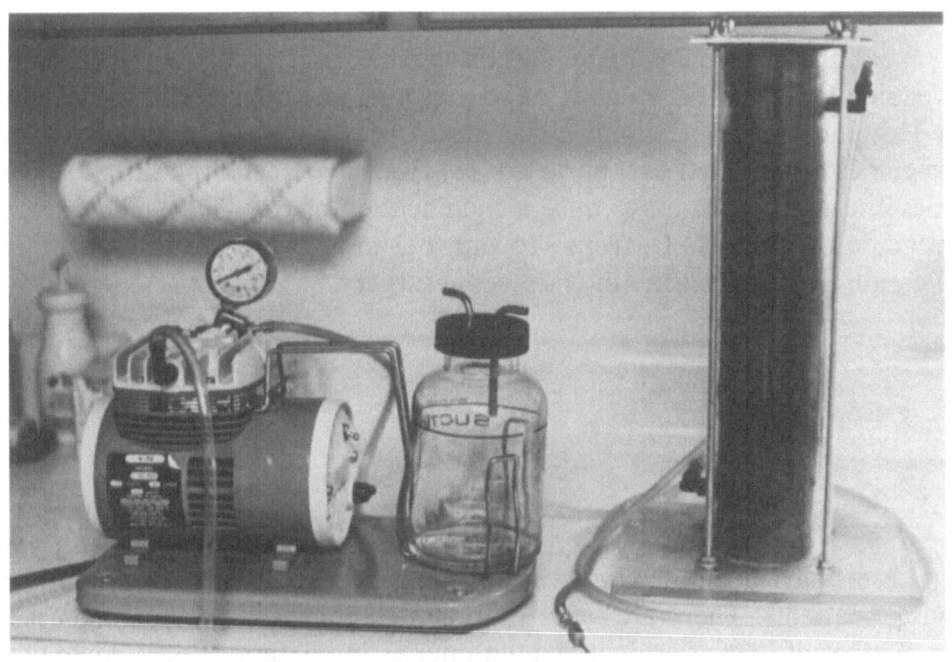

Figure 2.36. Inexpensive fiberglass filter.

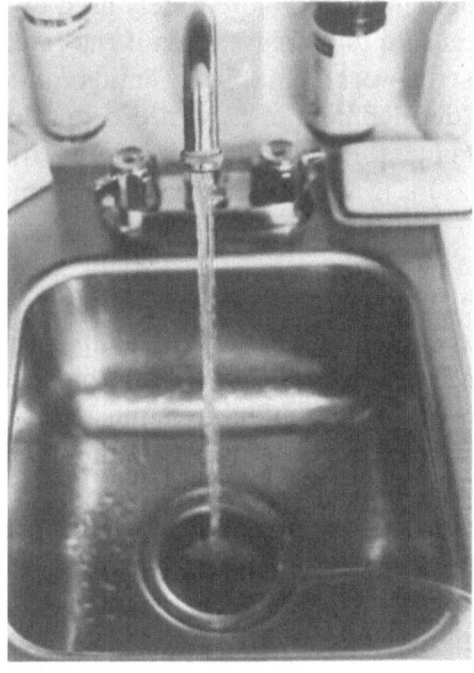

Figure 2.37. Water trap to remove vapors
and odors.

2.3.7.b. Waveguides The carbon dioxide laser requires a specialized waveguide or light pipe. Hughes Laboratory, in association with the American Hospital Supply Company, has developed the thallium-bromide-clad waveguide. Specialized exit ports are required to refocus the laser. Waveguides and light pipes may cause a modification of the TEM. The current waveguide ranges in O.D. from 125 μm to 2 mm. Advances in waveguides will create new possibilities in endoscopic surgery.

2.4. Laser Safety

2.4.1. General Information

Lasers have been used for therapeutic purposes for nearly 20 yr on thousands of patients. There are more than 20,000 clinically documented cases. The number of known or documented injuries in operations performed with lasers is less than 100, or 0.5%—a very respectable safety record. However, the total number of surgical lasers in use today, worldwide, is approximately 1000, and the total number of physicians using lasers in surgery (exclusive of retinal therapy) is less than 1000 worldwide. As surgical and therapeutic lasers become more numerous and more widely used by more physicians, the number of accidents is sure to increase, even if the rate remains the same.

To avoid increased governmental intervention in medical affairs, and to avoid restricting the development of new medical lasers and new beneficial applications of this unique form of energy, it is imperative that every present and future user of lasers in medicine apply this promising medical device with the most careful regard for the safety of patients, physicians, and medical personnel. Manufacturers must also bear their share of responsibility for the safety of medical lasers. They are now quite closely regulated by the federal government as well as by state and municipal regulations with regard to many classes of medical devices. As new and more sophisticated medical lasers become available, their manufacturers must carry the primary responsibility for educating the medical community in the safe and proper operation of their products.

Lasers are potentially dangerous devices. They are capable of concentrating large amounts of power or energy into very small, well collimated beams. They have an enormous potential for therapeutic benefit, as well as for destruction. Like any medical device, the laser must be used with skill, discretion, and common sense, and those who use medical lasers must always adhere to the following general rules:

1. Never operate any laser until you have read and understood the operator's manual furnished by the manufacturer.
2. Never fire any laser at any target until you know the complete path of the beam and are sure that no unintended targets lie in that path.
3. Never fire a therapeutic laser at any living target until you have been instructed by a competent teacher in both the correct operational procedures of the laser and the proper technique for application of the laser energy to the tissue to be treated.
4. Never use a laser for surgery until you have practiced its use on inanimate targets, cadaver parts, and/or laboratory animals.
5. Always take seriously the safety precautions specified by the manufacturer of the laser whenever you use it for any purpose.
6. Never use a laser on human patients until you have taken a course of instruction on laser surgery.
7. Always request that a qualified instructor for the manufacturer give you and your operating room service personnel training prior to using the laser on humans. Nurses have to be properly prepared for special surgery instrumentation care and only the minimum number of people required should be present in the operating room.
8. Always ask that a qualified operating room instructor in laser operation be present to advise you when you first use the laser on human patients. The laser must only be activated by the surgeon who is responsible for the safety system and has custody of the master key.

Remember that lasers, when properly used, are as safe as any device known to man. Do not be frightened by the laser; use it wisely and correctly. Anything can be dangerous if used improperly: pure water is lethal if used as a dialysis fluid for a kidney patient.

2.4.2. Hazards of Medical Lasers

The hazards of medical lasers jeopardize patients as well as the medical personnel who apply laser therapy. In general, there are three major categories of hazards:

1. Injury by primary action of the laser beam
2. Injury by secondary effects of the laser beam
3. Electrocution by high voltage within the laser

Hazards 1 and 2 threaten both patients and operators. Hazard 3 threatens only the operators or those who service the laser. Injuries resulting from the primary action of the laser beam can be caused by a direct beam or by its reflections. Injuries from secondary effects are usually caused by the action of the direct beam on materials in its path.

2.4.2.a. Injury by Primary Action of the Laser Beam

1. Damage to eyes
2. Damage to skin and underlying tissue
3. Damage to tissue of an unintended target (i.e., excessive, uncontrolled)

2.4.2.b. Injury by Secondary Effects of the Laser Beam

1. Burns caused by ignition of flammable materials
2. Mechanical trauma caused by explosion of flammable gas
3. Thermal trauma to healthy tissue adjacent to the intended target zone
4. Mutagenic effect of healthy tissue adjacent to the intended target zone
5. Toxic or pathogenic effect on healthy tissue caused by smoke or vapor from the intended target zone

In addition, an accurate air exchange system has to be present and functioning in order not to accumulate toxic laser-active gas (CO_2–N_2–He). Disconnection of power for all nonoperational equipment is recommended. A recently developed resin power checker at the focusing head can be useful.[5]

When using the operating microscope, the surgeon is in no danger since the glass optic components of the microscope located between the eyes and the beam's path fully protect him from the CO_2 laser energy. Neither the operator's hand nor flammable objects, including certain surgical preparation solutions, should be exposed. Plastic or rubber anesthetic tubes must be protected with a coating that will reflect and fissue any CO_2 laser energy, since such tubes constitute a serious hazard of explosion.[6-8] Cotton wet gloves, plastic speculums, or dulled metallic (chrome-covered) instruments are recommended.

2.4.2.c. Protecting the Patient's Eyes from Laser Radiation   The carbon dioxide laser beam is invisible at its wavelength of 10,600 nm. The beam reflects from metallic objects and the corneal epithelium (defined as a critical organ) absorbs totally even the reflected beams (Fig. 2.38). It can be, therefore, severely damaged by a thermal mechanism.[9-11] Therefore, the patient and all personnel in the operating room, when the laser apparatus is

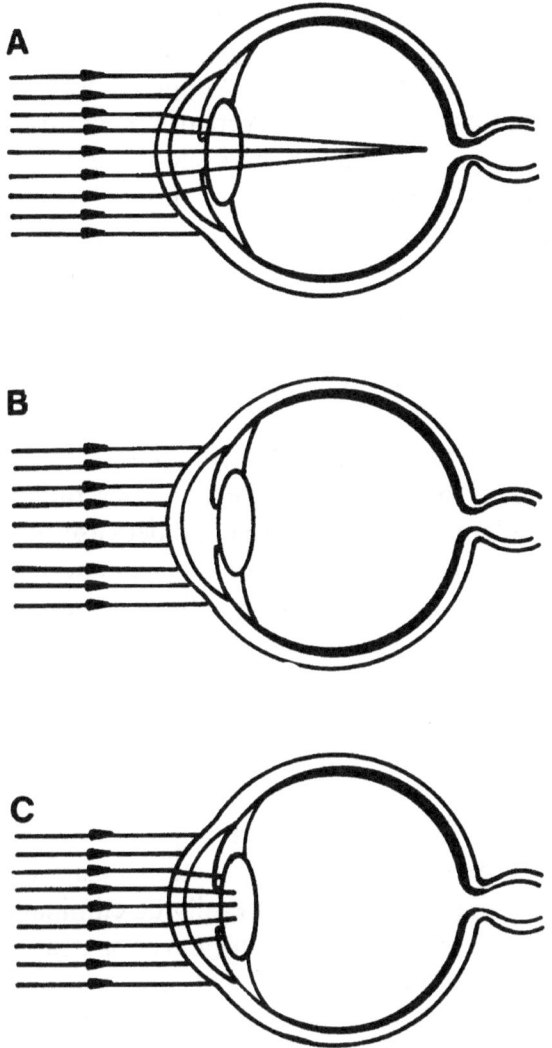

Figure 2.38. Ocular absorption is wavelength-dependent. (A) Retinal: visible, near infrared; (B) corneal: far infrared, medium ultraviolet; (C) crystal lens: near ultraviolet, medium infrared.

connected to the electrical main supply, must wear plastic or glass eye protection of proper optical density[12,13] in order to prevent accidental corneal damage. Even the visible HeNe laser beam can cause eye injuries.

If the patient is conscious (not under general anesthesia) during laser treatment, he or she should be required to put on the same protective eyewear that the attending medical personnel are using. However, if the patient is under general anesthesia, place protective eyewear of some suitable kind over the patient's eyes, and tape it securely in place. If a far-infrared laser is being used anywhere on a patient's head, neck, or upper thorax, tape the patient's eyelids shut, cover the lids with several layers of wet cotton or gauze, and be sure to remoisten these pads frequently with clean water or sterile saline. If the patient is conscious while the far-infrared laser is being used anywhere below the midthorax, require the patient to put on the same eyewear used by the attending medical personnel. These measures may seem unnecessarily strict; however, a conscious patient can move suddenly, and a laser beam can be reflected into the patient's eyes by a metal instrument. Eye damage caused by laser radiation is usually irreparable.

2.4.2.d. Damage to Skin and Underlying Tissues Damage to superficial tissues of the body by direct or reflected laser radiation is usually a much less serious problem than damage to eyes, because skin and underlying tissues will regenerate. Injury by laser beams to skin and underlying tissue is usually accompanied by pain; pain causes reflexive muscular action which usually withdraws the exposed part from the beam. Burns can be produced by high power densities or photosensitization can occur at low power density.[14] Thus the manual shutter at the laser head has to be opened at the end for all positioning on the target area.

2.4.2.e. Protecting Skin and Underlying Tissues For both patients and attending medical personnel, if there is a clear hazard of inadvertent skin exposure to a laser beam (and this cannot easily be eliminated because of the particular circumstances of the application), cover or wrap the site(s) at risk with rumpled heavy-gauge aluminum foil and tape it in place. In the case of far-infrared lasers (e.g., CO_2) put several layers of water or saline soaked gauze or cotton on the skin under the foil. Avoid any clothing or skin coverings which can easily be ignited if struck by infrared laser beams, design your surgical application of the laser to minimize the risk of inadvertent skin exposure, and conduct the surgery with skill and common sense.

Injury caused by explosion or combustion of flammable materials can be avoided by adhering to careful rules of operation. You should never operate an infrared laser in the presence of flammable anesthetics, or combustible gases, vapors, or liquids. Nor should you fire an infrared laser at any solid, liquid, or gas which is combustible in air, or which is in contact with medical oxygen. Always protect healthy tissue, if possible, by covering it with gauze or cotton soaked in sterile water or saline solution. The high absorption of water for laser energy at this wavelength range offers full protection. The reflective beam is usually harmless because it diverges beyond the point of the focus; however, the beam should not be directed outside the operating area.

Cover the margins of the operative fields with rumpled aluminum foil. Use neurosurgical cottonoid patties, if possible, to protect healthy tissue adjacent to intended target sites, because these patties have strings attached which allow them to be withdrawn when they become dried out. Also, never use an infrared laser in the mouth, larynx, trachea, or esophagus when an endotracheal tube carrying oxygen is present, unless the endotracheal tube is of the all-metal variety or, if elastrometric, is carefully wrapped with aluminum sensing tape (available from Radio Shack). Wrap it full-length with 50% overlap. You should always require that a patient upon whom you are using an infrared laser to treat vaginal, vulvar, or rectal lesions have the lower bowel evacuated prior to laser surgery to avoid ignition or explosion of rectal gas. Never fire an infrared laser at any tissue which has been moistened with alcohol or a volatile solvent.

2.4.2.f. Toxic or Pathogenic Effect of Smoke or Vapor from the Intended Target   When infrared lasers are used at high power densities to cut or vaporize tissue, the solid residues of these tissues will burn when they pass through the laser beam in air, causing a thick, malodorous smoke. In theory, malignant cell particles might be contained in the fumes restulting from tumor vaporization. In scrupulously structured experiments by Bellina et al.[15], the smoke plume from a malignant lesion being vaporized by a CO_2 laser beam has never been found to contain any viable malignant cells. Use a suction tip of adequate size and of nonflammable material, with a suction system of adequate capacity, to remove the smoke and vapor, as close to the laser impact site as possible to allow good visualization of the operative field. There is no evidence for possible direct carcinogenic properties of any laser beams used in medicine today, as with gamma or roentgen radiations.

The CO_2 surgical laser can be used with absolute safety if one is aware of the potential dangers and follows the precautions described here and in the manufacturer's guidebook. Extended details for safety precautions are available in the *American National Standard for the Safe Use of Lasers* (*ANSI*)[16] which was written by an organization of experts to provide information on current operating standards for lasers.

Finally, in some centers laser surgery is still regarded as experimental and a special consent form has to be signed by the patient. The Food and Drug Administration (FDA) cleared the CO_2 laser energy transfer system for use in human subjects in 1976. Thus, CO_2 laser instruments are no longer considered to be investigational tools and should, therefore, be considered routinely when one is selecting instruments for microsurgery.

2.4.3. Government Regulations for Laser Safety

2.4.3.a. Federal Regulations Federal regulations are promulgated and enforced for the use of lasers by the Bureau of Radiological Health (BRH) of the FDA. It is expected that at some time in the future the Occupational Safety and Health Administration of the Department of Health and Human Services will also promulgate a set of standards and rules, primarily for lasers used in commerce and industry.

The Bureau of Medical Devices of the FDA also has some jurisdiction over the use of lasers, namely those used in medical applications. The governing document for regulation by the BRH is the *Federal Register,* Volume 40, Part II, of July 31, 1975: "Laser Products—Performance Standards." The BRH classified all lasers into Classes I, II, III, and IV, according to their power levels of accessible radiation. Class I lasers are incapable of emitting radiation at levels considered to be hazardous; they are exempt from any controls.

All lasers currently in use in medical applications for direct therapy are of sufficient power output to be put into Class IV (most hazardous). There are presently no upper limits of power output for Class IV, and hence no Class V. Any laser having accessible radiation above the limits for Class III is put into Class IV. The BRH regulations require that certain warning labels be put on the outside of lasers.

A light and/or acoustical signal should be placed on the door of the room where the instrument is located to indicate when the laser is in use. The door should be kept closed while the laser is in use. There are CAUTION labels for Class II and Class IIIa and DANGER labels for Class IIIb and Class IV lasers.

Attached to the laser:

DANGER
VISIBLE AND INVISIBLE LASER RADIATION
AVOID EYE OR SKIN EXPOSURE TO DIRECT OR SCATTERED RADIATION
CLASS IV LASER PRODUCT

Outside the door of the laser controlled area:

DANGER
CO_2 LASER
RESTRICTED ACCESS

Outside the operating room:

DANGER

CO$_2$ LASER

RESTRICTED ACCESS WHEN LIGHT IS ON

BRH regulations also require that the aperture(s) of the laser, through which the coherent radiation is emitted, be clearly marked with the legend LASER APERTURE, or something equivalent.

The Bureau of Medical Devices classifies lasers into three categories:

Class I includes those devices which are of long-standing use and whose established applications are widely known, where life support is not a function, and where general controls on manufacturing, labeling, and packaging are sufficient to ensure the safety of patients and users.

Class II includes those devices which must meet not only the general controls of Class I but also prescribed performance standards. They must be made under the federal requirements known as Good Manufacturing Practices. Life support is not a function. The argon laser for ophthalmic use and the CO$_2$ laser for use in otorhinolaryngology, gynecology, and related fields are put into Class II by the Bureau of Medical Devices. It is very probable that the CO$_2$ laser will be formally put into Class II, for virtually every surgical application for which it is used is now well documented.

Class III includes those devices which are used for life support or whose use in particular applications is still investigational. Such devices are subject to general controls, Good Manufacturing Practices, and Investigational Devices Regulations. These include operation of the devices under specific protocols by well qualified operators in institutions whose regulatory committees for such activities have granted approval for these investigations, and have obtained informed consent for the use of such devices upon human patients.

In general, federal regulations impose requirements upon manufacturing, product performance, periodic reporting, and record-keeping. The intent of these is to insure the safety and quality of laser products for medical uses. Some states impose regulations on the use of lasers while others do not. Those which do have regulations impose differing requirements upon both manufacturers and users of laser products. Some states, such as New York, specifically exempt lasers used for therapeutic purposes in medicine by licensed practitioners from the other laser regulations. As with most regulatory matters left to states, there is no consensus regarding laser regulations. Medical practitioners using lasers should inquire of their own state governments as to the applicable regulations, if any.

2.4.3.b. Local Regulations   Local regulations are even more diverse than those of the states. Whether or not they apply to lasers as generators of coherent radiation, they do usually require that lasers as medical devices meet certain standards, which are usually based upon two sets of industrial requirements promulgated by organizations dedicated to the safety of commercial, industrial, and medical products: *Underwriters' Laboratories*—UL 544, and *National Fire Protection Association*—NFPA 76B.

Some cities, such as Chicago and Los Angeles, require certification for each laser installed in a hospital, that it meets the prescribed safety regulations. Los Angeles requires recertification of every laser model each year. Virtually every hospital has a governing committee, which must approve each laser model brought into the hospital for conformance to standards such as electrical leakage (from UL 544). Often, this committee also sets the requirements as to who is qualified to operate the laser.

References

1. Polanyi TG, Bredemier HC, Davis TW, Jr: A CO_2 laser for surgical research. Med Biol Eng 8:541–548, 1970.
2. Bayly JG, Kartha VB, Steven WH: The absorption spectrum of liquid phase H_2O and D_2O from 0.7 μm to 10 μm. Infrared Phys 3:211–223, 1963.
3. Fava G, Emanuelli H, Cascinelli N, et al: CO_2 laser: beam patterns in relation to the surgical use. Lasers Surg Med 2:331–341, 1983.
4. Fidler JP, Law E, MacMillan BG, et al: Comparison of CO_2 laser excision of burns with other thermal knives. Ann NY Acad Sci 267:254–261, 1977.
5. Maeda R, Satoru L, Ninsakul N: Instrumentation development for safe operation with CO_2 laser, in Kaplan I, Ascher PW (eds): Proceedings III International Congress on Laser Surgery, Graz, Jerusalem, Academic Press, 1979, pp 47–56.
6. Snow JC, Norton HL: Lasers and anesthesia. J Am Assoc Nurse Anesthet 43:464–469, 1975.
7. Snow JC, Norton HL, Saluja TS, et al: Fire hazard during CO_2 laser microsurgery on the larynx and trachea. Anesth Analg Curr Res 55:146–147, 1976.
8. Vourch G, Tanneres ML, Freche G: Anesthesia for microsurgery of the larynx. Anaesthesia 34:53–57, 1979.
9. Cabal C, Caillard JF: Risques liés à l'utilisation du rayon laser. Arch Mal Prof 36:545–546, 1975.
10. Sliney DH, Frazier BC: Evaluation of optical radiation hazards. Appl Optics 12:1–24, 1973.
11. Mackeen D, Fine S, Feigu L, et al: Anterior chamber measurement on CO_2 laser corneal irradiation. Invest Ophthalmol 9:366–371, 1970.
12. Fuller TB: The physics of surgical laser. Lasers Surg Med 1:5–14, 1980.
13. Department of Army and Navy: Control of Hazard to Health from Laser Radiation. Washington D.C., TB MED. 279/NAV MED. P-5032-35, 1969.

14. Goldman L, Rockwell RJ, Fidler JP, et al: Investigative laser surgery: safety aspects. Biomed Eng 4:415–418, 1969.
15. Bellina JH, Stjernholm R, Kurpel JE: Biochemical analysis of carbon dioxide plume emission from irradiated tumors, in Bellina JH (ed): Gynecologic Laser Surgery, Proceedings of the International Congress on Gynecologic Laser Surgery and Related Works. New York, Plenum Press, 1981, pp 17–25.
16. American National Standards Institute Inc. (ANSI). Committee on the Safe Use of Lasers: American National Standard for the Safe Use of Lasers. Z 136.1. New York, 1979.

3

Bioeffects

3.1. Introduction

The coherent monochromatic CO_2 laser beam can be precisely focused through an optical lens system (of appropriate material) so that high cross-sectional energy density can be achieved at the focal point in a spot of less than 1 mm. The high-energy laser beam passes through air and is absorbed as it hits liquid or solid objects, so that it can be used for precise surgical work for tissue incisions, vaporization, and coagulation. The reflectivity of the laser decreases as the wavelength increases for all substances other than surface-polished metals at wavelength of 10.6 μm. Because of its 80–90% water content, body tissue acts as a black body and will rapidly absorb this energy. For this reason, CO_2 lasers can be used in surgery. The energy of a continuously emitted CO_2 focused laser beam creates an incision by tissue vaporization. The defocused beam has a lower energy density and produces rapid thermal increase, with gradual fluid vaporization, dehydration, and carbonization causing the cells to shrink and having a coagulative effect.[1,2] The shape of the crater of the vaporized tissue and of the adjacent necrotic zone is in direct relation to the transverse electromagnetic mode (TEM) of the laser beam.[3]

For comparison, a 230-mm layer of water is required to absorb 90% of the radiation of the argon laser, while only 60 mm of water absorbs 90% of the radiation from the Nd-YAG laser. In contrast, only 0.1 mm of water is required for the carbon dioxide laser beam. Because of the high tissue water content, the CO_2 laser beam is absorbed by a very thin layer of tissue, and precise control of the depth of destruction is thus possible during surgery.

3.1.1. Experimental Studies

The thermal properties of the carbon dioxide laser were investigated with multiple analytic models.[2] The analysis was divided into two phases:

1. Human cervical sampling
   a. Cytologic analysis
   b. Histologic analysis
   c. Scanning electron microscopic (SEM) analysis
2. Heat transfer analysis
   a. Theoretical model
   b. Experimental model

The cytologic, histologic, and standard scanning electron microscopic studies were carried out from 1976 to 1978. Fourteen cases of severe cervical dysplasia to carcinoma in situ (CIN III), confirmed by histopathology, were chosen for this study.

A standard quantity of CO_2 laser energy was applied to the cervical epithelium. The standard energy was 250 W/cm^2 applied for 0.1 sec (i.e., 25 J/cm^2). If the lesion was large, multiple exposures at the same quantity of energy were used to eradicate the cervical disease.

3.1.2. Clinical Studies

3.1.2.a. Cytologic Analysis Cytologic samples were obtained daily on every other patient so as to give a complete review of healing from the first day of treatment to the 21st day. All samples were submitted for analysis by standard cytopathological techniques.

The cytologic pattern immediately after treatment revealed elongated cells resembling fibrocytes, whose histogenesis made it possible to define them as columnar cells by comparing them with previous biopsy specimens. Changes appeared to be the result of thermal coagulation, with lengthwise destruction of the stromal cells. Epithelial cells were absent; only carbon residue remained.

On the first day following treatment, a large number of acute inflammatory cells were visible. However, by the seventh to ninth days, this reaction subsided, and many multinucleated epithelioid cells were noted. The appearance of these giant cells heralds the rapid squamous cell replacement phase. By the 21st day, the cytologic smear returned to normal.

3.1.2.b. Histologic Analysis   Histologic samples were obtained on the first day of treatment, the 10th day after treatment, and the 21st day after treatment. Tissue samples were taken with a Jako microlaryngeal biopsy forceps and were examined by standard histopathological techniques.

The histologic pattern, immediately after treatment, revealed a total absence of epithelium. The lateral demarcation of tissue removal was sharp and perpendicular to the basal cell layer; adjacent normal epithelium remained undisturbed. Thermal injury could be observed for an additional 50–100 μm and terminated abruptly in a plane bordering the stroma. Occasionally, a small amount of carbon residue was noted in the bottom of the shallow crater formed by the laser impact.

On the 10th day, the histologic pattern was one of normal, reepithelialized tissue. Below the surface of the new epithelium, multinucleated giant cells should be seen. Cellular maturation, polarity, and cytoplasmic–nuclear ratios were remarkably normal.

Mature squamous epithelium was noted on the 21st day. The cellular polarity, maturation, and cytoplasmic–nuclear ratios were normal. There was usually an absence of inflammatory cells in the adjacent stroma. Tensile strength of this new tissue appeared to be normal.

All energy is predominantly absorbed by the water in the first 100 μm of tissue in an exponential fashion according to Beer's Law. A second zone of injury may occur and varies proportionally with the time exposure of power over the tissue.[4] This zone, however, has a maximum width of 200 μm and is less than 500 μm in depth as a result of tissue protein denaturation by heat.[4,5] With ultra-high-speed color cinematography, Hall[6,7] demonstrated that in the first 30 μm of tissue, 90% of the energy is transferred as heat to adjacent tissue. This results in boiling of intra- and extracellular water; as cellular temperature approaches 100°C, steam forms and the cells expand and then explode. The measurement of the velocity at which the steam expands from the point of laser impact has revealed that pressure exerted on adjacent tissue by cell disruption is small and unlikely to cause damage by shock waves or the splattering of viable malignant materials to adjacent sites. This kind of disruption of tissue architecture and the ablation of the tissue debris from the wound result in a three-dimensional incision and tissue removal. At a power output of 20 W, approximately 10 mm^3 of tissue can be vaporized in 1 sec.

There is no selective absorption of the CO_2 laser beam by tissues with different color and pigmentation as there is with some surgical lasers that emit shorter wavelength radiations. In fact, for the laser producing visible light the absorption coefficient is strongly dependent on the color of the tissue. For example, the blue-green light of the argon laser is readily absorbed by hemoglobin. In addition, the scattering coefficient or damage to surrounding tissues is larger for visible lasers than for infrared-wavelength lasers, such as CO_2. For the CO_2 lasers, the lateral-and backscattering coefficient is negligible.[8] Nevertheless, the thermal effects of the CO_2 laser beam are different for various tissues. The choice of power output, therefore, has to be related to the tissue characteristics, the amount of tissue to be removed, and the speed of the incision.

Capillaries of dermal and subepithelial tissue (0.5–1 mm in diameter) revealed thrombosis when irradiated with the CO_2 laser. This small zone of coagulation necrosis provides a relatively bloodless wound, since capillaries and small vessels are sealed. In contrast, most vessels that are 2 mm or larger will need to be clamped and ligated.[9–11]

Since long-term exposure leads to high heat conduction, short-term exposure of the CO_2 laser beam can be used for the destruction or removal of superficial lesions of small microscopic dimensions, and low power density (150–200 W/cm^2) is effective for coagulation of small bleeding vessels and fragile tissues. High power densities (1000–2000 W/cm^2) can decrease the required time exposure and, consequently, remove larger masses with reduced thermal damage to the adjacent tissues. The speed of tissue vaporization, hence the speed of crater extension, is directly influenced by the power density variations multiplied by the effective beam diameter. Actually the higher the speed, the lower the total thermal damage.

Although the margins have a small nonviable zone, as demonstrated by histologic studies,[2,12,13] the laser impact site shows no zone of ischemia. Histochemical and biochemical studies showed that cellular enzymes, during the healing process, behave in a normal fashion.[14,15] Moreover, pain is minimal because of the small extent of contiguous tissue damage. Therefore, the healing process develops without any problems in soft tissue, especially mucosa.

3.1.2.c. Scanning Electron Microscopic Analysis Tissue samples were obtained with a Jako microlaryngeal biopsy forceps, on the day of treatment, the 10th day after treatment, and the 21st day after treatment, then submitted for analysis by standard SEM techniques.

The SEM pattern immediately after treatment, at 25 J/cm^2, revealed a shallow crater in the form of an oblate hemispheroid (Fig. 3.1). The peripheral borders were slightly elevated. The rim of this crater showed fused microridges and loss of intercellular bars. The heating effect was greatest on the plane orthogonal to the axis of the crater. The adjacent cellular surface

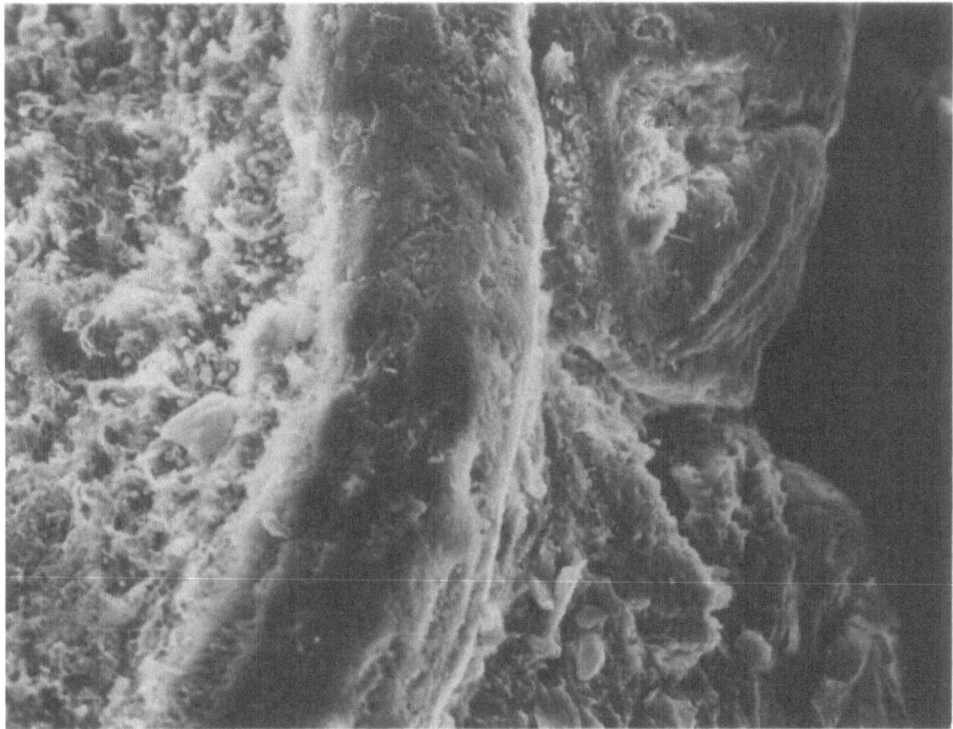

Figure 3.1. Scanning electron micrograph: laser impact site of 25 J/cm². Vaporization created an oblate hemispheroid geometric configuration ($\times$ 200). (Reproduced with permission: Bellina JH, Seto YJ: Pathological and physical investigations into CO_2 laser–tissue interactions with specific emphasis on cervical intraepithelial neoplasm. Lasers Surg Med *1*:47–69, 1980.)

returned to a normal architectural pattern within 100 μm from the crater surface. Previous electron microscopic and histochemical studies illustrated special sensitivity of the epithelial cells, showing a necrotic zone of 200–250 μm, whereas desmosome collagen fibers and erythrocytes were found structurally preserved 30–50 nm away from the thermal cut.[16–18] Analysis of the internal portion of the crater revealed complete absence of epithelial elements (Fig. 3.2). The underlying supporting stroma showed few entrapped red blood cells.

SEM analysis on the 10th day demonstrated a remarkably intact surface epithelium. Large flat squamous epithelium, with microridge formation and early intercellular bar formations, was noted (Fig. 3.3). Microvilli were seen in 39% of the scanned cells. The epithelium again revealed poor cohesiveness and large tissue plaques could be seen. The plaques were avulsed during preparation, indicating low tensile strength.

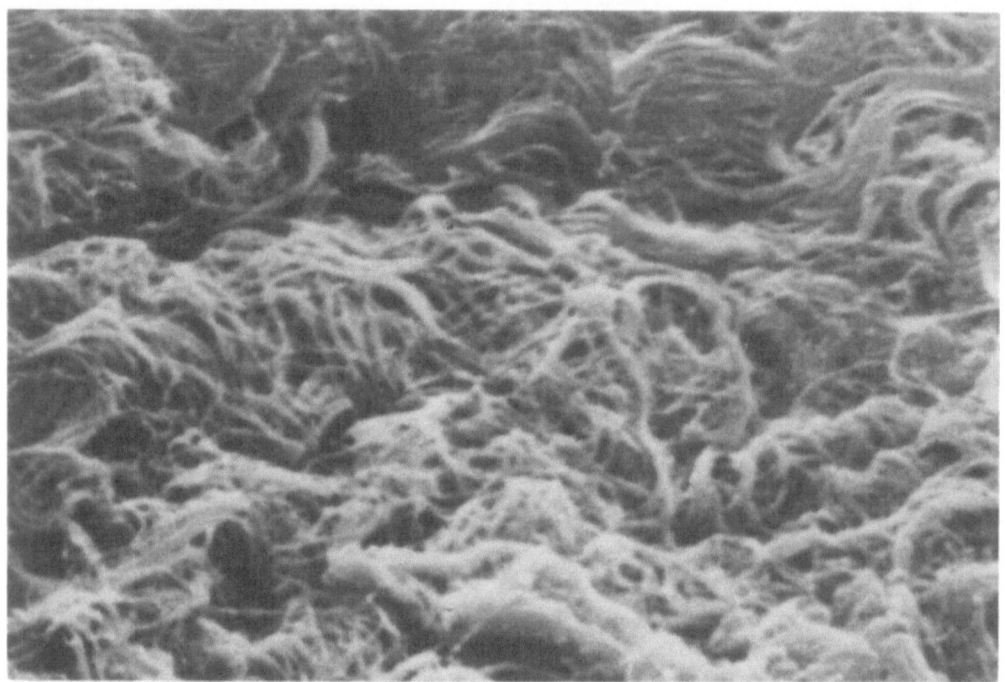

Figure 3.2. Scanning electron micrograph: internal cavity of laser impact site. Absence of epithelium cellular elements is noted ($\times$ 1500). (Reproduced with permission: Bellina JH, Seto YJ: Pathological and physical investigations into CO_2 laser–tissue interactions with specific emphasis on cervical intraepithelial neoplasm. Lasers Surg Med *1*:47–69, 1980.)

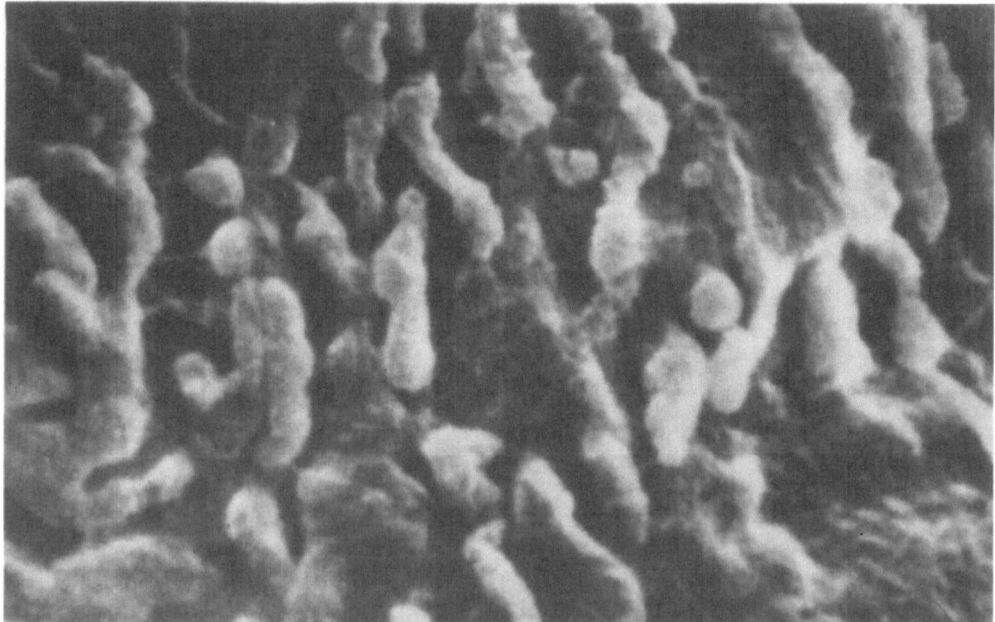

Figure 3.3. Scanning electron micrograph: epithelial regeneration 10 days after laser treatment. Metaplastic epithelium is present ($\times$ 3000). (Reproduced with permission: Bellina JH, Seto YJ: Pathological and physical investigations into CO_2 laser–tissue interactions with specific emphasis on cervical intraepithelial neoplasm. Lasers Surg Med *1*:47–69, 1980.)

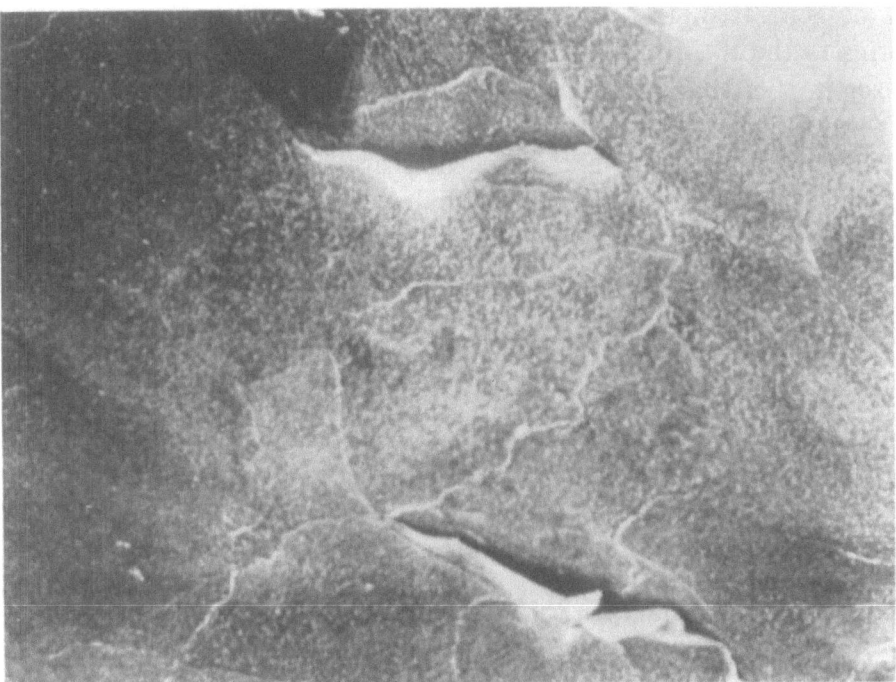

Figure 3.4. Scanning electron micrograph: epithelial regeneration 21 days after laser treatment. Normal, mature epithelium is present ($\times$ 1200). (Reproduced with permission: Bellina JH, Seto YJ: Pathological and physical investigations into CO_2 laser–tissue interactions with specific emphasis on cervical intraepithelial neoplasm. Lasers Surg Med *1*:47–69, 1980.)

On the 21st day after treatment, the surface topography appeared to be normal. Mature epithelial cells, with well defined microridges, prominent cellular bar formation, scant microvilli, and small nuclei convexities, were noted throughout the surfaces studied (Fig. 3.4). The tensile strength appeared to be normal, as free plaque formation was not present.

3.1.2.d. Clinical Findings Healing of laser-treated tissue is apparently a function of the size of the treated area and the depth of cellular destruction. Intensive cytologic, histologic, and SEM studies suggest that the water content of the laser-treated cells affects the heat transfer within them. The superficial squamous cells have a relatively low water content. The deeper intermediate, parabasal, basal, and stromal cells have progressively higher water content. Thus, one would expect the tissue destruction to be greatest for any given power in the superficial layer and to diminish rapidly as the stromal layers are approached. If, in theory, the energy transport is greatest in the X–Y axis and least in the Z axis, an oblate hemispheroid would be generated. In actuality, a shallow crater, whose internal volume conforms to the theoretical oblate hemispheroid, was observed by SEM at the laser impact site. As the energy is rapidly dissipated in the cells with higher water content, adjacent tissue necrosis is minimal to absent. Thus, as observed, few macrocytes and fibroblasts are present during the healing phase. This may account for the minimal scar formation and rapid healing time.

3.1.3. Theoretical Analysis and Experimental Verification

3.1.3.a. Theoretical Analysis of Heat Transfer—General   To explain some of the clinical observations delineated above, a theoretical model of CO_2-laser-produced heat transfer in tissue was developed. The theoretical mode, admittedly still relatively crude, was judged to be more realistic than most of the models proposed in the current literature.

For the theoretical analysis, we adopted and generalized the multilayer skin model of Stohivijk and Hardy. We assume an N-layer tissue model in which the $i = 1$ layer was eqivalent to the first epithelial layers of Stohivijk and Hardy.[19] As illustrated in Fig. 3.5, the model depicts varying thicknesses and different thermal properties for each layer. The total thickness (L), of the entire tissue (i.e., $L = N \Delta z_i$), however, was assumed to be large enough that the tissue temperature at the Nth layer would not be affected by the laser heat input at the $i = 1$ layer. This assumption was equivalent to having restricted the laser input to finite laser energy and finite impact time.

Other assumptions required by this model were that (1) thermal properties of tissue within each layer are homogeneous and isotropic, and (2) submucosal cooling via blood flow is absent.

The N-layer tissue model results in N second-order differential equations with $2(N + 1)$ boundary conditions to be simultaneously solved. Invoking circular cylindrical coordinate systems (r, θ, z) and observing a symmetry, the N differential equations are given symbolically:

$$\frac{1}{r} \frac{\delta}{\delta r} r \frac{\delta T_i}{\delta r} + \frac{\delta^2 T_i}{\delta z^2} - \frac{1}{k_i} \frac{\delta T_i}{\delta t} = \frac{A_i}{K_i} \tag{1}$$

where the subscript $i = 1, \ldots, N$ denotes the ith layer, and k_i and K_i are the thermal diffusivity and conductivity, respectively. $T_i (r, z, t)$ is the temperature at some point (r, z) and time (t) at the ith layer, and $A_i (r, z, t)$ is the heat source at point (r, z) and time (t), which is determined by the energy distribution in the laser beam and the absorption, scattering, and extinction coefficient of the ith layer tissue. The $2(N + 2)$ boundary conditions are:

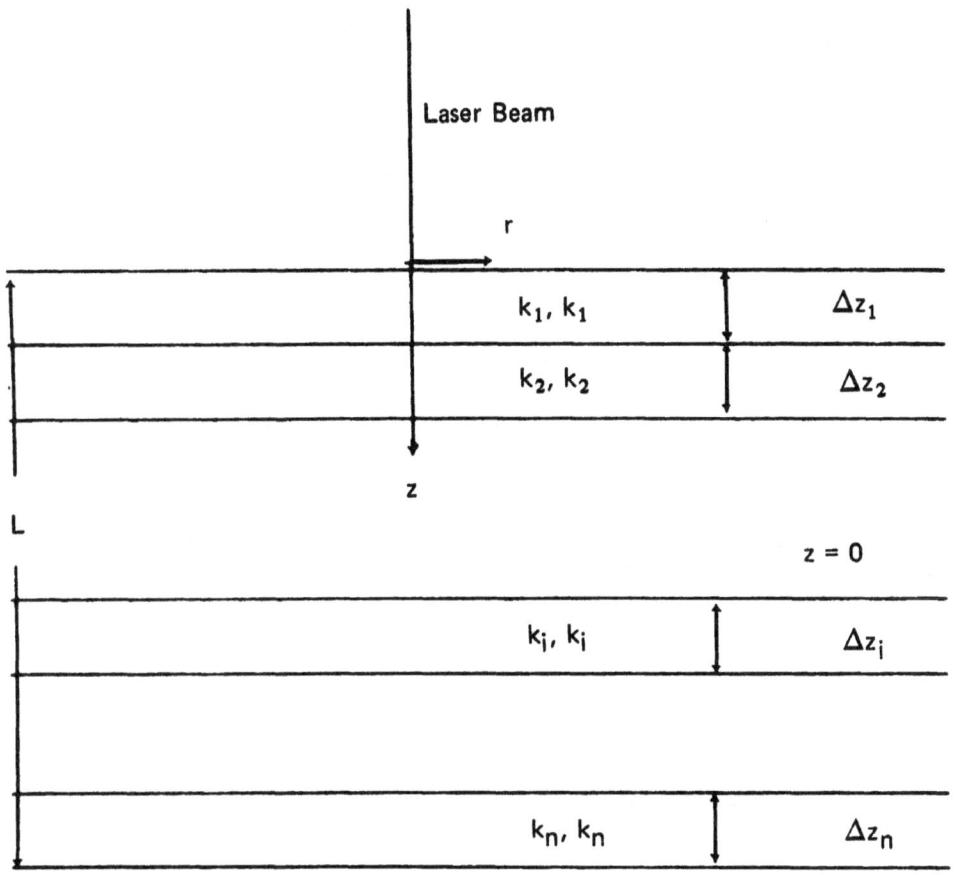

Figure 3.5. *N*-layer tissue model. Each layer $Z_i \ldots Z_n$ is given a mathematical representation that approximates its biological properties. (Reproduced with permission: Bellina JH, Seto YJ: Pathological and physical investigations into CO_2 laser–tissue interactions with specific emphasis on cervical intraepithelial neoplasm. Lasers Surg Med *1*:47–69, 1980.)

$$T_i = T_i + 1 \text{ at } Z = \sum_1^i \Delta z_m$$

$$A_i + \frac{K_i}{k_i}\frac{\delta T_i}{\delta Z} = \frac{K_i + 1}{k_i + 1}\frac{\delta T_i + 1}{\delta Z} + A_i = 1 \text{ at } Z = \sum_1^i \Delta Z_m \quad (2)$$

$$T_n = \text{constant}$$

$$T_0 = \text{constant}$$

$$\frac{1}{k_1}\frac{\delta T_1}{\delta Z} = -\frac{A_1}{K_i} + \frac{H}{K_1}(T_1 - T_0)$$

where H is the tissue surface radiation cooling coefficient.

Applying the Hankel transform for *r*-variation and the Laplace transform for *t*-variation and using matrix manipulation, Eqs. (1) and (2) could be solved with an *N*-fold iterative method. In principle, within the constraints of the assumption, the solution becomes more representative of human tissue as *N* increases. For large *N*, the iterative method requires a computer for numerical solution.

3.1.3.b. Theoretical Analysis—Closed-Form Solution The iterative method, as presented above, facilitates numerical solution to arbitrary degrees of accuracy. Numerical solutions, however, are possible only on a case-by-case basis where tissue properties are specified. To extract analytical general information, one needs a closed-form solution. For $N = 1$, [i.e., $z_1 = L$, providing that L is large so that at $z = L$, $T (L, r, t)$ is constant] a closed-form solution can be readily deduced from its general solution. Without loss of generality, one may assume a TEM mode laser beam with gaussian distribution and an infinitely short extinction length. The $N = 1$ solution for an impulse source formation is found to be

$$G(r, z, t) = I_0 \frac{2d^2k}{\pi k} \frac{\exp-(z^2/4kt)}{4kt} - \frac{H\pi}{2} \exp(H_z + H^2 kt)$$

$$\text{erfc} \left(\frac{z}{4kt} + \frac{H}{2} 4kt \right) \exp \frac{(-r^2/4kt + d^2)}{4kt + d^2} \quad (3)$$

where erfc (x) is the complementary error function of x. Since there is only one layer, the subscript i has been dropped. Equation (3) is called Green's function because it is the response to an impulse function, i.e., the absorbed laser energy at $z = 0$ being an impulse:

$$A(r, 0, t) = A(r, 0) \delta (t)$$

For TEM_{00} mode, assuming the laser beam is centered at $r = 0$, the gaussian distribution yields:

$$A(r, 0) = I_0 e^{-(r^2/2d^2)}$$

where d is the half-power width of the laser beam, and I_0 is the intensity absorption at $r = 0$.

Green's function is useful in its application to obtain temperature distribution for any temporal variation of the laser energy. If the laser temporal variation is $\theta(t)$—i.e., $A = A(r, 0)\theta(t)$—the temperature distribution in the tissue can be obtained through the following convolution integral:

$$T(r, z, t) = \int_0^{t'} \theta(t')g(r, z, t - t')dt' \tag{4}$$

On the other hand, Green's function is convenient in that if the extraction of information at a higher level of generality is needed, it is necessary just to examine Green's function without having to carry out the integral in Eq. (4).

3.1.3.c. Experimental Verification   The experiments on heat conduction in tissues were performed using tissue samples from excised abdominal walls of Sprague–Dawley rats. The temperature in the tissue was monitored using three Yellow Spring 507 miniature thermistor probes. Because of variations in individual thermistor characteristics, the probes were not electrically interchangeable. A drive circuit for each probe, consisting of a simple resistance bridge, was constructed in such a way that the values of the resistors were adjusted to yield comparable voltage output versus temperature characteristics. For measurements, the output voltages of the probes were recorded simultaneously by a two-beam, dual-trace (a sum of four traces) Tectronix RM565 oscilloscope. Permanent records were obtained by an oscilloscope-mounted Polaroid Land Camera.

The depth of each probe in the tissue was measured by a tubular micrometer. The micrometer was mounted vertically on the head of a microscope stand which supported the tissue samples. This micrometer has a sensitivity of 0.0127 mm and a needle point. The depth of a probe inside the tissue was determined by first taking the micrometer reading while the needle was at the tissue surface. The needle was then inserted into the tissue, and another reading was taken at contact with the thermal probe. The difference in the two micrometer readings represented the probe depth.

The lateral distance of each probe head from the edge of the crater formed by the laser firing was measured by a traveling micrometer microscope. The complete objective eyepiece system of the traveling microscope could move horizontally by a micrometer to the microscope stand supporting the tissue sample. The objective–eyepiece system had a crossed-hair alignment. One reading of the micrometer was recorded when the crossed hairline was aligned with the crater edge. The object eyepiece was then moved laterally until the hairline coincided with the tip of the probe, then a second reading was recorded. The difference between the two readings represented the horizontal location of the probe. This instrument was also used in measuring the size of the crater. The sensitivity of the micrometer was 0.005 mm (Fig. 3.6).

With the above-described experimental set-up, temporal variations of temperature at three different locations in tissue can be simultaneously

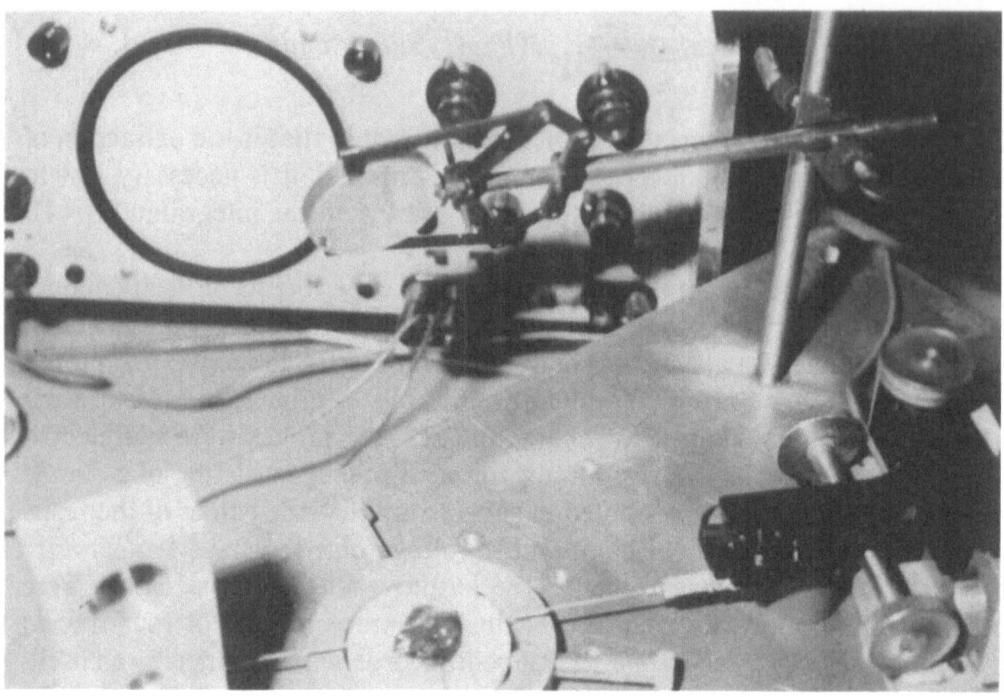

Figure 3.6. Experimental apparatus for the thermal measurements: Oscilloscope, thermal probes, tissue sample, and beam reflector. (Reproduced with permission: Bellina JH, Seto YJ: Pathological and physical investigations into CO_2 laser–tissue interactions with specific emphasis on cervical intraepithelial neoplasm. Lasers Surg Med *1*:47–69, 1980.)

recorded. The recordings of such temporal responses for any given laser energy can be compared with theoretical responses as calculated from Eqs. (3) and (4) by appropriate substitution of probe locations in Eq. (3).

Since precise values of diffusivity and conductivity for rat abdominal wall are not known, the following values for averaging tissues were used in the theoretical calculation:

$$k = 0.001 \text{ cm}^2/\text{sec}$$

$$K = 0.25 \text{ W/cm} - °\text{K}$$

The focused laser beam was set at 10 W for a half-width of $d = 0.05$ cm at the surface of the tissue, and the laser impact time was set at 1 sec; that is:

$$\theta(t) = \begin{cases} 1, & 0 < t < 1 \\ 0, & t > 1 \end{cases}$$

The laser power for each impact was incorporated in the power absorption parameter I_0 by assuming 100% power absorption in tissue.

A comparison of theoretically predicted to experimentally measured temperature responses in more than 50 subjects yields quantitative and statistical agreement. Quantitative differences between theoretical and experimental responses are attributable to the choice of diffusivity and conductivity values and to the accuracy of experimental measurements. A typical comparison of responses is shown in Fig. 3.7.

3.1.3.d. Summary of Theoretical Findings   The second term in Eq. (3) is interpreted as a surface radiation cooling term. If one assumes no surface cooling effect (i.e., $H = 0$), the entire second term can be omitted. For extraction of general information in cases where no forced air surface cooling is involved, examination of the first term in Eq. (3) suffices. The following is a summary of the analytical characteristics of temperature responses in tissue under typical laser impacts:

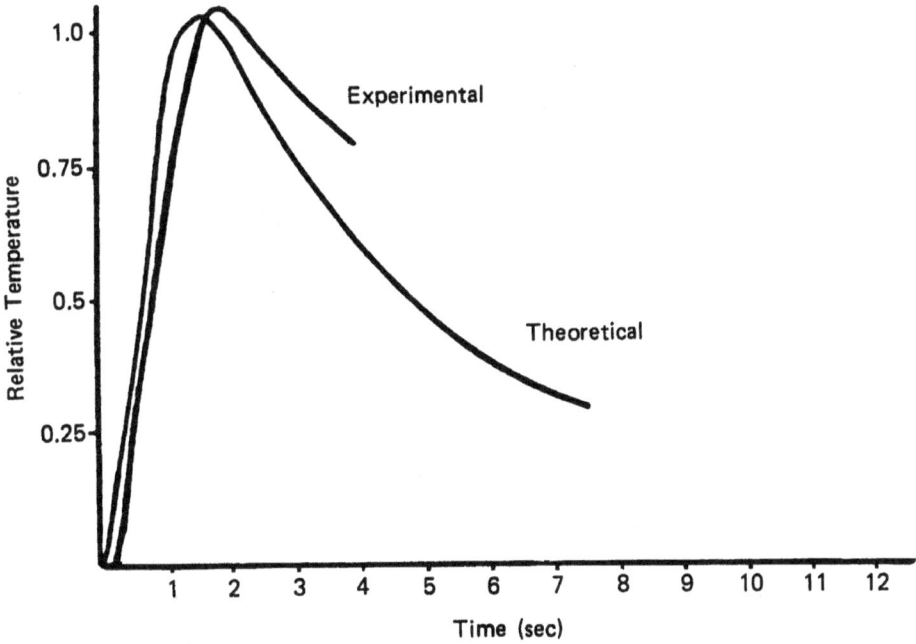

Figure 3.7. Graphic illustration of experimental data compared to theoretical data. (Reproduced with permission: Bellina JH, Seto YJ: Pathological and physical investigations into CO_2 laser–tissue interactions with specific emphasis on cervical intraepithelial neoplasm. Lasers Surg Med *1*:47–69, 1980.)

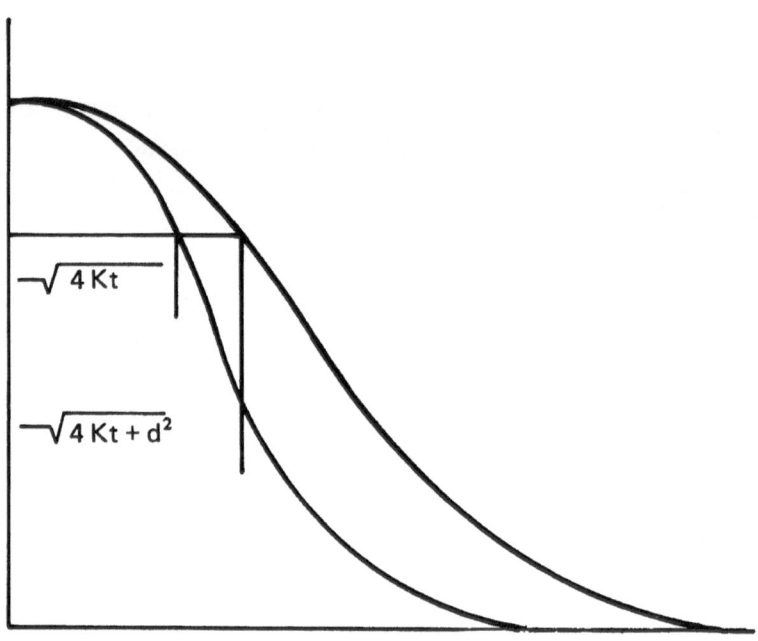

Figure 3.8. Gaussian distribution of thermal decay of laser induced tissue heating. (Reproduced with permission: Bellina JH, Seto YJ: Pathological and physical investigations into CO_2 laser–tissue interactions with specific emphasis on cervical intraepithelial neoplasm. Lasers Surg Med *1*:47–69, 1980.)

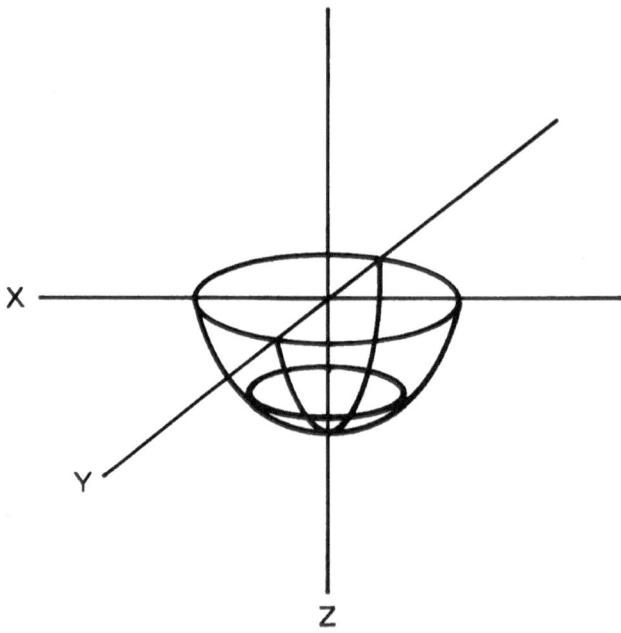

Figure 3.9. Measured thermal pattern of the carbon dioxide laser, oblate hemispheroid. (Reproduced with permission: Bellina JH, Seto YJ: Pathological and physical investigations into CO_2 laser–tissue interactions with specific emphasis on cervical intraepithelial neoplasm. Lasers Surg Med *1*:47–69, 1980.)

1. The analytical model quantitatively predicts heat transfer responses in tissue as verified by detailed experimental comparisons.
2. At any given time, the laser-induced temperature distribution decays radially outward from the point of impact. The decaying temperature function obeys a gaussian distribution function rather than simple exponential decay (Fig. 3.8).
3. For the same distance from the point of impact, at any given time $t > d^2/4k$, a point lying on the surface of the tissue will have a temperature higher than a point lying directly under the laser's point of impact. An alternative interpretation of this observation for $t > d^2/4k$ is that the equal temperature surfaces would take oblate hemispheroidal shape as shown in Fig. 3.9. This is far different from deep cutting temperature distribution in tissue as given by Bodecker and colleagues.[20] For comparison, their equal temperature surfaces are resketched in Fig. 3.10. The temperature difference between a surface point and a point directly under the impact point at equal distance rapidly decreases as time progresses beyond $t > d^2/4k$. This means that equal temperature surfaces in tissue will ultimately approach concentric hemispheres.

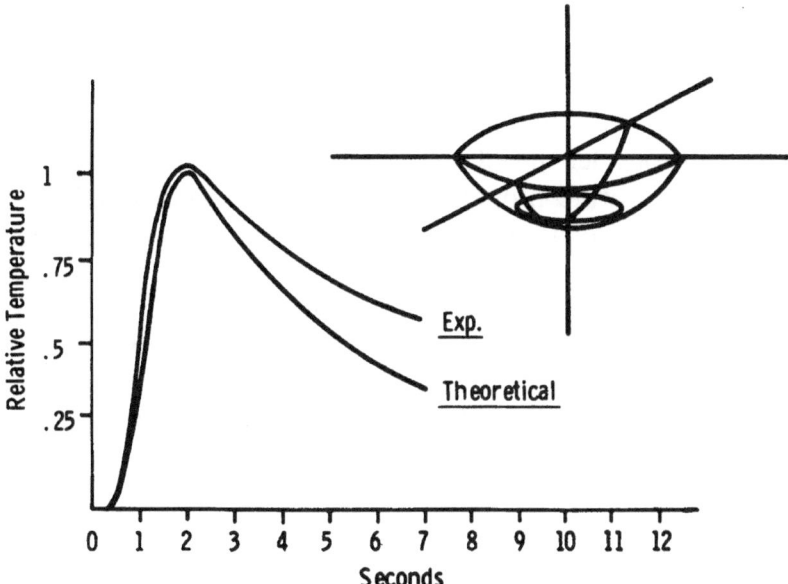

Figure 3.10. Comparison of theoretical and experimental measurements are in agreement with a hemioblate spheroid geometry. (Reproduced with permission: Bellina JH, Seto YJ: Pathological and physical investigations into CO_2 laser–tissue interactions with specific emphasis on cervical intraepithelial neoplasm. Lasers Surg Med *1*:47–69, 1980.)

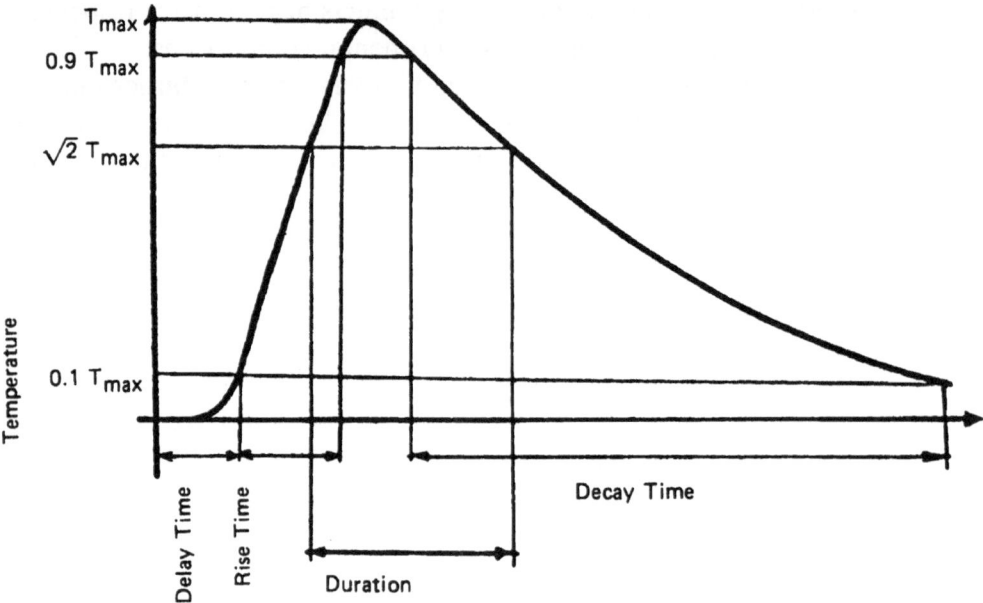

Figure 3.11. Maxwellian distribution function illustrates temporal variation pattern as measured in the experiments. (Reproduced with permission: Bellina JH, Seto YJ: Pathological and physical investigations into CO_2 laser–tissue interactions with specific emphasis on cervical intraepithelial neoplasm. Lasers Surg Med *1*:47–69, 1980.)

4. At any given point in tissue, the temporal variation of temperature resembles a Maxwellian distribution function (Fig. 3.11).
5. One can consider the CO_2-laser-induced heat conduction in tissue as a radially outward-propagating temperature pulse much like a potential pulse propagating along a nerve system. At points near the point of impact, the pulse has a sharp rise time, high peak temperature, and relatively long decay time. As the pulse propagates outward, the peak temperture decays as described below, and the sharp curve shape of the pulse becomes flattened. By examining Eq. (3), one can deduce that the speed of the pulse is inversely proportional to the distance from the point of impact, that is:

$$\tilde{V}p \propto \frac{1}{r} \qquad \tilde{V}p \propto \frac{1}{z}$$

Thus, the temperature pulse is seen to propagate relatively rapidly at the vicinity of the impact point, but the speed is reduced as it propagates outward.
6. The model predicts approximately that the peak of the temperature

pulse is, at any point, inversely proportional to the cube of the distance between that point and the laser impact site. This holds as long as $4kt > d^2$.

3.1.3.e. Conclusion The analytical model in our study predicted that (1) an oblate hemispheroid configuration of constant temperature surfaces in tissue results from impact of an ideal CO_2 laser system; (2) the temperature distribution decays radially outward from the point of impact in a gaussian form; and (3) the surface or lateral thermal pulse peak, T_p, decreases inversely proportionately to the cube of the distance traveled.

The SEM observations of laser impact sites reveal an internal cavity whose geometric configuration is an oblate hemispheroid. The limit of the lateral thermal cellular damage is finite and well-demarcated. This phenomenon is explained by the rapid reduction of the peak temperature as it travels radially outward, $T_p \sim 1/r^3$. The SEM observations appear to confirm the predicted thermal pattern.

Histologic evidence of limited stromal necrosis conforms to the heat-transfer properties predicted in the model and measured in our experiments.

Thus, it is our conclusion that the rapid reepithelialization noted by cytologic, histologic, and SEM analysis is due to the thermal interaction patterns of the CO_2 laser (Fig. 3.12).

Minimal stromal damage results from laser application and, as the heat radiates in a lateral fashion, the greatest thermal damage occurs in the epithelial layer. This layer heals rapidly in a centripetal and reserve cell fashion. As the application of CO_2 laser energy to tissues creates minimal adjacent tissue necrosis, replacement of the epithelium occurs without extensive phagocytosis. This is in contradistinction to hot cautery or other volumetric destructive modalities. The zone of injury created by the laser is minimal to absent at 50 μm or less in thickness. The zone of injury and necrosis created by other treatments varies from millimeters to centimeters in thickness.

In conclusion, we have attempted to explain the rapid reepithelialization occurring on the cervix following laser vaporization. We believe that the biophysical properties of this infrared energy can and do advance our understanding of the tissue healing phase.

3.2. Plume Emission Analysis

As previously discussed, the 10.6-μm wavelength is exponentially absorbed by the water molecule. Absorbed photons at this wavelength can

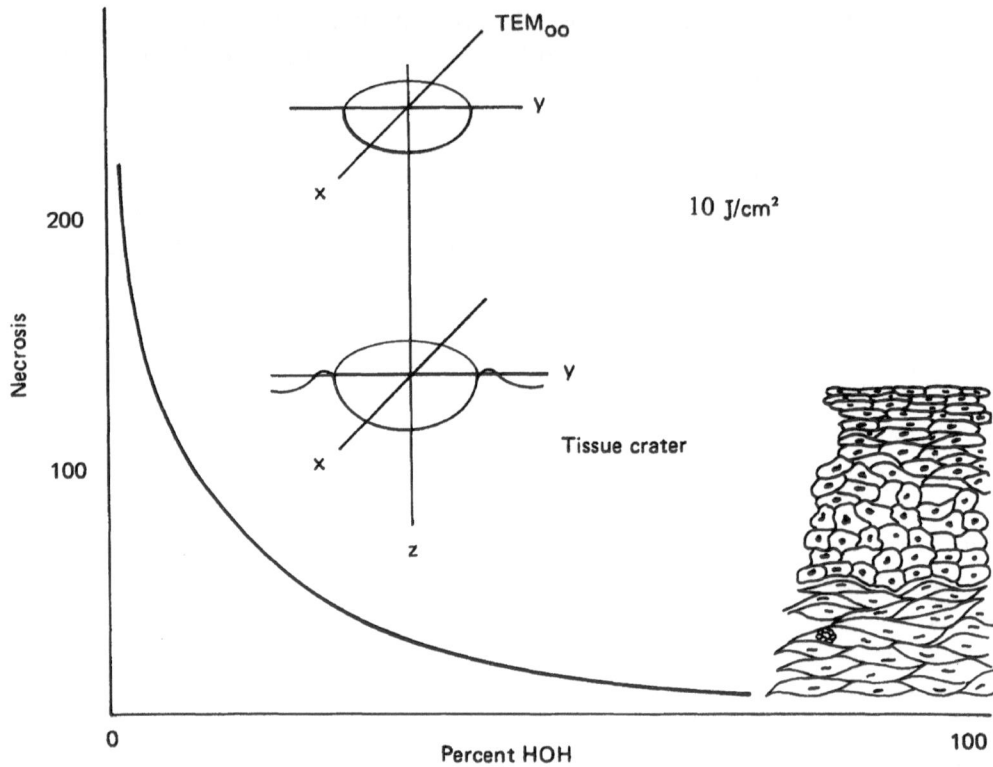

Figure 3.12. Biothermal effects of laser gave impetus to rapid healing of the epithelium. The oblate hemispheroid thermal configuration explained the residual tumor problem. Minimal stroma damage results from the laser. To avoid residual disease, the stroma must be removed to a depth of 2 mm. (Reproduced with permission: Bellina JH, Seto YJ: Pathological and physical investigations into CO_2 laser–tissue interactions with specific emphasis on cervical intraepithelial neoplasm. Lasers Surg Med *1*:47–69, 1980.)

transfer their energy (*hν*) through vibrational shifts in the triatomic water molecule, thereby creating heat. The rapid temperature elevation of intracellular water results in cellular wall disruption. Cellular water vaporization produces a plume containing intracellular components which are further heated by the 1500°C radiant beam. The major question concerning the surgeon and patient is the possibility of DNA transfer to the surgeon's lungs or the splattering of vapor containing oncogenic DNA from the wound site. We undertook a study to analyze both problems carefully.

Hoye, in his work with pulsed laser systems, described viable tumor cells in the laser plume.[21] Oosterhuis, using trypan blue vital stain, described what he considered to be nonviable (morphologically intact) cells after CO_2 laser irradiation of melanotic lesions.[22] However, the in vivo inoculum in Oosterhuis's study failed to produce a melanotic tumor. Serial passage of the debris in tissue culture showed no cellular propagation.[23]

The study was designed to investigate the plume debris at the molecular level, using techniques described by Stjernholm.[24] The degree of enzymatic function was assessed by the ability of the debris to utilize [^{14}C]glucose for energy metabolism. Additional studies were performed to detect possible DNA replication or RNA transcription using [^{3}H]thymidine and [^{3}H]uridine.

Tumors from patients infected with papovavirus were used as the tumor model. This virus is sexually transmitted and results in a wartlike growth known as condyloma acuminata. The virus has also been identified as the etiologic agent for laryngeal papilloma usually seen in young children.[25] It is hypothesized that vaginal transmission to the aerodigestive tract of the infant occurs at parturition. In women, coital exposure to this virus results in a genital papillary growth within 60–90 days of exposure. As this virus is a DNA virus, it is a good tumor model, with known transmissible traits in the human. If the debris contained viable biological material, then the surgeon and patient could be at risk for tumor development.

After appropriate analysis, all samples failed to demonstrate viability. Evaluation of metabolic activity using [^{14}C]glucose showed no activity. Similarly, labeled nucleosides failed to demonstrate replication or transcription activity. The presence of intact but dehydrated cells suggested the possibility of intact cytoplasmic or nuclear pathways. However, in this study[26] no cytoplasmic or nuclear activity could be detected. If a hazard exists, it may appear after long-term exposure.

Previous research[27] demonstrated the denaturation of DNA molecules by the laser, so that phagocytic cells would not incorporate the entire particle, which could represent a potential danger for neoplastic recurrence during the healing process. Goldman[28] has studied this question for more than five years and has found no evidence linking laser-exposed tissue to the development of malignancies.

3.3. Photoacoustic Properties

Photoacoustic properties of lasers are very important in dealing with oncogenic tumors. Should an acoustic wave be generated with sufficient strength to displace a tumor cell, then rapid metastases could occur.

Using a Michelson interferometer, the impact of CO_2 photons was measured as the displacement of a pivoted mirror. The interference pattern generated by a properly balanced pivotal mirror resulted in a shift of interference

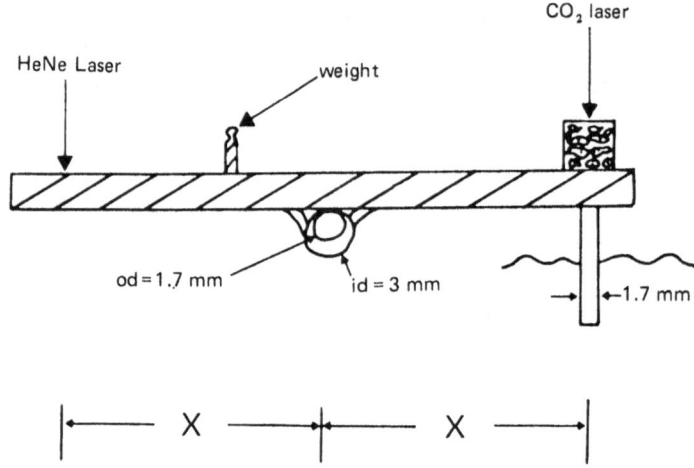

Figure 3.13. Balanced mirrors of interferometer record the incidental change as a result of photon impact.

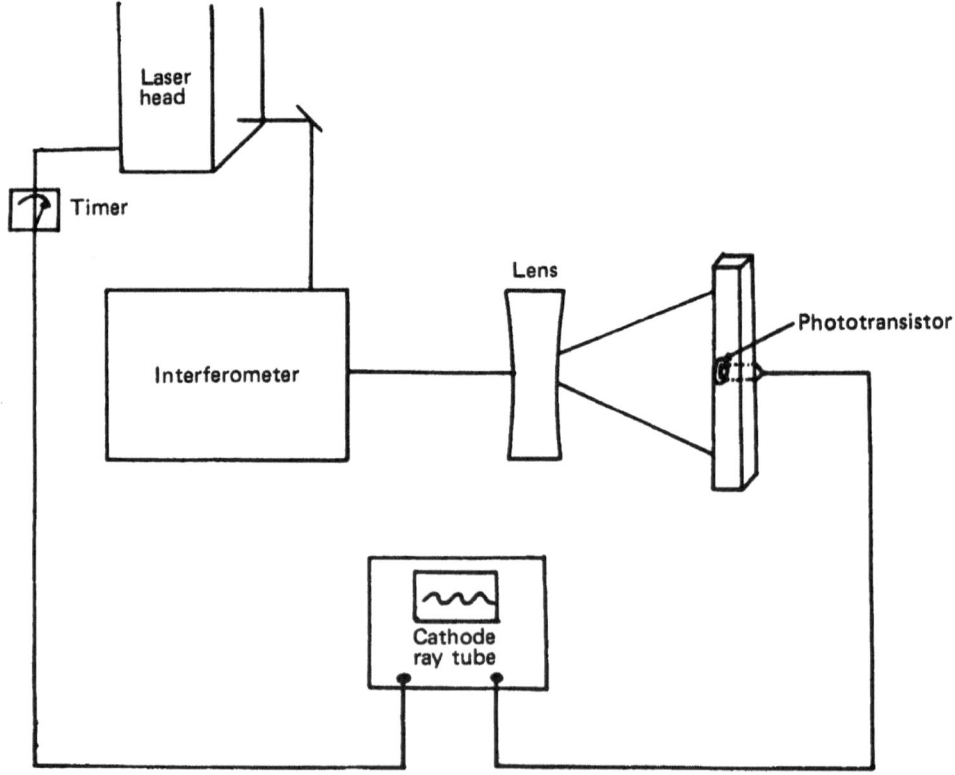

Figure 3.14. Experimental design for measuring photon moment.

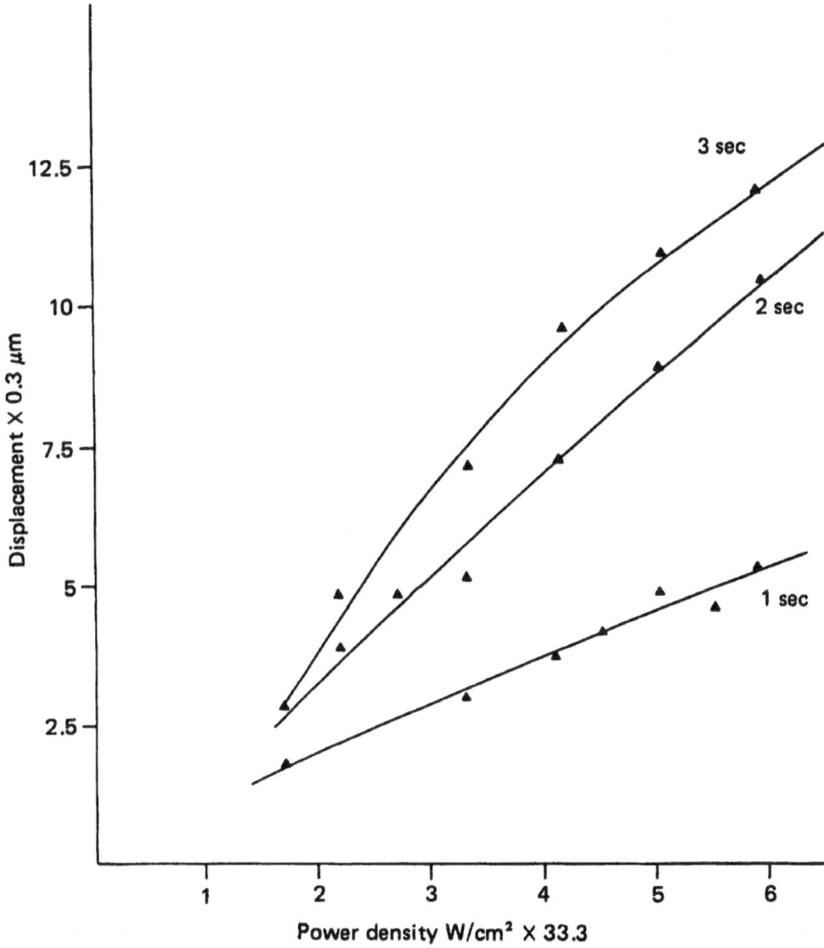

Figure 3.15. Experimental data on black-body movements revealed that wet paper had maximum motion due to water jet vaporization phenomenon while tissue had least amount of moment.

fringe pattern (Fig. 3.13). This shift was recorded via the phototransistor and displayed on a cathode ray tube (Fig. 3.14).

The experimental study investigated black-body absorption, wet-paper absorption, and tissue absorption. The final conclusion was that the photon moment was negligible and constant at 60 Hz as related to the 60-Hz cycle of the laser. The effect on wet paper was largely the result of water vaporizing, the downward force resulting from the ejected vapor. The maximal displant was negligible, <0.15 μm. This photon moment was slightly increased when the time of exposure was increased. We concluded that the photon moment in vivo is less than for a black body but significantly less than for wet paper (73.3 μm) (Fig. 3.15). Thus, acoustic wave or photon impact

101

should be of negligible clinical significance. Additional studies are needed using holograms to document vibrations in each direction of impact, preferably real-time, double-exposure holograms.

3.4. Photon–Tissue Interaction

The argon laser (λ = 0.488–0.515 nm) was used to evaluate tissue photobiology as a function of (1) power density, (2) energy density at constant velocity, and (3) delayed tissue photobiodynamics as a function of (1) and (2). Rabbit fallopian tubes were used as models. Our interest was not only in the initial incision effect of this wavelength, but also, and more importantly, in the return of organ function over time.

The animals were divided into three test groups, each containing 10 animals. Group I was treated with a power density of 1000 W/cm^2 at a linear velocity of 1.0 cm/sec (energy density, 100 J/cm^2). Group II was treated with a power density of 1000 W/cm^2 at a linear density of 1.5 cm/sec (energy density, 75 J/cm^2).

From each group, two animals were sacrificed at days 0, 5, 10, 15, and 20. Tubal segments 1.5 cm long were taken for analysis and placed in 10% formalin. The tissues were dehydrated and embedded in Paraplast®. Sections from 5 to 8 μm in thickness were affixed to albumin-coated slides, stained with van Gieson's solution, and counterstained with Gray's Celestine Blue. When this preparation is used, cellular nuclei stain blue to blue-green, collagen stains magenta, muscle stains brownish yellow, and keratin and erythrocytes stain brilliant yellow.

3.4.1. Experimental Design

A Spectra-Physics Model 770 argon photocoagulator was used as the wavelength source. The laser was focused to a diameter of 0.10 cm at the tissue irradiation site. A mechanical device constructed by the investigators was used to produce a constant linear velocity over the test tissue site. To insure precise dimensions of the linear cut, a mask was constructed which allowed passage of the incident energy for a fixed distance of 1 cm. The device was also constructed to hold the focal distance of the laser at a constant distance from the tissue.

3.4.2. Results

The findings were similar at all three linear velocities although the changes were more marked when the linear velocity was 2.0 cm/sec. Initially (day 0), a thermal effect is seen at the impact site involving the serosa and underlying muscularis. The capillaries of the underlying submucosa were contracted and filled with hemolyzed erythrocytes. By day 5, the site of injury showed a zone of fibrosis in the serosa and muscularis and thrombosis in the capillaries of the submucosa. By days 10–15, there was fibrosis in the serosa, atrophy and fibrosis in the muscularis, atrophy of the submucosa, and hyperplasia at the site of the injury. By day 20, the changes were accentuated, with fibrosis of the serosa and muscularis, dilated large venules, collagen and hemorrhage in the serosa, with increased fibrosis in the submucosa and hyperplasia of the mucosa. The mucosal hyperplasia was contra-coup in nature (i.e., appeared most extensive directly opposite the site of laser irradiation).

3.4.3. Discussion

When the known effects of photon–tissue interaction were explored, it was found that photobiological effects can be divided into two major categories; linear effects and nonlinear effects. Linear effects are comprised of the direct or observed heating, vaporization, and plume phenomena. The non-linear effects are more theoretical but may help to explain some of our experimental results. Nonlinear effects can include in situ generation of elastic waves by (1) radiation pressure, (2) electrostriction, (3) self-trapping, and (4) stimulated Brillouin scattering. Nonlinear effects can also include in situ generation of ionizing radiation by (1) multiphoton effect, (2) harmonic generation, (3) stimulated Raman scattering, and (4) electric breakdown.[29]

In both nonlinear pathways the end product or observed effect is heating by either photon absorption or electron absorption, resulting in tissue vaporization. However, the by-products of nonlinear pathways may give rise to secondary tissue effects in the form of ionization, plasma production, and in situ generation of ionization radiation from UV to X rays. Their effects may or may not be of biological significance.

The thermal effects of laser photobiology have been amply elucidated, with major references to the CO_2 wavelength of 10.6 μm, by many authors.[2,12,17,20] To draw conclusions, we shall compare and contrast the known properties of the carbon dioxide wavelength of 10,600 nm to the argon wavelength of 488 nm. Furthermore, we shall use certain mathematical models to validate our observations. The formulas are self-explanatory and do not require an extensive mathematical background.

When one compares the thermal effect of the argon wavelength to the CO_2 wavelength, the first discrepancy appears in the tissue absorption coefficiency. The adipose tissue absorption coefficient is 1.5 cm^{-1} at 488 nm and that for skin is 60 cm^{-1}, whereas most tissue at 10,600 nm has an absorption coefficiency of $\leq$200 cm^{-1}. Using the absorption coefficiency in Beer's exponential law of absorption:

$$I = I_0 \exp(-\alpha Z) \tag{5}$$

where α represents the absorption coefficient of the tissue at the laser wavelength, it becomes readily apparent that α of 1.5 cm^{-1} when compared to α of 200 cm^{-1} will result in a greater penetration of the argon laser when compared to the CO_2 laser. In fact, the incident CO_2 laser energy is 90% absorbed by less than the first millimeter of fat while >1 cm will be required to absorb 90% of the argon incident laser energy. Thus, it becomes apparent that even a sharply focused argon laser will theoretically have a potential for distant photon penetration.

Next, considering the quality of energy necessary to vaporize a tissue, one is again struck by the fact that a simple inspection of a balanced energy equation reveals another major discrepancy.

Using the balanced heat equation:

$$X = \frac{(1 - R)pnt}{ApJ(L + c\Delta T)} = \frac{(1 - R)4PT}{\pi d^2 pJ(L + c\Delta t)} \tag{6}$$

where the absorption depth of the tissue is assumed to be 0.02 cm, R is the reflectivity of rat skin (at 10,600 nm this is less than 5%), P is the average laser power (W), A is the area of the focused laser beam $(\pi d/4)^2$ (cm^2), p is the density of the tissue (1.2 g/cm^3), n is a gas law constant derived from the formula $I = I_0 \exp(-\alpha Z)$, J is Joule's constant (4.185 J/cal), L is the latent heat of the tissue (540 cal/g), c is the specific heat of the tissue (0.86 cal/g°C), ΔT is the temperature rise to the vaporization point (100°C − 36.5°C = 63.5°C), t is the time to vaporize the small volume to the absorption depth (sec), T is the total time of exposure ($T = nt$), d is the focused laser spot diameter (cm), and X is the nz total depth of the incision (cm).

The value of R (reflectivity) is greater for argon ($\gg$1) when compared to that for CO_2 ($\ll$1). As R is in the numerator, the value of X or energy required to vaporize a given quality of tissue, will be increased in direct proportion to an increase in R as long as all other variables are held constant. Indeed, this is the case with the argon/CO_2 "X" evaluation. Thus, the argon laser should require a greater power output to achieve the same vaporization volume when compared to the CO_2 laser. However, experimentally, when power densities were held constant, the vaporization volume reported by Boggan et al.[30] was slightly greater in the argon test group. In their experiments, power densities were corrected by beam diameter rather than input power. Thus, the greater or lesser the surface area of impact, the greater or lesser the effects of reflectivity R.

There is a theoretical minimal surface at which R becomes negligible. However, as the focus becomes minimal, the other effects come into existence. In nature, all substances are bound by atomic interactions. The forces binding atoms are electromagnetic fields defined in V/cm. When the field strength surrounding a molecule exceeds 10^6 V/cm, an instantaneous massive redistribution of the electrical system can occur with production of free electrons, ionized atoms, and possible X rays from bremsstrahlung (i.e., plasma formation).

To determine if, in medicine, the argon or CO_2 laser could achieve this electromagnetic field strength, solve the following equation:

$$E = 2W \frac{\mu_0}{\epsilon_0} \tag{7}$$

where $\mu_0/\epsilon_0 = 37.6 \, \Omega$, W is the power density (W/cm^2), and, E is the electric field strength (V/cm).

Solve for E or $E = 27.4 \, (w)^{1/2}$, and then substitute for E, 10^6 V/cm. In solving, we now discover that both the argon and CO_2 laser at 1.3×10^9 W/cm^2 could produce undesirable ionization effects. Thus, if we can develop power of 1.3×10^9 W/cm^2, stimulated Raman and Brillouin scattering and field stripping effects become possible. However, to develop power densities of this order of magnitude, we must either develop very powerful input voltages or critically focus the laser to a very small diameter. Theoretically, a laser could be critically focused to a diameter equal to the wavelength of the exacting media. However, the mirror properties of the laser optical cavity (Fabry–Perot resonant cavity), prevent this focus minimum. This is referred to as diffraction limitation.

The emission from a diffraction-limited laser can be focused to a diameter approaching the order of magnitude of its wavelength. The equation for this focusing is defined by:

$$d_{\text{TEM}_{00}} = \frac{2.44f\lambda}{D} \tag{8}$$

where $d_{\text{TEM}_{00}}$ is the diameter at the tissue, λ is the laser wavelength, D is the diameter of the laser beam exiting from the optical cavity, and, f is the focal length of the lens.

Using the ideal "f number" ratio of $f/0 = 1$, the minimum is $d_{\text{TEM}_{00}} = 2.44\lambda$, and we can calculate the minimum-focused "diameter." The CO_2 laser can be focused to a theoretical spot size of 25,864 nm, while the argon laser can be focused to a theoretical spot size of 1190.72 nm.

Now, using these diffraction-limited minima-focused "diameters" we can solve for the power requirement of each laser to generate field strength in excess of 10^6 V/cm by using a power density formula:

$$\text{PD} = \frac{100 \times \text{watts of output}}{(\text{diameter of "spot size" in millimeters})^2} \tag{9}$$

This power density formula is an approximation to correct for a beam profile of gaussian distribution (i.e., TEM_{00}). Using this method, we discover that our CO_2 laser power supply would require an output of 8696 W while the argon laser power supply would only require 18.43 W of output. There are no CO_2 lasers existing in medicine today with power supplies of this order of magnitude, but power outputs of 18 W could be achieved with argon. Thus, nonlinear effects are no longer theoretical when an argon laser focal spot size approaches 1.2 μm. There is currently, however, no medical system that can deliver this spot size in the argon wavelength.

Thus, the theoretical properties of nonlinear reactions should not be encountered at power densities from 1×10^3 to 5×10^6 W/cm^2 with either the argon or the CO_2 laser, as most undesirable effects begin near power densities at 1.3×10^9 W/cm^2, which could generate electromagnetic fields of 10^6 V/cm.

However, in our experiments we noted tissue reaction in excess of those expected. In evaluating the mathematical models, we noted the major area of discrepancy to be in the absorption coefficiency of both lasers. The argon-reflective properties are probably minimal when focused below 100 μm but at 1 mm must be taken into consideration. The CO_2 laser is not reflected.

We are left with but one explanation for our experimental results; absorption and scattering of the argon photon causes additional photobiological effects. The results, noted in our study, revealed delayed tissue changes associated with fibrosis. These changes are believed to be related to direct heating effect of the argon wavelength on tissue through vibrational energy translation and photochemical chemical changes not fully elucidated. The first effect of healing has a well defined geometry and a random healing pattern due to scatter and reflected argon photons.

In our fallopian tube model, the primary pigmentation is from the hemoglobin molecule, and secondary pigmentation is from the myoglobin molecule. Argon photons are strongly absorbed by the hemoglobin and oxyhemoglobin molecules. The hemoglobin molecule acts as the limiting factor in absorption and scatter. The fallopian tube is relatively transparent to 488 nm except for its angioarchitecture. A focused argon laser will cut by Eq. (6), but by Eq. (5) deeper photon penetration due to the lower absorption coefficient must result. Intercellular reflection will occur where reflection is in excess of the absorption. One can postulate that scattering of the argon photons to distant sites could lead to additional tissue changes. Indeed in our set of experiments additional photobiological effects were noted. Delayed necrosis appeared to be directly related to an intravascular microcoagulation.

We hypothesize that at the primary focus vaporization occurs, with a resulting scatter of 488-nm photons. The scatter photons are distributed in the surrounding tissue on a more or less random basis depending on the incident angle of the primary argon beam, cellular reflectivity, absorption, and the angioarchitecture of the organ. As is the case with certain organs, critical vascular supplies are of the terminal capillary type with limited collateral circulation.

Should an intravascular event lead to a rise in plasma temperature, endothelial damage could result in a microvascular clotting event. As the principle mechanism for photon energy dissipation is thermal, "hot" erythrocytes could heat and damage the endothelial surfaces. These "hot" or damaged erythrocytes would be immediately swept away from the injury site by the plasma flow. Thus, early review of tissue would not demonstrate tissue or vessel damage. However, as the endothelial layer is avulsed by additional trauma from passing erythrocytes and lysozyme activity, intracellular thromboplastin could start a process of clotting. Should this intravascular clot be in a critical pathway, one with minimal to no collateral circulation, terminal arteriole necrosis would result. This process was observed in our model. The immediate injury was of a limited and well defined area. However, by the 10th day, delayed intravascular clotting was noted, with tissue necrosis developing as late as the 15th day. Large wedges of tissue necrosis suggested a terminal arteriole occlusion, healing and repair occurring thereafter until the 21st day of study.

In the set of experiments by Boggan et al.,[30] cerebral tissue was exposed for very short intervals (0.2 sec) to the argon and CO_2 wavelengths. The effects of scatter were minimal due to the very short exposure of peripheral hemoglobin to scattered photons. In fact, their set of experiments showed no apparent delayed effects. When the argon laser was used to cut neural axons, the delayed effects were evident, but only indirect in the healing process. They found that nerves cut with the continuous wave (cw) argon "healed faster." In contrast, the CO_2-laser-cut nerves showed "delayed healing" and took a prolonged interval to achieve normal tensile strength. Is it possible that the "rapid healing" and tensile strength were the results of an increase in tissue destruction stimulating an increase in fibroblastic activity? Other argon tissue experiments revealed an increased proliferation of fibroblastic activity.[31] A more appropriate test of axon recovery would be the return of normal function. In fact, experience with experimental animal models as well as human subjects reveals this return to normal function to be due apparently to the reduction in reparative collagen deposition. The greater the collagen deposition in the healing phase, theoretically the greater the probability of poor organ function. This is particularly true with fallopian tubes, whose function depends not only upon the return of normal neural function but also on tissue flexibility and mobility.

These results are thought to be the first evidence of the existence of nonlinear effects of argon wavelength on tissue. We believe that the vascularity and collateral circulation of the vascular tumors and retinal diseases on which the argon laser was primarily used in the past prevented these observations. Similarly, in otorhinolaryngology the relatively avascular tympanic membrane and ossicles failed to reveal this delayed phenomenon.

Of importance was the discovery of mucosal hyperplasia. This phenomenon suggests a photochemically induced response of this cell layer. It is also most interesting to note that the hyperplasia is discrete in location and appears to be in those sites directly exposed to a high density of photons.

In conclusion, surgeons employing new techniques of laser surgery must be cognizant of the possibility of delayed effects from various wavelengths. As new instrumentation is developed, variable operating beam diameters will become available. However beam diameter alone will not solve all the problems facing the laser surgeon. A careful study of all beam diameters and new techniques is very important to laser surgery and the surgeon.

References

1. Bellina JH, Polanyi TG: Management of vaginal adenosis and related cervico-vaginal disorders in DES-exposed progeny by means of carbon dioxide laser surgery. J Reprod Med *16*:295–296, 1976.

2. Bellina JH, Seto YJ: Pathological and physical investigations into CO_2 laser-tissue interactions with specific emphasis on cervical intraepithelial neoplasm. Lasers Surg Med *1*:47–69, 1980.
3. Fara G, Emanuelli H, Cascinelli N, et al: CO_2 lasers: beam patterns in relation to the surgical use. Lasers Surg Med *2*:331–341, 1983.
4. Verschueren RC: The CO_2 Laser in Tumor Surgery. Amsterdam, Van Gorcum, 1976, pp 38–47.
5. Mihashi S, Jako GJ, Inoze J, et al: Laser surgery in otolaryngology. Interaction of CO_2 laser and soft tissue. Ann NY Acad Sci *267*:263–291, 1976.
6. Hall RR, Hill DW, Beach HD: A carbon dioxide laser. Ann R Coll Surg Engl *48*:181–188, 1971.
7. Hall RR, Beach HD, Baker E, Morison PC: Incision of tissue by carbon dioxide laser. Nature *232*:131–132, 1971.
8. Toaff R: The carbon dioxide laser in gynecological surgery, in Kaplan I (ed): Proceedings of the First International Symposium on Laser Surgery, Tel Aviv, Israel, November 1975. Jerusalem, Academic Press, 1976, pp 129–132.
9. Bellina JH: Gynecology and the laser. Contemp Ob/Gyn *4*:24–34, 1974.
10. Hahn GA: The carbon dioxide laser in gynecology. Phila Med *74*:344–347, 1978.
11. Yahr WZ, Strully KJ: Blood vessel anastomosis by laser and other biomedical applications. J Assoc Adv Med Instr *1*:1–4, 1966.
12. Hall RR: The healing of tissue incised by a carbon dioxide laser. Br J Surg *58*:222–225, 1971.
13. Hishimoto K, Rockwell RJ, Epstein RA, Fidler JP: Laser wound healing compared with other surgical modalities. Burns *1*:13–21, 1974.
14. MacLean AB, Sharp F, More IAR, Murray EL: Histochemistry of laser destruction of human cervical tissue in Kaplan I, Ascher PW (eds): in Proceedings of the III International Congress on Laser Surgery, Graz, 1979.
15. Helwig EB, Jones WA, Hayes JR, Zeitler EH: Anatomic and histochemical changes in skin after laser irradiation. Fed Proc (Suppl 14) *24*:83–91, 1965.
16. MacLean A, Sharp F, More IAR, Murray EL: Cervical tissue interaction: transmission electron microscopy and histochemical aspects, in Bellina JH, et al (eds): Gynecologic Laser Surgery. Proceedings of an International Congress on Gynecologic Laser Surgery and Related Works. New York, Plenum Press, 1980, pp 151–164.
17. Ben Bassat M, Kaplan I: An ultrastructural study of the cut edges of skin and mucous membrane specimens excised by carbon dioxide laser, in Kaplan I (ed): Laser Surgery. Jerusalem, Academic Press, 1976, pp 95–100.
18. More IAR, MacLean AB, Sharp F, Murray EL: Transmission electron microscopy of laser destruction of human cervical tissue, in Kaplan I, Ascher PW (eds): Proceedings of the III International Congress on Laser Surgery, Graz, Tel Aviv, Israel, OT-PAZ, 1979, p 254.
19. Stohivijk JAS, Hardy JD: Skin and subcutaneous temperature changes during exposure to intense thermal radiation. J Appl Physiol *20*:1006–1013, 1965.
20. Bodecker V, Bechholz J, Drake KH, Groteluschen B: Influence of thermal effects on the width of neurotic zones during cutting and coagulating with laser beams, in Kaplan J (ed): Laser Surgery I. Proceedings of First International Symposium on Laser Surgery Israel, November 5–6, 1975. Jerusalem, Academic Press, 1976, pp 101–108.
21. Hoye RC, Ketcham AS, Riggle GC: The air-bounce dissemination of viable tumors by high energy neodymium laser. Life Sci *6*:119–125, 1967.

22. Oosterhuis JW (ed): Tumor surgery with the CO_2 laser, in Studies with the Cloudman S91 Mouse Melanoma. Veenstra-Visser, Grooninger 1969, pp 30–38.
23. Oosterhuis JW, Verschveren RCJ, Eibergen R, Oldhoff J: The viability of cells in the waste products of CO_2 laser evaporation of Cloudman mouse melanomas. Cancer *49*:61–67, 1982.
24. Stjernholm RL: Metabolism of glucose, acetate and propionate by human plasma cells. J Bacteriol *93*:1657–1661, 1967.
25. Cook TA, Cohn AM, Brunschwig JP, et al: Wart viruses and laryngeal papillomas. Lancet *1*:782, 1973.
26. Bellina JH, Sternholm RL, Kurpel JE: Analysis of plume emissions after papovavirus irradiation with the carbon dioxide laser. J Reprod Med *27*:268–270, 1982.
27. Goldman L: Laser surgical research. Ann NY Acad Sci *168*:649–663, 1970.
28. Goldman L: The laser in the current cancer program, in Goldman L (ed): Third Conference on the Laser. Ann NY Acad Sci *267*:324–328, 1976.
29. Goldman L, Rockwell RJ, Jr: Laser reactions in living tissue, in Goldman L, Rockwell RJ Jr (eds): Lasers in Medicine. New York, Gordon and Breach 1971, p 201.
30. Boggan JE, Edwards MSB, Davis RL: Comparative neural tissue toxicity of argon and carbon dioxide surgical lasers, in Atsumi K, Nimsaku N (eds): Laser—Tokyo '81. Proceedings of the 4th Congress of the International Society for Laser Surgery, Tokyo, Japan, Inter Group Corp, 1981, p 11.
31. Kanna JS, Hutschenreiter G, Haina D, Waidelich W: Effect of laser power density laser radiation on healing of open skin wound in rats. Arch Surg *116*:293–296, 1981.

4

Applications in Gynecology with Emphasis on the Cervix

4.1. Introduction to Laser Surgery

The bioeffects of the CO_2 surgical laser have been described; it is now necessary to examine the advantages of this new surgical tool which have allowed the development of its practical applications in surgery, and how its biophysical properties may be used advantageously (Table 4.1). The surgeon can easily learn this new technique with training and practice. When one uses a knife, the depth of incision is controlled by the pressure applied to the scalpel. In contrast, using a laser instrument is a unique experience: the tissue is not touched and the desired effects are obtained by varying the biophysical parameters (Table 4.2) in freehand surgery as well as microscopic surgery. Precise power and beam spot size settings, appropriate speed of incision, and control of secondary burn effects from the heat energy of the beam by cooling methods are necessary for optimizing laser techniques. In spite of the disadvantage cited in Table 4.3, the precision of the laser instrument allows more conservative surgery and the characteristic of the hemostatic incision, with its self-sterilizing operative field, must be considered of essential importance in modern general surgery and especially useful for gynecologic applications (Table 4.4). The broad spectrum of continuous power output setting and exposure time allows the surgeon high flexibility of application. Laser surgery usually requires a combination of coagulation, excision, and vaporization techniques.

111

Table 4.1.   Advantages in Surgery with CO_2 Laser Application

Reduced operative time
Reduced hospital stay
Minimal operative and postoperative complications
Reduced postoperative pain
Minimal adjacent tissue damage
Lymphatic and small blood vessels are sealed
Microscope-integrated system allows for precision microcutting
  of tissues or exact vaporization of tumors

Table 4.2.   Basic Concepts for CO_2 Laser Surgical Application

Stationary beam (cw)	Moving beam (cw)
Volume of tissue to be ablated is function of the energy and the exposure time	Depth of ablation is proportional to power density and beam spot diameter
Depth of ablation is power-density- and time-dependent	Depth of ablation is inversely proportional to lasing speed
At constant power density, depth is time-dependent	At constant lasing speed, depth is proportional to power output
	At constant power output, depth is inversely proportional to lasing speed

Table 4.3.   Disadvantage of Laser Surgical Application

Loss of proprioception sense (absence of physical contact)

Table 4.4.   Specific Indications for CO_2 Laser Application in Gynecology

Intraabdominal
  Pelvic neoplasia
  Fallopian tube obstruction
Cervical
  Viral disease
  Cervical intraepithelial neoplasia
Vaginal
  Viral disease
  Vaginal intraepithelial neoplasia
Vulvar
  Viral disease
  Vulvar intraepithelial neoplasia
  Dystrophia
Perineum
Anus
Breast

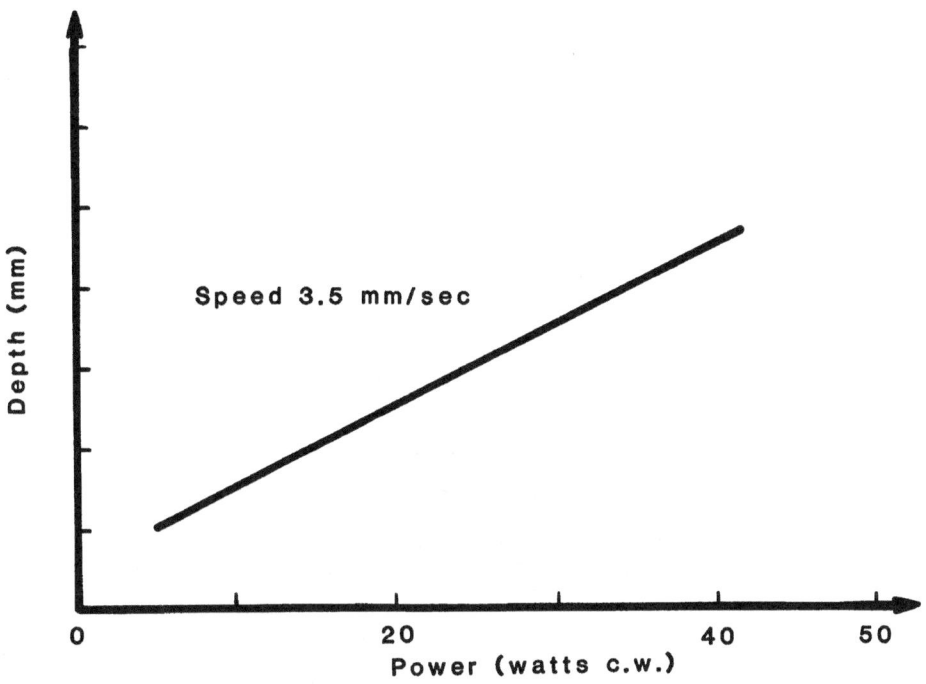

Figure 4.1. At constant lasing speed, the depth of penetration is proportional to the power.

The technology of laser surgery provides the surgeon with an impressive, versatile tool which permits the removal of small areas of neoplastic tissue, even in the most inaccessible anatomic regions, or the complete destruction of large neoplastic masses (i.e., tumor debulking) and separation of tissues with precise margins. The CO_2 laser energy necessary for tissue mass destruction appears to be directly related to the volume of the mass.[1] The power density determines how much tissue will be destroyed or how deep the incision will be (Fig. 4.1). The speed of movement of the laser determines the amount of energy which is transmitted to the tissue. The longer the beam is focused on one spot, the greater the amount of energy that will be delivered to the tissue. The more vaporization of the tissue that occurs, the deeper will be the destruction of that tissue (Fig. 4.2). Excisional laser surgery is reported with increasing frequency. Some laser procedures report results superior to conventional scalpel surgical procedures. High power density is required for excisional laser application (i.e., 1400–3000 W/cm^2). Spot diameter, which can be reduced to a fraction of a millimeter, is used for rapid cutting, with minimal thermal tissue damage, and consequently reduced healing time. Particular advantages have been reported[2] for the excisional

113

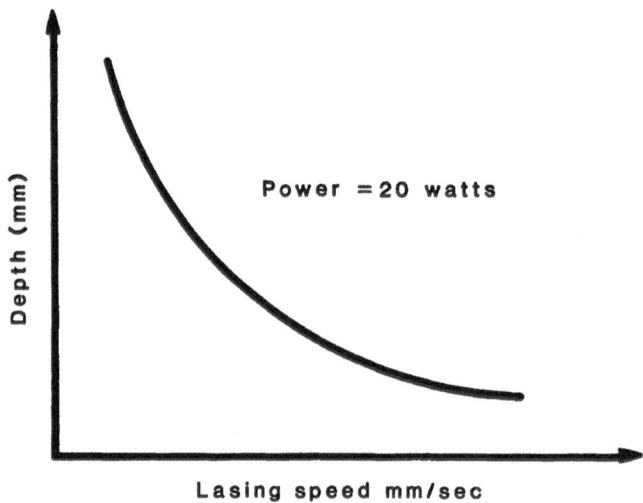

Figure 4.2. At constant power, the depth of penetration is inversely proportional to the square of the lasing speed.

application of postirradiated thoracic and vulvar tissue. Chronically inflamed, infected, or rigid tissues are generally difficult to cut through. In these cases the CO_2 laser provided satisfying technical results. No delay was reported in the healing process even when grafts for reconstructive surgery were performed after laser excision.

The coagulative property of the defocused laser beam with a larger spot size and reduced power density seals the lymphatic channels as well as the small vessels (<2 mm diameter), thereby obstructing the path for metastatic tumor cell migration and preventing lymphorrea and bleeding.[3] Thus, it allows the surgeon to remove vascular tumors and highly vascularized tissues, and to cut or resect parenchymal organs by varying the power settings and focal distances, and by using both focused and defocused beams. Moreover, the absence or near-absence of bleeding during surgery creates a bloodless field that enables the surgeon to pinpoint abnormalities clearly, which benefits the patient and avoids blood transfusions.[4] Under these conditions, it is possible to operate on high-risk patients with hemophilia or hemopathies or on those who are on anticoagulant therapy. Other categories of high-risk patients that are suitable for laser surgery include cardiac patients with pacemakers, because they do not run the risk correlated with electrical discharge interferences, nor do electrical disturbances occur during cardiographic and encephalographic monitoring.

Another of the advantages of laser surgery is in treating infected tissue. Since laser surgery and the "no-touch procedure" are self-sterilizing, bacteria are destroyed by the high temperature of the beam directed over the tissue, making this method the ideal technique for treating infected lesions.[5-7] Since CO_2 laser heat destroys conventional fiberoptics, no endoscopic application is available to date for CO_2 laser surgery. Argon and Nd-YAG lasers, however, can be used for this purpose.[8-10] American[11] and Japanese[12] researchers are currently working to develop new fiberoptic laser models. In fact, laser technology improves continuously, and as new delivery systems become available, lasers will be applied more effectively and efficiently.

4.2. Clinical Applications in Gynecology

In recent years, economic pressures have given rise to a change in social behavior that is playing a definite role in the natural history of the reproductive female. Today, with the ever-increasing pressure to sell by sex, our young women are being subjected to subtle and overt demands to "become a total woman." This change, coupled with the preferred use of the birth control pill over the condom as a contraceptive, has led to higher incidences of venereal disease. The protective sheath that once inhibited or prevented physical transmission of disease is no longer at work, and this has aided in the dramatic increase in benign and premalignant cervical, vaginal, and vulvar disease. The changes encompass viral and oncologic pathologic processes. The process is now being observed in our young women of 13–14 years of age. The problem of management becomes immense when dealing with a premalignant cervical pathology in a prereproductive female.[13] The conventional approach of conization can lead to sterilization, cervical stenosis, and obstetrical complications. New and better modalities are needed to preserve female reproductive ability better. The problem of the costs must be weighed against the real advantages in terms of early and late complications and recurrence rates of disease. The social commitments of the new biomedical technology are approached by diminishing the drawbacks related with old procedures. Laser technology has demonstrated the capabilities of replacing the old systems.

4.3. General Considerations of Applications in Cervical Intraepithelial Neoplasia

When the laser was first adapted to surgical procedures, one of the first medical specialties to embrace the technique was gynecology. At the onset physicians primarily used the CO_2 laser for treating cervical intraepithelial neoplasms with favorable, documented results. Even though the principal application of CO_2 laser gynecologic surgery appears to be in premalignant and neoplastic diseases, other common benign gynecologic diseases can be successfully treated. From a technical point of view, two main types of possible operative procedures can be distinguished, which will be discussed in detail: (1) the vaporization mode, with or without microscopic aid (i.e., free hand) and (2) the excisional mode, with or without microscopic aid (i.e., free hand). These modes have different indications with regard to the disease entities one is going to treat. Moreover, both modes can be used for the treatment of superficial, intravaginal, or intraabdominal lesions.

Microscopic procedures are available for all applications with the laser and it allows the ablation of tissue to a precise depth, even in areas which are inaccessible by conventional surgical procedures. Furthermore, in most cases, it is not necessary for the patient to be hospitalized nor are the untoward effects of general anesthetics a risk.

End-stage laser therapy should be attempted only by a skilled surgeon; in untrained hands, as with any surgical tool, the CO_2 laser is potentially hazardous to the patient, surgeon, and ancillary personnel. Therefore, when it has been established that laser surgery is the appropriate mode of treatment, the following prerequisites must be fulfilled before using the technique:

1. The physician must be knowledgeable in gynecologic pathology and must be experienced in colposcopic examinations; accurate geometric evaluation of the lesion and the approach to treatment with the laser are dependent upon such background skills.
2. Precise and detailed technical knowledge of the powerful energy source is equally important.
3. The physician must understand the biophysical principles of laser–tissue interaction.
4. The physician must be well trained in the applications of basic laser microsurgical techniques.
5. The physician must have a thorough understanding of the instrument and the hazards that can be associated with laser surgery.
6. Guidelines for preparation of laser patient and appropriate preoperative therapy have been developed and should be followed rigidly.
7. The postoperative follow-up examination schedule is a critical part of the treatment for the patient and the physician as well.

4.4. Cervical Applications

Since cervical disease is considered the most frequent lesion of the female genital tract, especially in young women, preliminary epidemiologic and pathologic tests are necessary before treating the condition.

4.4.1. Epidemiology

Recent reports[13,14] have shown that the overall mortality rate for carcinoma of the cervix has significantly decreased in the screening areas during the past three decades, whereas the incidence rate of women recognized as having the precursors of the disease has increased considerably.[15] The precancerous, noninvasive lesions occur approximately nine times more commonly than cancer of the cervix. The data and rescreening studies (Fig. 4.3) of Christopherson[16] also suggest a higher incidence of the early disease. However, the modern association of the cytologic and colposcopic diagnostic methods allows earlier diagnosis,[17] and effective therapy can be consequently applied before a life-threatening form of the disease develops (Table 4.5). Furthermore, the age-related incidence rate peak of curves of premalignant and in situ lesions of the cervix has demonstrated a decrease in the age at which it appears (Fig. 4.4).[18-20]

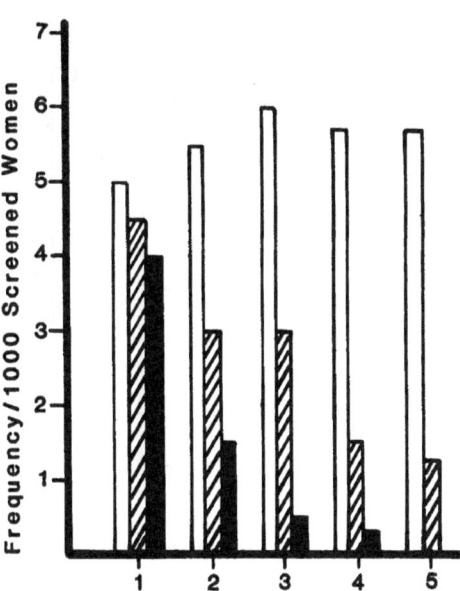

Figure 4.3. Frequency of disease per 1000 women; □, dysplasia; ▨, carcinoma in situ; ■, squamocarcinoma invasive.

**Table 4.5.   Ideal Management of CIN,
VIN, VAIN**

Accurate diagnosis
Easy execution of therapy
Low morbidity
Low cost
Preservation of sex and fertility functions
Successful long-term results

Besides the previously mentioned epidemiologic studies, the results of basic biochemical research support the thesis that cervical cancer can be considered a sexually transmitted disease. Sperm cells[21-23] and viral particles[24-27] are considered among the most common etiologic factors. Thus, the earlier the age of first sexual intercourse, the earlier the appearance of cervical dysplastic disorders.[19,23,28-30]

4.4.2. Pathology

The ecto- and endocervical mucosa can be considered a steady-state system, with changes in the position of the junction relating to physiological and pathologic conditions (Fig. 4.5).

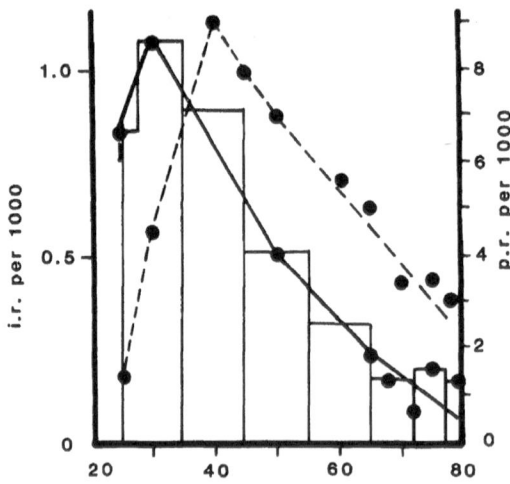

Figure 4.4. Prevalence (●————●) and incidence (●— — —●) rate of disease per 1000 women.

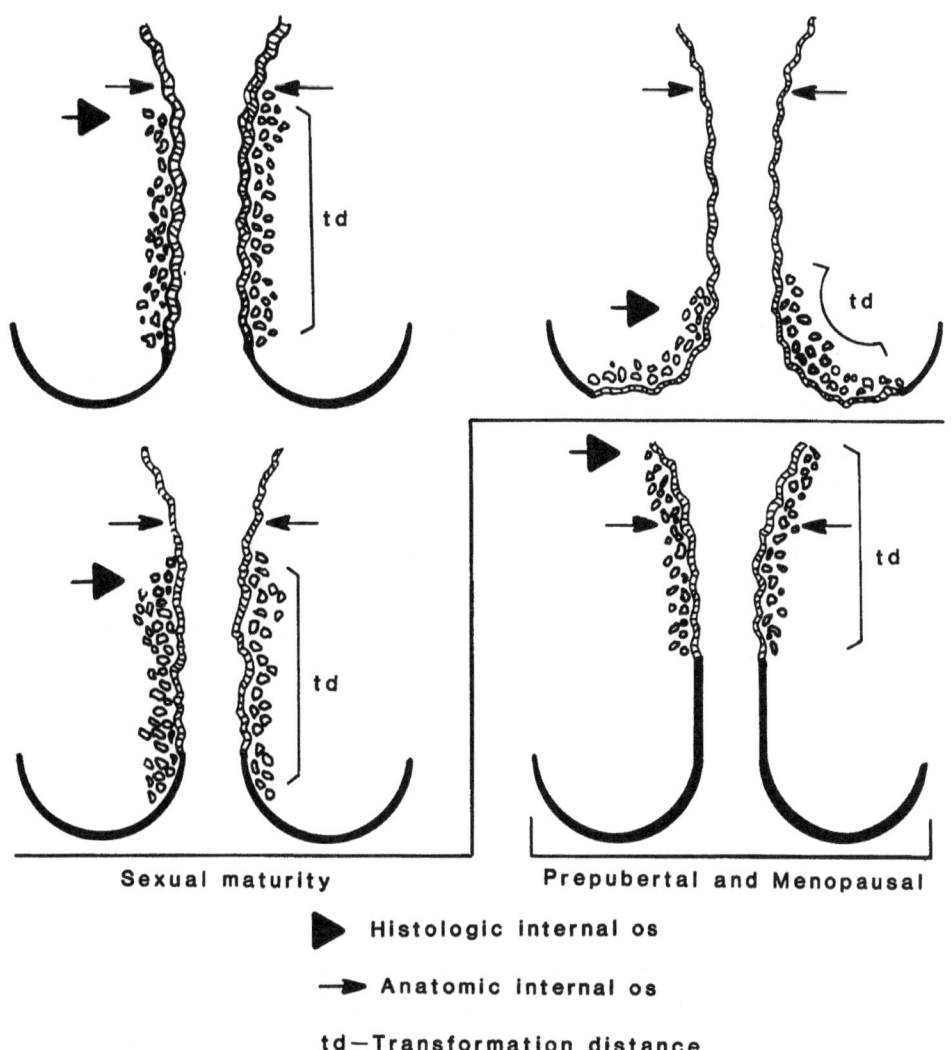

Sexual maturity   Prepubertal and Menopausal

▶ Histologic internal os

➤ Anatomic internal os

td—Transformation distance

Figure 4.5. Anatomical distribution of endocervical glandular tissue with respect to age.

It is considered a regular anatomic condition, even if not usually found, for the squamous epithelium to meet the columnar epithelium at its last gland, at exactly the external uterine orifice.

Ectropion or ectopia occurs when the frontier of the two epithelia has shifted downward on the ectocervix, while the length of endocervical mucosa from the isthmus to the last gland remains constant.[31]

Entropion, frequent in advanced postmenopausal women, occurs when squamous cell epithelium moves upward into the cervical canal.[32]

The distribution of endocervical glands follows the shift of columnar epithelium. Furthermore, the squamous cell epithelium can partially cover the endocervical mucosa and glands, not only in its ectopic portion, but also in the cervical canal. Metaplasia originates from the reserve basal cells which are located in the stroma under the endocervical columnar cells.[33,34] These reserve basal cells can proliferate under chemicophysical stimulation. The dysplastic process can occur during both the dynamic transition and the proliferation of the metaplastic (i.e., squamous) cells,[35] and it usually occurs at the squamocolumnar junction and border and in the squamous exocervical epithelium.[36] In the so-called glands and in the area below the isthmic part of endocervical mucosa, the dysplastic processes may develop more slowly[37,38] and the dysplasia does not overcome the early phase in a multifocal fashion, as demonstrated by electron microscopic studies.[39-41]

The alterations of the differentiation of the cervical epithelium, as a continuous pathologic process[42-45] are precursors of in situ and invasive[46,47] carcinoma, irrespective of the speed of evolution.[48,49] The spectrum of the pathologic process progresses from mild to moderate to severe dysplasia and then to carcinoma in situ and invasive cancer. The term **cervical intraepithelial neoplasia** (CIN) has been used to describe any degree in the entire spectrum (Fig. 4.6).[44,51] Spontaneous regression of dysplastic disorders can occur.[49,50] Topographically, cervical intraepithelial neoplasia can occur in the squamo-

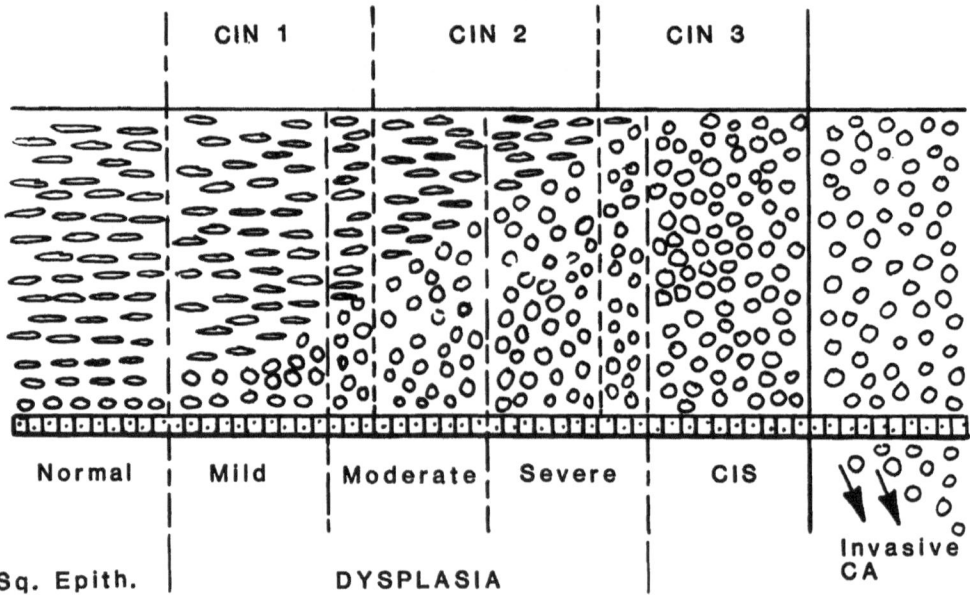

Figure 4.6. Cervical intraepithelial neoplasia (CIN) includes all degrees of dysplasia and carcinoma in situ.

120

columnar and ectocervical portions or in the endocervical canal, and tends to involve the entire thickness of the epithelium.[52] Multicentric development has also been recognized. The endocervical extension of the dysplastic disorders has been frequently demonstrated to be directly related to age.[53]

Cervical intraepithelial neoplasia, which involves the endocervical extension, can easily be detected by cytologic examination. A colposcope-directed biopsy is mandatory for accurate histopathologic diagnosis. This will determine the degree of cellular changes in order to establish a correlation with cytology and to classify the lesion as being mild, moderate, or severe dysplasia or **carcinoma in situ** (CIS).[54] The colposcopic examination can localize the lesion as a "transformation zone," but cannot determine the extension beyond the external uterine orifice.[55] The normal mucosal depth in the fertile age is 1.2–3.5 mm, and ranges from 3 to 6 mm during pregnancy at the third quarter.[56,57] In addition, the possibility of glandular involvement in dysplastic lesions to a depth of more than 5 mm has been reported,[52,61,62] and cellular changes can be present in the basal layer. Almost 70% of the cases of cervical dysplasia had glandular involvement, while glandular involvement was noted in 87% of the cases of carcinoma in situ[52,59]; therefore, the depth of destruction must be the same in every case. Furthermore, since the extension of CIN can be considered a large field of disease beyond the microscopic lesion, a 5-mm margin of tissue should be destroyed adjacent to the transformation zone.[52,58–60] These observations are important when considering conservative management of cervical malignant disease. Anderson[61] (and Przybora[52]) studied the histologic penetration of CIN in extirpated specimens. Three hundred forty-three conization specimens, with 15 sections per cone, were examined for a total of 5250 sections. A linear-graduate measurement was used to determine the depth of the deepest crypt. The measurements were taken perpendicular to the target line on the surface epithelium. The mean depth of glandular involvement was 1.24 mm, and the mean depth of uninvolved crypts was 3.38. Thus, a theoretical destruction to 2.92 mm (± 1.96 S.D.) would approach 95% eradication.

Although 99.7% of the cases do not have crypt involvement greater than 3.8 mm beneath the surface of the cervix,[61] the exact gland extension and the exact depth cannot be determined with certainty. Therefore, somewhat deeper destruction or removal, involving the layer below the lamina propria, is necessary in order to insure destruction of any potential gland extension. This work defined the theoretical depth limits of cervical intraepithelial dysplasia.

Anderson's work, coupled with the studies on surface extension, led to the hypothesis that if one eradicates an area 5 mm beyond the surface borders and to a depth of 5–7 mm, to correct for the 3.8 mm (± 3 S.D.), then

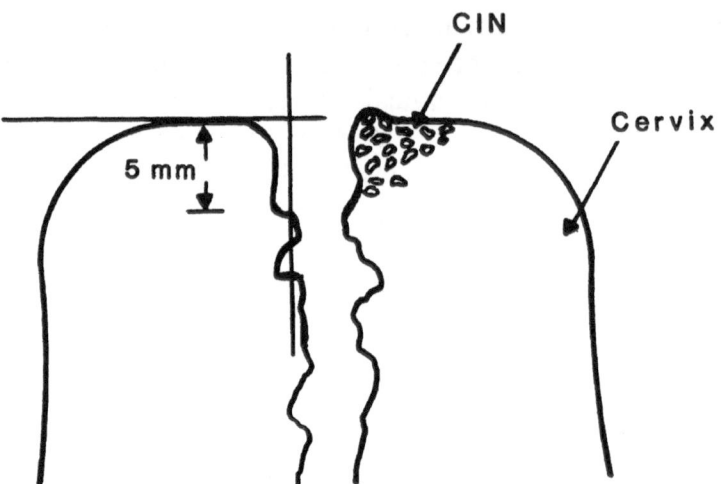

Figure 4.7. Depth of destruction must be 5–7 mm below a line tangent to the cervical epithelium; CIN, cervical intraepithelial neoplasia.

one could expect to approach a 99% "cure rate" (Fig. 4.7). Failure to do so will leave residual lesions.[63] The key words to the arguments are *beyond the boundary* and *below the lesion*. This requires that the surgeon be totally competent in colposcopy, that he have taken a colposcope-directed biopsy, and that the histology be in agreement with the cytology and the colposcopic appearance.

These assumptions may seem trite, but they are the hallmark of success or failure with any treatment mode. If you treat (1) without knowing the extent of the lesion in three dimensions, (2) without knowing the histology, and/or (3) using a system that does not remove or eradicate the *total* lesions, then by definition you have failed. This failure may not always be evident in CIN, as the natural history of this disease may give the appearance of a false success, since dysplastic lesions are known to involute spontaneously. This, along with the difficulty in grading the dysplasia, gives rise to error in accurate diagnosis. If a slide was read as CIN III and in fact was a CIN I, the probability of failure or invasion is slight. Conversely the CIN I, misdiagnosed and undertreated, could lead to an invasive carcinoma. CIN lesions, given the appropriate environment and time, can lead to invasive carcinoma. The statistical probability of a CIN I progressing to invasive carcinoma is slight, but real, whereas the statistical probability of a CIN III lesion progressing is much greater (Fig. 4.8). From the time-dependent and disease-dependent graph you can appreciate this phenomenon. The probability of CIN I, over five years, becoming invasive is less than that for a CIN II over three years, but it still exists. Likewise the CIN III has a much greater probability of progressing to an invasive lesion.

This is a probability phenomenon; thus, we must strive for "cures" and reduce the probabilities. Therefore, we need a system which can treat CIN I, II, and III on an outpatient basis effectively, relatively painlessly, and with reduced short-term and long-term complications, and which is acceptable to the patient.

The above argument is quite important when one considers the variability in histologic diagnosis made from the same slide by various observers. Recently we concluded a two-year study[64] in which highly respected gynecologic pathologists were asked to review a set of cervical biopsy specimens. The conditions imposed reflected the "real-life" situation faced by each practicing gynecologist: a patient has an abnormal cytology; colposcope her cervix and obtain a biopsy specimen from the appropriate site; then evaluate the slide and render a verdict. The question is *Is it a just verdict?* To answer, we submitted the same slide to the same pathologist twice (at a >6-month inter-

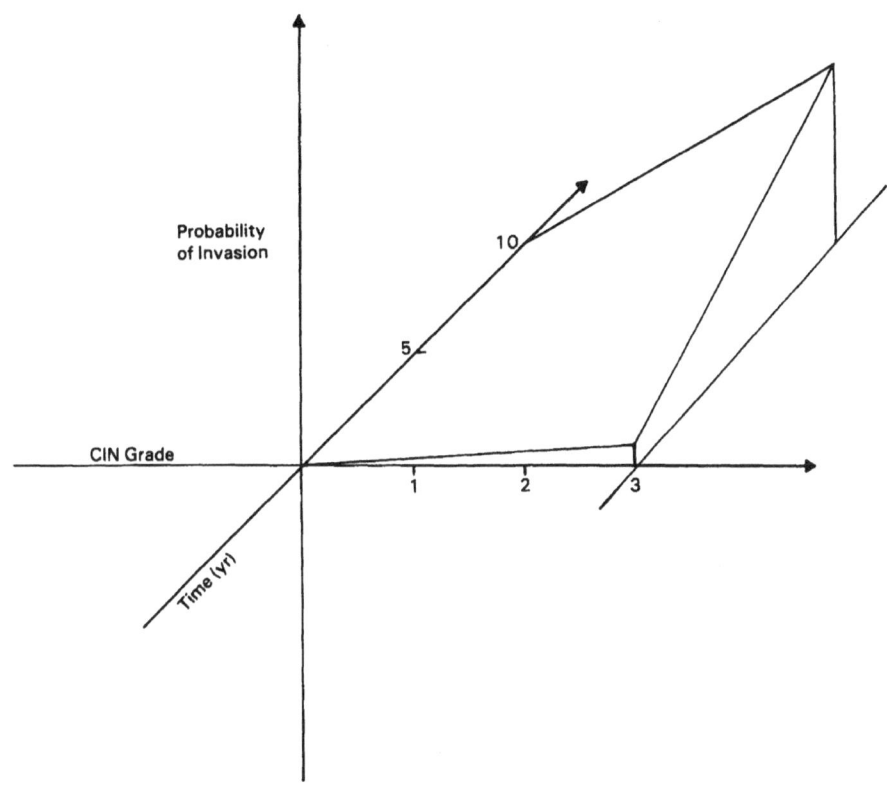

Figure 4.8. Time vs severity in probability of invasive carcinoma.

Table 4.6. Interobserver Agreement of Diagnoses at First Reading

Observer combinations	Identical classification		Classifications within 1 grade		Classifications more than 2 grades different		Correlation of diagnoses (r)
	No.	%	No.	%	No.	%	
A-B	13	50	19	73	7	27	0.51
A-C	10	38	22	84	4	16	0.75
A-D	13	50	22	84	4	16	0.46
B-C	19	73	24	92	2	8	0.65
B-D	13	50	20	76	6	24	0.55
C-D	10	38	20	76	6	24	0.34
Overall	78	50	127	81	29	19	

Table 4.7. Consistency of Diagnoses between Observations for Each Pathologist

Pathologist	Identical diagnoses		Within 1 grade		2–3 grades disparate		Correlation of first and second diagnoses (r)
	No.	%	No.	%	No.	%	
A	20	77	23	88	3	12	0.71
B	18	69	25	96	1	4	0.72
C	19	73	24	92	2	8	0.81
D	17	65	25	96	1	4	0.70
Overall	74	71	97	93	7	6.7	

Table 4.8. Colposcopic Terminology[a]

Normal colposcopic findings
    Original squamous epithelium
    Columnar epithelium
    Transformation zone
Abnormal colposcopic findings
    Atypical transformation zone
        White epithelium
        Punctuation
        Mosaic
        Keratosis (leukoplakia)
        Abnormal blood vessels
    Suspect cervical carcinoma
Unsatisfactory colposcopic findings
Other colposcopic findings
    Vaginocervicitis
    True erosion
    Atrophic epithelium
    Condyloma, papilloma

[a]The nomenclature for colposcopy was approved by the Committee on Terminology of the Second World Congress of Cervical Pathology and Colposcopy, October 1975, Graz, Austria.

val) and then to three additional gynecologic pathologists in the same fashion. Table 4.6 shows the interobserver agreement in diagnosis at first reading and Table 4.7 shows the consistency of diagnosis between 'observations for each pathologist.

Immediately, there is an awareness of the variety of diagnoses and the severity of discrepancies between diagnoses by the same and different observers. Thus, the gynecologists, until the pathologists can produce more reliable data, must treat for maximum cure while attempting to preserve reproductive function with the least amount of treatment complications. This is where the CO_2 laser appears to have a significant place in the management of CIN.

4.4.3. Preoperative Analyses

Diagnosis of the disease must be accompanied by knowledge of the topography of the lesion and, since a high incidence of endocervical extension involvement and misdiagnosis has been reported,[52,65,66] the following criteria must be met before treatment is undertaken:

1. Cytologic examination is the preliminary test and is necessary to determine the degree of cellular changes. The Papanicolaou cytologic test can detect abnormal cervical, vaginal, and, occasionally, endometrial disorders.
2. A colposcopic biopsy specimen will determine the ectocervical topography of the lesion(s). Since colposcopic terminology must be clearly defined to avoid ambiguity, for the purposes of this text, the authors have chosen to use the terminology of the American Society of Colposcopy and Cervical Pathology (Table 4.8).
3. Histologic studies of the biopsy specimen and of the endocervical curettage are considered a fundamental part of the evaluation process. In this way, invasive lesions can be diagnosed with 92.5% accuracy.[69,70]

For the sake of clarity, the following terms shall be considered synonymous:

> CIN I: Mild dysplasia
> CIN II: Moderate dysplasia
> CIN III: Severe dysplasia and carcinoma in situ

Furthermore, we shall define **disease** as any abnormal cytologic or histologic pathology exclusive of atypical, secondary to bacterial infection. Finally, CIN cannot be classified as "cured" unless the results of cytologic, colpos-

125

copic, and histologic examinations, when indicated, remain normal for more than 25 months. Rigid classifications ensure that statistical calculations are meaningful and not merely numbers which reflect manipulation of the variables.

Today, invasive carcinoma cannot be treated by CO_2 laser methods; a less conservative treatment is necessary. "Warty dysplasia" is considered to be frequently associated with a cervical dysplasia,[27] thus, in this case, it should be treated similarly. This term is indicative of the viral changes seen in conjunction with a papovavirus infection, suggestive of condylomatous changes.

Moreover, an endocervical curettage should be performed routinely following the colposcopic assessment, even if the upper limits of the lesion are seen, in order to determine the endocervical extension. In fact, although treatment of CIN with limited endocervical canal extension has been reported using a contact hysteroscope,[67] there is not sufficient evidence to date to consider that this extensive mode of treatment be given primary consideration.

All preoperative parameters must be in complete agreement: *Cytology + Colposcopy + Histology.*

If we do not have a *correct* preoperative diagnosis, we *must not* and *cannot* proceed with therapy. The failure of physicians to follow the above "law" is the reason for articles recently reported in our literature regarding invasive carcinoma following conservative management.[66,68]

To omit any of the steps—cytology, colposcopy, or biopsy—could constitute malpractice. Abnormal or atypical Pap smears treated, without colposcopy or biopsy, by cryosurgery have been demonstrated to lead to ineffective results and failures.[71] In fact, the College of Obstetrics and Gynecology Committee on Gynecological Practice has issued the following statement on the use of cryotherapy to treat CIN III:

> The Committee on Gynecological Practice believes that patients with potential CIN should be fully evaluated with endocervical curettage and cervical biopsies prior to any treatment. Until additional information is available, the Committee has serious concerns regarding the use of cryotherapy in the presence of CIN III. [September 8, 1978 (*ACOG Newsletter,* November 1978)]

In conclusion, when conservative management is desirable, or when surgery is contraindicated and when the diagnosis has been made based on a correlation among cytologic, histologic, and colposcopic tests, and when the patient is considered to be reliable with regard to regular follow-up visits, laser surgery can be performed confidentially.

Table 4.9. Patient Selection for Cervical Procedures

Age	Conditions	Suggested treatment
Reproductive age (< 40yr)	Desires children; ectocervical lesion	CO_2 vaporization (conservative)
	Desires children; lesion extended into cervix	Conization (CO_2 laser or cold knife)
	Does not desire children; ectocervical lesion	Individualized (conservative to hysterectomy)
Perimenopausal age (> 45yr)	Does not desire children; ectocervical and/or endocervical lesion	Individualized (conservative to hysterectomy)

Preoperative evaluation: identify all lesions with colposcope:

1. Cervix
2. Vagina
3. Urethra
4. Vulva
5. Rectum

Obtain histologic confirmation.

4.4.4. Patient Selection

If the patient is of childbearing age, treatment with the CO_2 laser should be considered. As illustrated in Table 4.9, if the lesion is only in the ectocervix, then the vaporization procedure can be used. If the lesion extends into the endocervix but its boundaries are completely visible, then a conization is performed. For women who do not desire children or who are over 45 years of age, the treatment regimen needs to be individualized. If the lesion is amenable to conservative treatment with the CO_2 laser, the patient must be willing to comply with the follow-up schedule.

4.5. Technical Approach to CIN Lesions

4.5.1. Microsurgical Procedures

The surgical CO_2 laser has the exclusive capabilities of being suitable for vaporization techniques, or it can be used as an effective method for excising cervical tissue to obtain a cone biopsy specimen of any size. The physician must possess exact knowledge of the cell population at risk, as well as of cervical anatomy and pathology, and he must especially have a complete understanding of the method of destruction with regard to the geometrical distribution of the lesion. It can be useful to calibrate the instrument for microsurgical procedures on cervical tissue by using surgical specimens, cutting in the fashion of a conization and scrutinizing for the depth of destruction. All laser treatment for cervical lesions can be carried out under direct colposcopic visualization and by micromanipulation of the laser beam.

The treatments can be performed on either an outpatient or an inpatient basis. Colposcopy units should be available where patients can be referred for such examinations. The proliferative phase of the menstrual cycle is considered to be the most suitable for both the diagnostic and the therapeutic procedures. Before a detailed description of the two microsurgical procedures and their specific indications is presented, it is useful to point out the exact meaning of the terminology used.

The term **laser conization** has been used for different procedures performed on the cervical tissue. Actually, if a completely visible area of CIN is deeply destroyed by vaporization, then, in a certain sense, a limited conization has been done. Furthermore, a more extended vaporization–conization can be performed by destroying a cone-shaped volume of tissue upward into the endocervical canal. Using this procedure, there is no specimen available for pathologic examination. Thus, a third type of conization can be performed with the CO_2 surgical laser by using the focused beam as a scalpel and obtaining a cone biopsy specimen when there are indications that a more detailed pathologic examination is required.

4.5.2. Instruments, Equipment, and Patient Preparation for Cervical Microsurgery

The basic set-up for laser surgery consists primarily of the laser and suction apparatus (Fig. 4.9). Instruments include gloves, Jako microlaryngeal biopsy forceps, cotton balls, a plastic or nonflammable speculum, acetic acid, Lugol's solution, and sponge forceps. Plastic is used because it reduces the hazards posed by the laser beam being reflected off metal surfaces. Acetic acid is used as it permits the physician to identify the diseased area precisely. The mildly acidic solution, with its mucolytic agent, removes cervical mucus and engorges the epithelial cells, increasing the density of the nuclei. Cotton balls are used to dry the surface of the cervix. All instruments and equipment should be set up prior to bringing the patient into the operating room. The patient is then brought in, placed on an operating room table, and encouraged

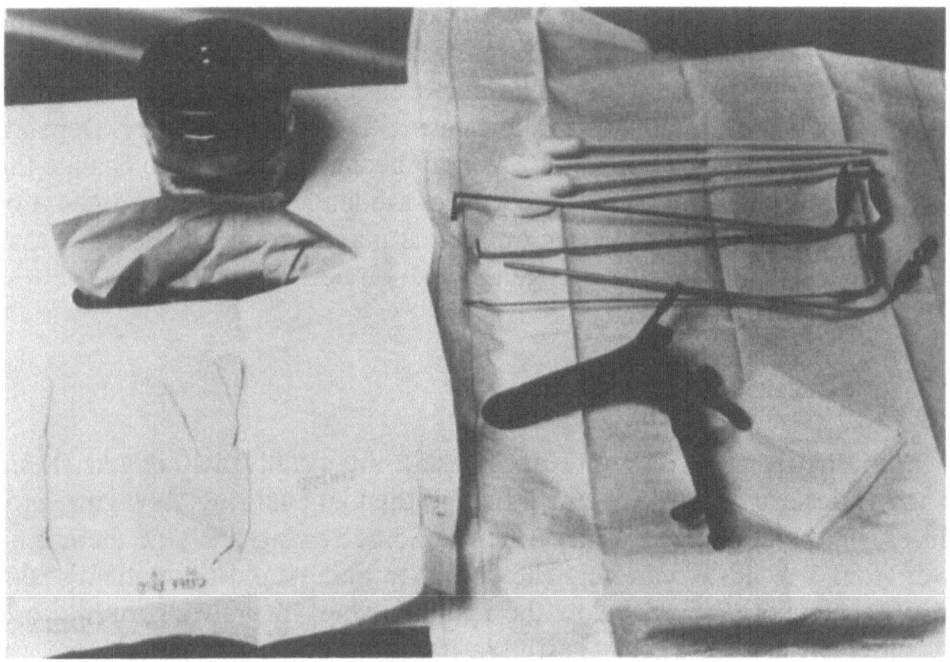

Figure 4.9. Basic tray for office laser surgery.

to relax. A full explanation of the procedure, along with active attention to the patient's concerns and a response to those concerns, will usually decrease the patient's anxiety about the impending surgery. The patient is placed in the dorsal lithotomy position. The cervix is exposed by inserting a bivalved speculum that has a nonreflective surface or is made of nonflammable plastic. A suction apparatus must be attached to evacuate the vapor plume generated by the laser–tissue interaction. The cervix is then cleaned with 3% acetic acid and the colposcope, with laser attached, is positioned for firing.

At this point, the physician will reevaluate the preoperative findings, redetermine the exact limits of the lesion, and take colpophotographs. It is preferable to record all preoperative colpophotographs in cases where a residual, recurrent, or new lesion has occurred. These permanent documents allow the surgeon to evaluate the technical approach. Should the original lesion be in the same location as the residual, then he can be sure that the lesion was not vaporized to the correct depth, while a lesion on the periphery would indicate that an appropriate margin of excision was not ablated. Both errors are correctable, but only with permanent records can the surgeon document a competent self-assessment program. Once the cervix has been cleaned, colposcoped, and photographed, the procedure can begin.

The physician, sitting at the foot of the examination table, visualizes the target area with the colposcope, and, based on his previous decision as to type of operation, begins the surgery. The nurse directs the suction cannula into the operating field to remove the vapors caused by the laser surgery. Depending upon the length of the procedure, it may become necessary to change the CO_2 cylinder in the laser. When procedures are long, an excessive amount of vapor is produced and the suction apparatus may become clogged. All that is necessary in this case is to change the suction bottle.

4.5.3. Anesthesia

Some patients may require anesthesia, but usually neither anesthesia nor analgesics are required for work behind the hymenal ring, in vaginal procedures, or for cervical laser treatments. Some testing shots at increasing power from 5 to 20 W can help the doctor to understand the patient's sensitivity for pain. However, below the hymenal ring, for vulvar, urethral orifice, and perineal operation, anesthesia is required because these areas are more sensitive. In such cases local, regional, or general anesthesia may be required. For the conization procedure, a paracervical block may be necessary. This can be determined by testing the patient's sensitivity with short bursts of laser energy prior to surgery.

4.6. Vaporization Procedure

Cervical vaporization is usually performed at 20–25 W of energy output, which corresponds to a power density of approximately 500–1200 W/ cm^2 when the beam spot diameter is 1.5–2 mm. Since the higher the power density, the faster the beam has to be moved in order to avoid uncontrolled tissue boundary destruction, the high-power-density mode should not be used until skillful control of the manipulation has been achieved.

Actually, lower power densities or pulsed emission modes increase the risk of recurrences[67,76] because of incomplete destruction of the basal layer of the cervical lesion in the same plane. The continuous operating mode is preferable in order to obtain a greater depth of destruction and to yield the most easily controlled and gentlest form of tissue removal. The rules of application are given in Table 4.10.

Laser vaporization is performed by initiating at a margin of safety of 5 mm from the visible borders of the lesion and the transformation zone.

Table 4.10. CO_2 Laser Cylinder Vaporization of CIN: Rules of Application

Physical	
Instruments	Laser CO_2, colposcope, micromanipulator, suction device, caliper
Power output	20–25 W
Power density	800–1400 W/cm^2
Spot size	1.5–2 mm diameter
Focal length	275–400 mm
Operating mode	Continuous
Clinical	
Conditions	No invasivity; identify complete boundaries of lesions, verify with histology, do not treat endocervical extensions
Depth of destruction	6–7 mm
Width of destruction	
Marginal	4–5 mm beyond the visible border of the lesion (transformation zone outlined with Schiller test)
Internal	Angle of reflection (create a cylinder vaporization not cone geometry)

The endocervical canal is then circumscribed using the continuous power mode (Fig. 4.10A). Next, the outer limits of the transformation zone are identified and circumscribed in a similar fashion (Fig. 4.10B).

When this topographic outline is completed, Lugol's solution is applied to the entire upper vagina and ectocervix. This staining will help to clarify any remaining lesions. If these are present, the additional pathology should be outlined. The beam can be directed by the micromanipulator concentrically or by quadrants (Fig. 4.10C) but it is necessary that the beam be swept across the area twice and that the lines be in a mutually perpendicular pattern so that, layer by layer, the desired critical depth can be uniformly treated.

The preferred path is a raster of *X-Y-Z* (Fig. 10D–F). This procedure is continued until the desired depth is achieved. This rapid movement has a twofold effect. The first is that the core temperature of the cervix remains normal (a rise in cervical core temperature results in uterine contractions and discomfort), and the second is that the rapid movement reduces the heat transfer to surrounding normal tissue (this aids in a rapid healing phase).

A word of caution: Acute cervical bacterial or parasitic infections should be pretreated appropriately; otherwise, bleeding and discomfort may be increased.

Once the inflammatory process subsides, management of the dysplasia can be continued. The major question is *How do I know that I am 7 mm below the surface epithelium?* Sharp[77] has developed a system of drill holes which appears to have merit. However, by inserting a small needle marked

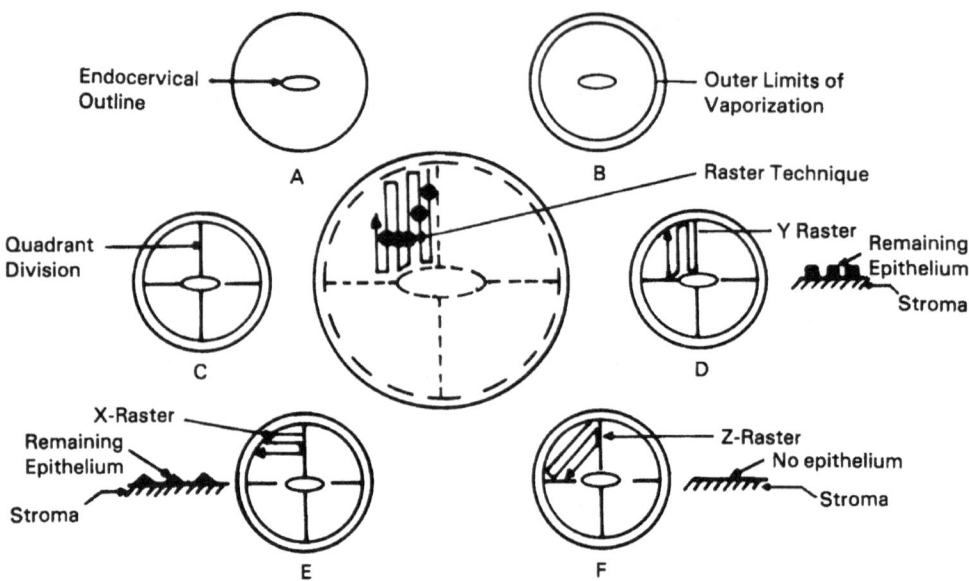

Figure 4.10. Vaporization conization. (A) Outline endocervical canal; (B) outline outer limits of transformation zone; (C) divide cervix into quadrants (center) and overlock beam diameter during raster X-Y-Z: (D) Y-raster; (E) X-raster; (F) Z-raster. (Reproduced with permission: Bellina JH: The carbon dioxide laser in gynecology, Part II, in Leventhal JM (ed): Current Problems in Obstetrics and Gynecology, Vol. 5, Chicago, Yearbook Medical Publishers, 1981, pp 1–35.)

at 7 mm into the cervix, or by using a proper caliper with a micrometer, it is possible to determine exactly the depth of laser tissue destruction (Fig. 4.11). Once the desired depth is achieved, the rule is put in place and the measurement is read through the colposcope. The adjacent quadrants are then managed in similar fashion. The cylindrical crater is recalibrated until the surgeon is satisfied (Fig. 4.12). Should bleeding occur during the procedure, the following technique can be used to control most, if not all, cases. Upon first encountering a vascular droplet, immediately turn the laser to 800 W/cm^2 and burn out the area of bleeding. In 90% of the cases this is effective. Although high power densities of the laser beam will coagulate small blood vessels, and there is less bleeding than with a scalpel, vessels less than 1–1.5 mm in diameter can be more easily sealed by circularly applying the defocused laser beam at a lower wattage. Occasionally one must use a cotton swab containing ferrosulfate (Monsel's solution). This astringent will control 99% of the remaining bleeding, but, should it fail, microfibrillar collagen may be employed. When all else fails, use a suture.

Based on clinicopathologic considerations and previous experience,[63,78] a

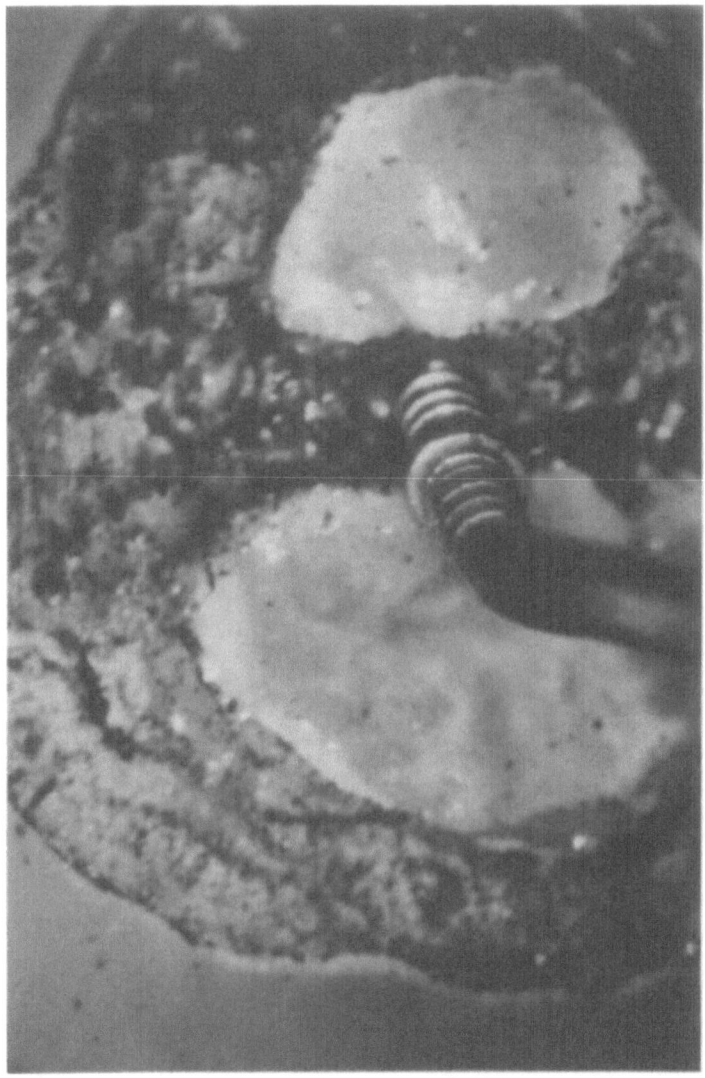

Figure 4.11. Cervical ruler to determine depth of destruction. (Reproduced with permission: Bellina JH: The carbon dioxide laser in gynecology, Part II, in Leventhal JM (ed): Current Problems in Obstetrics and Gynecology, Vol. 5, Chicago, Yearbook Medical Publishers, 1981, pp 1–35.)

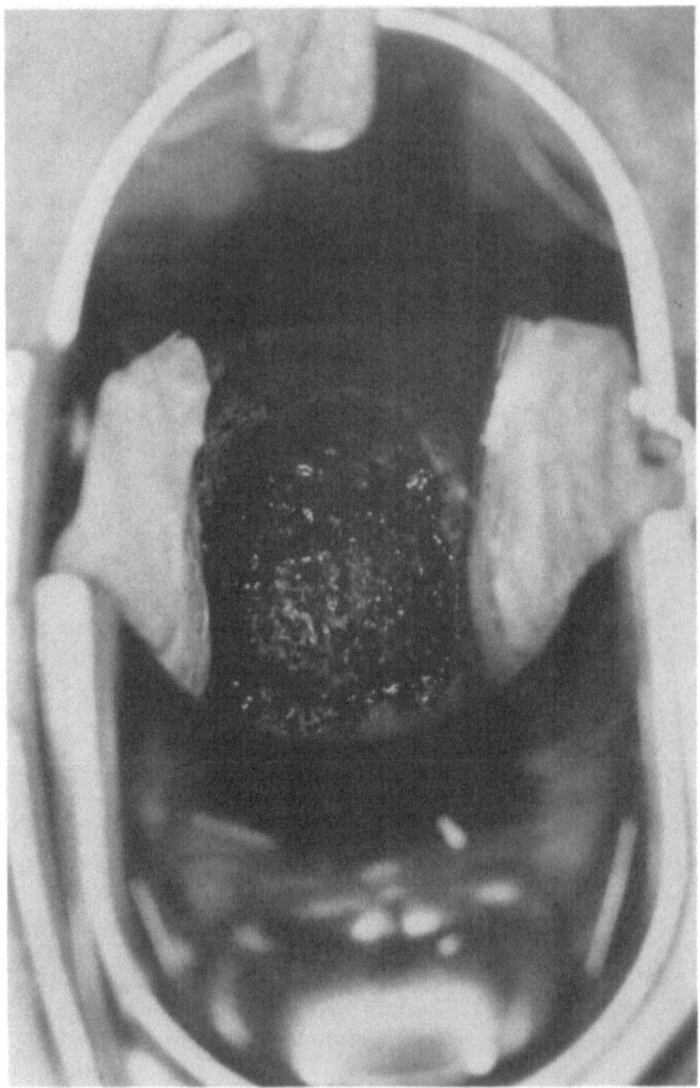

Figure 4.12. Completed vaporization procedure. (Reproduced with permission: Bellina JH: The carbon dioxide laser in gynecology, Part II, in Leventhal JM (ed): Current Problems in Obstetrics and Gynecology, Vol. 5, Chicago, Yearbook Medical Publishers, 1981, pp 1–35.)

depth of more than 4 mm and at least 6–7 mm is required in order to destroy the possible involvement of the cervical crypts. It must be emphasized that the microscopic or subjective elements for the evaluation for the depth of destruction can lead to inadequate treatment of the cervical lesions. In fact, the absence of mucus production does not correspond to total gland destruction, since in advanced lesions CIN involvement may totally replace the mucus-secreting columnar cells. Furthermore, the level of the lymphatic weeping, even though indicative of the subepithelial stroma penetration, does not insure that one has achieved complete crypt destruction. Finally, the progression of the destruction in depth may require a continuous adjustment of the colposcope focus; here it is suggested that the speculum be pushed against the vaginal fornices early in the surface phase focusing and thereafter that the speculum and the cervix progressively be brought together as well. In order to maintain the beam in focus at the desired level, the colposcope should not be moved. The whole procedure usually does not require more than 15–20 min. Once the diseased tissue has been removed, the procedure is concluded.

In order to differentiate a persistent lesion from a recurrent one, a terminal biopsy specimen from the base of the lasered area may be useful for histologic examination, especially at the border of the healthy tissue. Since the biopsy may be accompanied by bleeding, a properly quantitated depth of destruction can be considered as sufficient for completely eliminating crypt residual disease, and a proper width of destruction, including the metaplastic marginal areas, insures that there will be no proliferation at the borders.

4.7. Excisional Conization

Conization of the cervix is a surgical procedure that was described more than a century and a half ago.[79] Over the years, the indications and techniques for the procedure have varied. Although the operation was first employed as therapy for invasive cervical cancer, it rapidly became apparent that it was inadequate when used to treat an aggressive disease that had the capability for early lymphatic involvement. The emergence of modern concepts of the natural history and pathophysiology of cervical intraepithelial neoplasia has provided a logical application for cervical conization. This operation offers accurate diagnosis of the intraepithelial nature of cervical neoplasia, eradicates preinvasive neoplasia, and still preserves reproductive capability. Until relatively recently, total hysterectomy was the preferred procedure for therapy of CIN. Although there is no doubt that this approach to the disease will result in a cure in an overwhelming majority of cases, it is

Table 4.11. Conization (Cylinder) Procedure: Rules of Application[a]

Instruments	Laser CO_2, colposcope, micromanipulator, laser scalpel, suction device, caliper, pickups, scissors
Spot diameter	0.050–0.125 mm (laser scalpel)
	0.400–0.700 mm (micromanipulator)
Speed of incision	3.5 cm/sec
Power output	25–30 W
Power density	1400 W/cm²
Hemostatic measures	Pitressin infiltrations, lateral sutures (optional)

[a]Depth and width of the cylinder related to lesion topography (colposcopic determination, possible contact hysteroscopic evaluation).

certainly radical therapy for a premalignant condition which often affects young women.

The use of the laser to excise cervical tissue surgically has been neglected in the literature. J. Dorsey[80] first described this procedure and successfully demonstrated its applicability by performing serial biopsies on selected patients at the Greater Baltimore Medical Center. After this report, several additional authors described laser conization and results, both with microsurgical and free-hand techniques.[67,93] A preoperative Pap smear, colposcope-directed cervical biopsy, and endocervical curettage are currently performed. No additional equipment is required for these procedures. Thus, modern CO_2 laser instruments with medium power output, colposcopic attachments, and micromanipulator are sufficient. The rules of application are given in Table 4.11.

4.7.1. Technical Approach

The vast majority of these operations can be done as outpatient procedures using either paracervical or general anesthesia. Patients are allowed to go home 4 hr after completion of the operation. Excisional laser conization uses smaller focal spot diameter and higher power density than do cervical vaporization procedures.

It has been shown that lateral heat conduction from the laser impact site into the surrounding tissue increases with the time spent in lasing.[81,82] High power density and small spot size produce rapid cutting and very little thermal damage, thus, it follows that the rapid incision made by small spot size and high power density minimizes the heat effect in the cervical stroma. Since it is most important for the pathologist to interpret both the degree of the neoplasia and the involvement of the margins of the coned specimen, there must be little or no thermal artifact present to distort tissue. A spot size diameter of 1.5–1.7 mm and power density of approximately 1400 W/cm² will produce a satisfactory specimen with the proper operative technique.

After the preparation of the patient, supplementary procedures are needed in order to provide adequate mobility and proper cutting angles at the cervix. Thus, a weighted posterior vaginal retractor and a single-toothed tenaculum for grasping the cervix allow gentle retraction downward and toward the targeted portion of cervix.

Much of the hemostatic effect of laser surgery is produced by heat coagulation of the cut ends of small vessels in the surrounding stroma. With high power densities, the hemostatic effect of the laser beam is reduced. It is therefore necessary to use additional methods of hemostasis when performing an excisional laser conization.

Dorsey[80] reported that hemostasis can be adequately controlled by placing chromic 0 sutures at an appropriate depth, bilaterally, in order to occlude descending cervical vessels and accelerate the operation time. This method of excisional laser conization has been modified slightly since it was first described.[80,83] Lateral cervical sutures are no longer used for temporary hemostasis as, occasionally, there was delayed bleeding from the suture sites. Ten milliliters of a dilute solution of vasopressin (1.5%) injected into the cervical stroma in the approximate location of the laser incision will give excellent initial hemostasis.

It is important to plan the size of the cone carefully. Adequate margins at the borders of the visible lesion are necessary for pathologic interpretation. Since the incision width corresponds to the beam spot diameter (approximately 1.5 mm) and the thermal artifact is equal to 1 mm in histologic slides, the incision must be at least 2.5 mm from the free border. Actually, for performing a *radical conization* it is best to excise 5 mm from the border of the lesion, in order to obtain a biopsy specimen border which is free from the thermal artifact and suitable for diagnostic interpretation. At 5 mm from the outer margins of the lesion, the circumference of the cone is then outlined on the cervix using short bursts of laser energy at 25–27 W power setting and high power densities (Fig. 4.13A). The short bursts will also serve as indicators to the surgeon of the pain tolerance level of the patient, which, in turn, will provide guidelines for the selection of anesthesia. Relatively high power densities of 1110–1400 W/cm² allow one to excise cervical cone biopsy specimens with high-speed cutting so that the lateral heat and thermal artifact can be minimized.

A location for the apex of the cone may be determined either by sound-

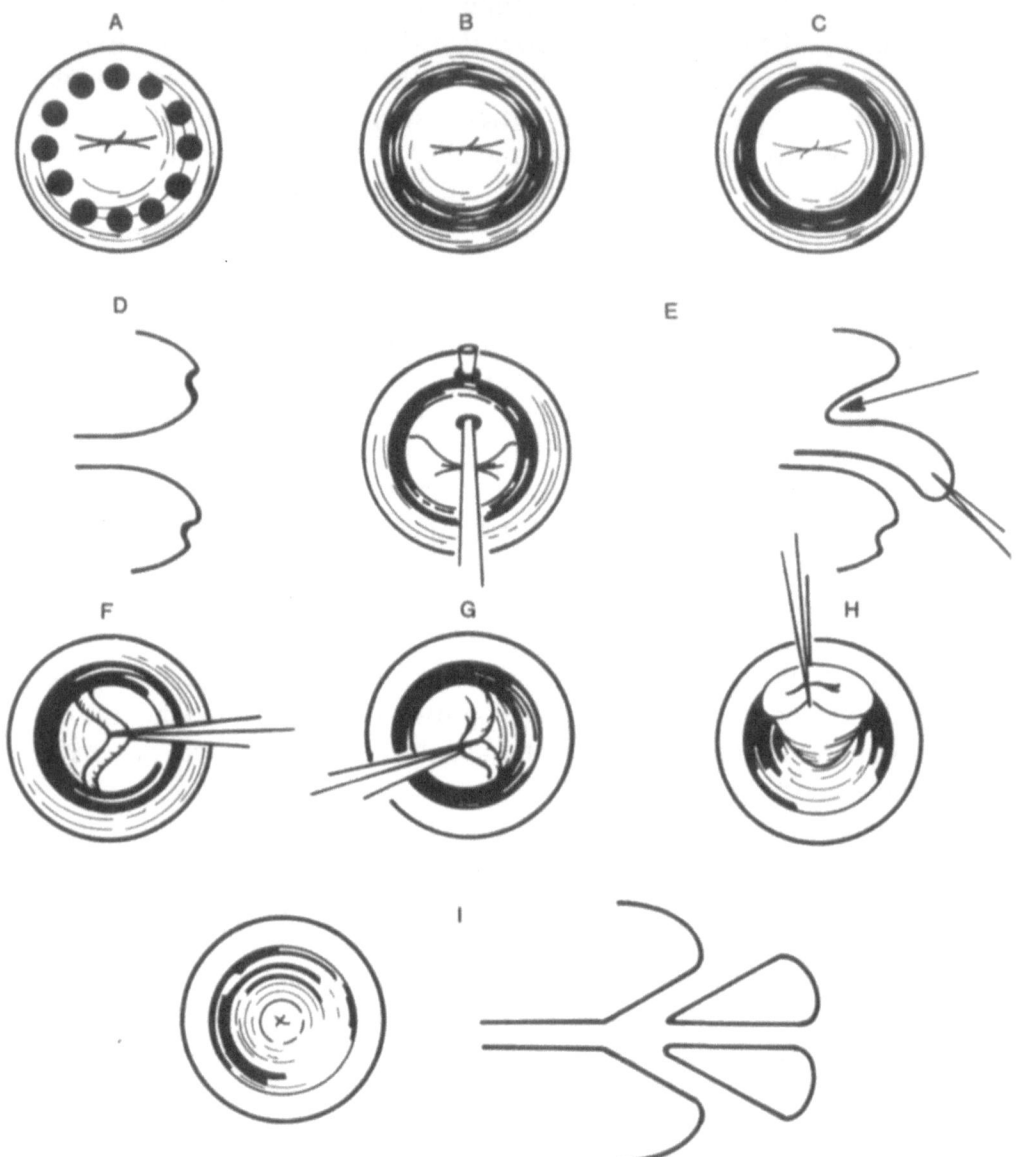

Figure 4.13. Laser conization procedure. (A)The outer margins of the cone have been marked by bursts of laser energy. (B,C,D)The incision has been made and deepened to 2 mm so that the cone specimen may be grasped with forceps. (E)The laser beam is angled towards the apex of the cone. Gentle traction on the specimen aids in laser beam cutting. (F,G,H)The specimen is developed in the four quadrants so that movement of the laser and colposcope is minimized. (I)The cone specimen is removed. The last few millimeters may be taken with a knife. The apex of the incision may be biopsied to show free margins. This cone bed is then lased with power density for hemostasis.

ing the cervix with a probe, in order to identify the internal os, or, more accurately, by using the contact endoscope to judge the appropriate location.

A continuous operating mode is used to incise the cervix circularly straight down into the stroma to a depth of at least 2 mm (Fig. 4.13B–D). That initial incision allows one to obtain a good lip of cervical stroma for grasping with the forceps and proceeding with the conization. Rather than continue to develop the circular incision equally throughout its circumference, we use a four-quadrant approach. The superior quarter of the incision is first deepened until the canal is entered at the anterior edge of the cone apex (Fig. 4.13E). The laser is then repositioned and the right, left, and inferior portions of the incision completed. The *four-quadrant approach,* similar to the vaporization technique, is recommended to continue the incision more easily through the stroma of the endocervical canal. As the incision penetrates into the depth of the canal, the developing cone is pulled medially, quadrant by quadrant, so that changes in the position of the forceps and the laser beam are minimal (Fig. 4.13F–H).

Because bleeding may decrease the efficiency of the laser energy, due to its absorption of the heat, it must be prevented by sealing vessels throughout the procedure by lower power densities of the defocused laser beam. Rarely, a triple 0 catgut suture is necessary for the control of bleeding from major arterioles.

Usually the apex of the cone that has to be approached is located several millimeters into the canal beyond the internal os. Since the diameter of the cone specimen decreases toward the apex and, consequently the distance from the central endocervical canal also decreases, the last few millimeters of the cone should be taken with cold knife or scissors in order to avoid the thermal artifact in a tissue of shorter diameter and to insure the pathologist a reasonable margin free of thermal damage (Fig. 4.13I). Furthermore, the "shrinkage effect" on the laser-excised cone must be taken into account, because the greater the cone, the more precise the microscopic interpretation of the specimen. The cone is removed with the knife so there is absolutely no thermal artifact present.

At this point, the power density is reduced by reducing the laser wattage and, if the surgeon desires, defocusing the laser beam. The cone is then lased for hemostasis. Lower power density, large spot size, and slow vaporization impart heat to the cervical stroma so that blood vessels and lymphatics are sealed. The end result of this operation is, therefore, very similar to the end result of a laser vaporization procedure for CIN (i.e., there is a cone-shaped cervical defect consisting of a laser stroma separating the squamous epithelium from the apical endocervical columnar epithelium). The average blood loss from the technique of conization is usually less than 5 cc.

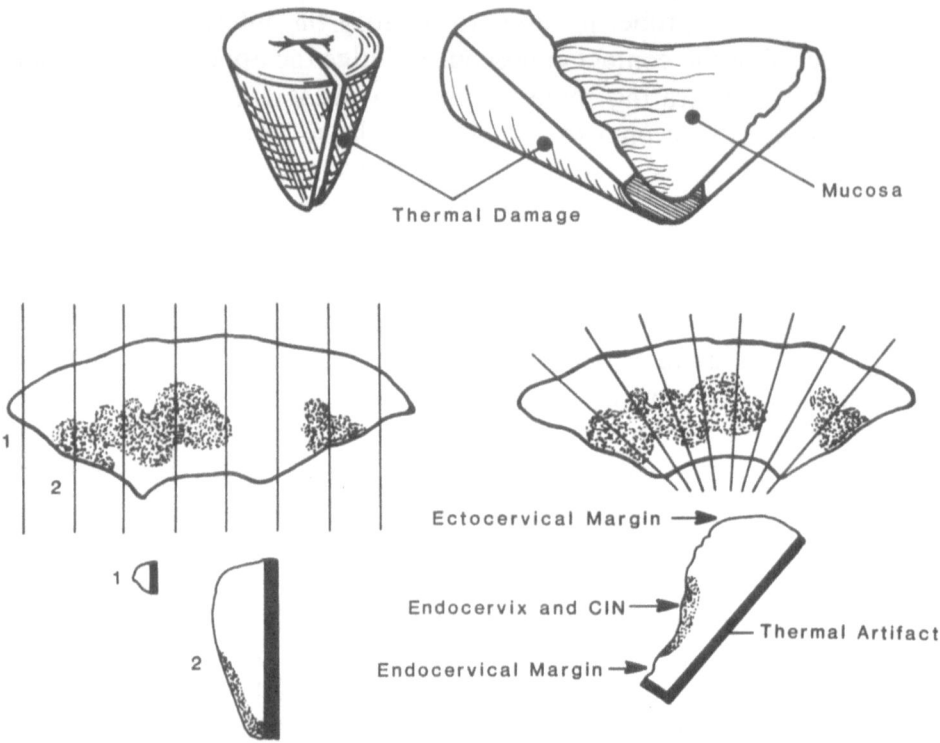

Figure 4.14. The cone specimen has been opened.The mucosal surface is sectioned so as to show the margins. If sections are taken vertically through the specimen, margins will be falsely interpreted. Section 2 would be interpreted by the pathologist as intraepithelial neoplasia involving the lower margin of the cone. Thermal artifact is shown on the stromal margin, but not on the mucosa of the cone.

4.7.2. Pathologic Examination

The conization specimen must be properly sectioned by the pathologist in order to evaluate the margins of excision. Any method of cutting the specimen which does not allow complete visualization of the apical margins of the cone will not yield the all-important information on the adequacy of the conization (Fig. 4.14).

4.7.3. Combined Procedures

Excisional laser conization is a technique which we have often combined with laser vaporization procedures. In women with intraepithelial neoplasia, where a large part of the portio vaginalis of the cervix as well as the endocervical canal is involved, excision of all dysplastic areas would remove a large volume of cervical tissue, producing an end result anatomically and physiologically similar to total cervicectomy. The endocervical extensions of these giant lesions can be evaluated and treated by an excisional conization of small diameter, but appropriate depth, while peripheral cervical and/or vaginal extension may be treated by laser vaporization.[84,85]

Again, the excisional conization must be suitable for pathologic evaluation of the apical margin, but the colposcopically visible ectocervical margin will be positive for neoplasia. Vaporization of this remaining cervical intraepithelial neoplasia, which has been thoroughly evaluated by biopsy, is then carried out to the appropriate depth. In this manner the endocervical canal is evaluated and, it is hoped, rid of the disease. The more peripheral lesion is vaporized and the normal functional architecture of the cervix is preserved.

The CO_2 laser affords a highly accurate microsurgical method of attack on CIN. If one uses a combination of the techniques of vaporization and excision, effective diagnostic as well as ablative operations may be combined for therapy of cervical vaginal intraepithelial neoplasia. In the hands of a trained colposcopist and laser surgeon, cure rates should exceed 95%.

4.8. Postsurgical Care

During the laser microsurgical procedure of vaporization or conization, if the surgeon is patient and allows the heat to dissipate from the tissue, the treatment will be very easily tolerated. If opportunely advised by the nurse in the pretreatment conference, the patient will not be surprised about the steam and the fumes emitted from the vagina. However, this event can be minimized by the suction device which eliminates the odor of burning tissue. Patients describe their sensation during laser treatment as a pinching heat which is felt only when high power densities are used.

Pain is minimal (i.e., uterine cramps) or nonexistent after laser treatment, even during pregnancy, and very few postoperative analgesics are needed. Some patients may have some spotting during the first 10 days postsurgically, but since bleeding is not usually a problem, neither intraoperatively nor after the treatment, vaginal packing is not used. In the rare case of bleeding, silver nitrate application can be used on an outpatient basis.

Morbidity associated with excisional conization has been low, and the only significant problem to date has been delayed postoperative bleeding. Most patients will develop minor amounts of vaginal spotting or bleeding; approximately 10% of women complain of bleeding which develops between the 4th and 10th postoperative days and is in excess of their usual menstrual flow. The pattern of this bleeding is intermittent and, almost invariably, it can be controlled by colposcopically directed application of silver nitrate to the small bleeding vessel. Sutures for an occasional bleeding vessel in the cervix are 3-0 chromatic catgut.

The patient is instructed to expect a watery discharge for 24–48 hr, or at maximum, during the first postoperative week. Sanitary napkins rather than tampons are recommended. No vaginal cream or douche should be used. The patient should avoid vaginal contamination or sexual intercourse for 4 weeks after surgery.

Lastly, since no pelvic infections have been reported, prophylactic antibiotics are not recommended.

4.9. Evaluation of Healing

The healing process is directly related to the amount of tissue destruction (i.e., the depth and surface of the treated area).[78,86,87] There is minimal to absent fibroblastic activity during the repair state, and thus the healed epithelium fails to show scar formation, stenosis, or adhesions. Therefore, large areas of cervical lesions can also be treated.

Previous papers[88,89] report early detailed follow-up of the first 50 patients who were treated by laser cervical vaporization. During the first 48 hr, maximal sloughing of the necrotic tissue was noted, and the discharge had an average duration of 24 hr (much shorter than after cryosurgical treatment) and in all cases it was related to the size of the surgical site. In the early phase, the base of the treated area appeared reddened and leukorrhea was present on the surface. Spotty bleeding was noted in 10% of cases, but in none of the patients was it necessary to resort to sutures or vaginal packing as there was no persistent hemorrhaging. The next 48 hr were characterized by peak of discharge and the beginning of remission of symptoms. After 8 days a clear, circumscribed, treated area with yellowish fibrin covering the reddened depression was seen. The border remained pink and no vascular hyperemia, bleeding, or leukorrhea was noted. A thin layer of squamous metaplastic epithelium was apparent after 10 days and a complete cover of young squamous epithelium appeared after 2 weeks. After 3 weeks healing was complete. By 21 days, most of the inflammatory cells had disappeared and the cytologic examination revealed primarily squamous epithelial cells. Finally, after 4 weeks, the treated area was not recognizable because the epithelium appeared normal.

Healing after laser conization is relatively rapid and presents some particularities when compared with healing after vaporization. Most patients experience spotting for 1 week to 10 days following conization, but no copious discharge is present. Delayed hemorraging can be avoided if hemostatic measures of vasopressin and lateral sutures are used.

Since no technical attempt is made to reconstruct the cervical wound, a large area of laser-incised cervical stroma forms, which separates the ectocervical squamous epithelium from the endocervical columnar epithelium high into the canal at the cone apex. The cervical wound appears clean after 1 week of the postoperative course and in the second and third weeks the colposcopic examinations reveal the crater to be covered by a thin necrotic inflammatory pseudomembrane, which disappears gradually during the fourth week. A delicate epithelium covers the entire wound and the margin of the ectocervical incision becomes smooth and rounded where the epithelium migrates on the incised stromal area. The reepithelialization of the crater consists primarily of the progressive proliferation downward of the columnar epithelium and the growth of the squamous epithelium upwards until a new squamocolumnar junction is realized.

Histologic examination of biopsy specimens from the margins confirms the normal evolution of mature squamous epithelium on the granulation tissue, while endocervical border specimens show the columnar cell dipping downward and is well established after the pseudomembrane disappears. The new squamocolumnar junction, which can be clearly visualized, is found close to the origin of the incision rather than deep in the crater.

4.10. Follow-up Examinations

After tissue healing examinations, in order to identify the persistence or recurrence of cervical premalignant or neoplastic treated lesions, a schedule of follow-up examinations is recommended after laser treatment. Additionally, we must define our limits when discussing residual disease, persistent or recurrent disease, and new pathology:

Residual disease: <12 months
Recurrent disease: 13–24 months
New disease: >25 months

Moreover, if no persistent disease has been identified by the second complete 3-month followup examination, the chance of identifying persistent disease after that time appears to be minimal.[90] If early colposcopic and cytologic follow-up within the fourth week reveals persistent disease (atypical changes), retreatment with further CO_2 laser vaporization at a radial distance of 2 cm or more from the previous border is indicated. It is recommended[15] that the cytologic examinations be repeated after 1 month, because there is the possibility of finding ambiguous pathology in the late healing phase.

It is suggested that the novice laser surgeon first perform a colposcopic examination after 3 weeks, then a monthly examination for 3 months and, thereafter, quarterly examinations until the end of the first year, after which time follow-ups can be performed every 6 months.[90] Other follow-up schedules that have been suggested[15,91] consist of only a quarterly cytologic and colposcopic examination during the first year, then every 6 months.

4.11. Current Research on CIN

To demonstrate the effectiveness of the CO_2 laser surgery for CIN, a survey of available reports from the literature was conducted. However, since the authors do not report completely comparable series, only partial conclusions can be drawn. Also, long-term follow-up is required to determine the ultimate value of CO_2 laser treatment.

In a series of 247 cases of CIN (67 of them were CIS) treated with laser vaporization, an overall persistence rate of 4.4% was reported[86,90] considering both benign and preinvasive disease. Dividing the treated cases into subsequent periods of 6 months, this paper reports a decreasing recurrence rate as far as the surgical experience progressed, approaching a 2% recurrence rate in the last period. The CIN subcategories do not show a significant difference in recurrence rate. Actually, mild dysplasia recurred at a rate of 2/45 (4.4%), moderate dysplasia at 4/147 (2.7%), and severe dysplasia and carcinoma in situ at 3/55 (5.5%).

Baggish,[88] in a series of 115 treated cases of CIN with age varying from 18–82 and a follow-up ranging from 8–24 months, reported an overall recurrence rate of 4.34%, whereas the majority of persistent disease was noted during the first year, primarily due to lack of experience on the part of the surgeon with regard to the depth and lateral extent of tissue destruction required.

Stafl[92] treated 42 cases of CIN and reported an overall 10% recurrence rate, which persisted within 3 months. He used a lower output (i.e., 7 W) with short exposure times.

Krantz[76] reported treating 73 cases of CIN; three patients were retreated in a 6-month follow-up for persistence.

Carter[93] described a series of 45 selected young patients, treated for CIN with a follow-up of more than 2 years. Clear colposcopic visibility of ectocervical lesions without extension into the canal and well defined boundaries of the CIN were the conditions for treating with CO_2 laser vaporization to a depth of approximately 5 mm. The overall recurrence rate was 6.6% after 2 years and seven cases of retreatment for persistent lesions in the early phase of the trial. After the surgeon became more familiar with the instruments, the margins of the evident area of lesion were better outlined, the time exposure was lessened, and a significant decrease in residual cervical disease was noted.

More recent reports of the same authors[94] reported a 10% recurrence rate in a series of 230 CIN-bearing patients with 5-year follow-up after CO_2 laser vaporization. The original treatment plan was modified by treating the entire transformation zone instead of only visible lesion. The continuous operating mode with a power density greater than 2000 W/cm^2 and a depth of destruction of 5–7 mm were recognized as definitive technical parameters for CO_2 laser surgery in order to optimize the clinical results.

Jordan[89] treated more than 400 cases of premalignant lesions of the cervix and vagina. Most had a follow-up ranging from 15 months to 3 years. Even though some of those patients were treated more than once for persistent disease, the overall recurrence rate was found to be less than 6%.

Burke[63] reported a study group of 60 patients and identified subgroups in which there was a major incidence of recurrence when improper technique and insufficient depth of destruction had been used.

Popkin[95] reported a 92% cure rate in a preliminary study of a series of 13 CO_2 laser-treated patients. The results of treatment were assessed by examining cone biopsy specimens 3–8 months after therapy.

Some of the above-mentioned series have been studied to analyze the results. Persistent disease rates following primary laser application appear to have a direct relationship to the depth of destruction in every series and for every grade of CIN (Tables 4.12–4.14). Some of the patients in all of those series required more than one treatment. This should not be considered to be a failure of the CO_2 laser treatment since the follow-up is adequate for detecting persistent lesions after a few months, and a second or even a third laser treatment can be performed which will usually eradicate the disease completely. With CO_2 laser treatment, one achieves the minor overall recurrence rates as seen in patients who were treated with the conservative methods.[88,96]

Tables 4.12–4.14 cite those investigators whose experiences reflect the

Table 4.12.   Persistent Disease Rates for CIN I Following Primary Laser Application by Depth of Destruction as Reported in the Gynecologic Literature

Depth (mm)	No. cases	Persistent disease rate (%)	Contributing author(s)[a]
1–2	6	50.0	Jordan
2–4	27	37.0	Jordan
5+	259	4.3	Baggish, Jordan Bellina, Wright

[a]Bellina J H (ed): Gynecologic Laser Surgery, Proceedings of the International Congress on Gynecologic Laser Surgery and Related Works, New Orleans, LA, Jan 1980. New York, Plenum Press, 1980.

Table 4.13.   Persistent Disease Rates for CIN II Following Primary Laser Application by Depth of Destruction as Reported in the Gynecologic Literature[a]

Depth (mm)	No. cases	Persistent disease rate (%)	Contributing author(s)
1–2	7	86.7	Jordan
2–4	18	38.9	Jordan
5+	307	6.2	Baggish, Jordan Bellina, Wright

[a]Follow-up range: 3–42 months

Table 4.14.   Persistent Disease Rates for CIN III Following Primary Laser Application by Depth of Destruction as Reported in the Gynecologic Literature

Depth (mm)	No. cases	Persistent disease rate (%)	Contributing author(s)
1–2	26	84.6	Jordan
2–4	60	66.7	Jordan
4–5	20	30.0	Jordan
5+	328	14.0	Baggish, Jordan Bellina, Wright

Table 4.15.   Summary of Persistence Rates at 5+ mm Depth[a]

CIN	Persistent disease(%)
I	4.3
II	6.2
III (includes CIS)	14.0

[a]Wright recently published a survey [Wright C V: Use of the CO_2 in treatment of CIN (abstact), in Popkin DR et al (eds): Second International Congress on Gynecological Laser Surgery, Montreal Quebec, Canada, May 1982. Plenum Press, 1982.] with meticulous preparation and following with a 98% cure rate, or 2% persistence.

Table 4.16. Guidelines for Reporting Treatment Success

Power density
Pulsed or continuous mode
Depth of destruction
Peripheral destruction beyond lesion borders
Disease category reported separately
Follow-up interval and mean
Patient disease rates for first and second retreatments

state of the art in laser management of CIN lesions. It becomes quite apparent that the depth of destruction continues to be the hallmark for a successful outcome (Table 4.15).

Even though other case reports are available in the literature, most of them report a limited number of treated cases, lack of standardized methods of laser calibration and of definition of the depth of penetration into the cervical tissue, and disregard the recording of the power densities used and of the long-term follow-up. They therefore do not allow up-to-date documentation of the real effectiveness of CO_2 laser treatment. In order to approach exact evaluation of comparable data, a guideline for reporting treatment success is suggested (Table 4.16).

No long-term results of the conization procedure have been reported to date in a treated series. Minimal discomfort for the treated patients and reduced intra- and postoperative bleeding have been emphasized in the Dorsey series[97] even in the 28 patients operated on as outpatients. Vaginal discharge has not been a problem nor have any clinically apparent systemic or local infections been noted.

A more recent series, presented at the last International Congress, reported generally positive results of the conization procedure. Grundsell and colleagues[98] reported a randomized study consisting of 110 treated patients. Bleeding complications were found in 1.8% in the laser group, whereas bleeding occurred in 14.6% of the group treated with the cold knife technique.

Technical differences have been also pointed out by Sadoul and associates[99] in a recent study of 40 treated cases, comparing CO_2 laser microsurgery and free-hand techniques. Conclusions are that the handpiece has been found to have several advantages when compared to the microsurgical method. Shortening of the operative time, perfect control of the hemostasis, cleaner and faster cutting, and fast healing time have been reported as the main advantages of CO_2 laser surgery.

4.12. Complications

Papers dealing with vaporization of CIN reported absence of significant complications following the treatment and the results have been very encouraging. Bellina's[90] series of 256 cases reports some cases of bleeding within the first 10 days after therapy. This bleeding was usually described by the patient as "spotting" or a flow similar to a light menstruation. Two patients required an outpatient application of silver nitrate to the laser wound for hemostatic effect. One patient required suturing of a small arterial bleeding point under anesthesia. No cases of pelvic infection have occurred. Antibiotics were neither prescribed prophylactically nor were they required following therapy.

Particular attention has been given to recent reports of the early and late complications associated with the use of CO_2 laser surgery.[100] In examining a series of 215 patients treated with CO_2 laser vaporization for CIN, out of 624 gynecologic surgical operations for various diseases, a total of 53 hemorrhagic complications have been found. No treatment was required in 47 of these 53 patients. In the six hemorrhagic complications considered to be major (two immediate and four delayed) vaginal packing or sutures were necessary.

Pain has been reported to be minimal, especially when the heat buildup was allowed to dissipate. There were no late complications such as scar formation (e.g., cervical stenosis) reported in the entire series. Similarly, no infections were reported.

Excellent repair without trophic sequelae, even after treatment of exten-

Table 4.17. Specific Advantages of the CO_2 Laser for Treatment of CIN

Easy to perform (both diagnostic and therapeutic procedure may be carried out with one instrument)
Minimal operative risk
Precise boundary destruction
Selective destruction depth
Minimal damage to healthy tissue
Minimal or absent side effects (pain, bleeding, infection)
Reduced quantity and duration of postoperative discharge
Rapid healing
Anatomic conservation of squamocolumnar junction
Functional conservation for sex and fertility
Reduced risk of recurrence
Treatment repeatability
Equally effective as removal technique (i.e., conization) in selected cases

sive areas, including colposcopic and cytologic follow-up, has been widely reported in the literature.[90,100,101]

4.13. Laser Technique versus Conventional Methods

Cervical disease can be treated with a number of surgical modalities, such as cryosurgery, diathermy, scalpel, and the CO_2 laser. Each modality has its advantages and disadvantages. The specific advantages of the CO_2 laser for treatment of CIN are given in Table 4.17. The use of the CO_2 laser as treatment for CIN will be compared with conventional surgical techniques in subsequent sections.

4.13.1. Laser Vaporization versus Cryosurgery and Diathermy

The same factors considered as advantages in CO_2 laser treatments are analyzed here in order to estimate their real effectiveness when compared to other conventional methods of conservative treatment for cervical premalignant or in situ neoplastic lesions.

Conization and hysterectomy are considered separately. In diathermy, cryosurgery, and CO_2 laser vaporization no operative specimen is taken for histologic confirmation; thus a previous biopsy, accurate colposcopic examination, and exact tissue ablation are required. Diathermy, to be effective, requires deep cauterization as well as the use of general anesthesia. Cryosurgery is performed at $-60°$ to $-80°C$, employing nitrous oxide or freon as the refrigerant. It is applied for 3–8 min, primarily employing the freeze-thaw–freeze technique. Tissue destruction is achieved by freezing or dehydrating the cellular water,[102] which results in damage to the cellular wall. Both cryosurgery and diathermy, by obstructing the operating field, make control of treated tissue in width and depth difficult and unselective, while CO_2 laser surgery can vaporize tissue to any desired depth.

The tissue damage extends much further for cryosurgery and diathermy and involves additional damage of adjacent healthy tissue. The wide area of necrosis is responsible for the edema, abundant sloughing, persistent discharge, and prolonged healing time—usually more than 6 weeks. With the CO_2 laser, there is less than 1 mm of adjacent tissue damage. Moreover, there is a potential high risk of infections, pain, and bleeding as major side effects when the scabs from diathermy slough. The extensive tissue repair moves the transformation zone into the endocervical canal and the tissue distortion associated with cryosurgery and diathermy treatment leads to frequent upward migration of the squamocolumnar junction, so that colposcopic examination during the follow-up period disallows evaluation of this critical zone. This does not occur following laser treatment. Moreover, stenosis, menstrual cycle changes, and dyspareunia occur frequently following cryosurgery, but less frequently after diathermy, but have never been reported after laser treatment.[78,100] Finally, an average failure rate of 18% has been reported[95,103,104] after cryotherapy for CIN II and III by several investigators, while others[105–107] have reported a 90% cure rate. One investigator[106] also reports uncertain interpretations of cytologic samples and histologic biopsy specimens during the follow-up period, because of the active regenerating epithelium and related cytologic changes.

A direct comparison of cryotherapy and CO_2 laser treatment performed by the same author has been reported.[108] A 17.2% failure rate (i.e., persistent lesions) after primary cryosurgery treatment was found in a series of 98 patients with different degrees of CIN. In a second group of 73 patients treated with the CO_2 laser, the overall persistence rate was 2.7%.

Even if it requires simple, safe, and inexpensive equipment, cryosurgery, since there is the possibility of undetected residual disease manifesting itself as invasive carcinoma,[68] can therefore be considered to be[109] misleading with regard to expectations for achieving success in treating CIN (Table 4.18). Furthermore, diathermy, though widely used, has to be recognized as having the untoward effects of massive destruction of normal adjacent cervical tissue. The extended necrosis area is 3–10 times larger than with CO_2 laser vaporization.[92] Considering the consequent sloughing, prolonged discharge, and possible bleeding following vascular injury, it cannot be viewed as an

Table 4.18. **Synopsis of Alternative Treatment Modalities for CIN without Endocervical Extension**

Variable	Type of treatment		
	Cryo	Diathermy	CO_2 laser
Precision of tissue ablation	−	±	+ +
Operatory risk	−	±	−
Healthy tissue damage	+ + +	+ +	+
Side effects	+ + +	+ +	±
Discharge duration (days)	10–20	7	3–4
Healing time	Very slow	Slow	Rapid
Anatomic and functional conservation	±	±	+
Average recurrence rates (%)	10–40	10	4

Table 4.19. Persistence Rates of Destructive Modalities for Treatment of CIN

Technique	Persistence rates (%)
Cold knife conization	1–13
Hot cautery	2–60
Cryosurgery	12–48
CO_2 laser	<4

ideal treatment for cervical preneoplastic disease. In addition, deeper and more radical coagulation produced by diathermy requires general anesthesia, which increases the cost and risk to the patients.

Infertility problems after diathermy conization have also been reported. McVicar and Villocks[110] reviewed a series of 633 patients following diathermy conization: 214 wished to become pregnant, but only 74% of these were successful; more than 33% of this group experienced miscarriages or premature labor.

Finally, the reported failure rate of 10% or more with this treatment is too high to consider it as the treatment of choice.[111–114]

On the other hand, it must be remembered that, despite any method of treatment, conservative or radical, recurrences do occur[115–117] and a complete success in every case is not achievable at present. Moreover, there is evidence of multicentricity of CIN with involvement of the other parts of the female genital tract.[118] Thus it is suggested that an endocervical curettage and a 10-year follow-up be carried out before reporting the results of treatment for CIN. The persistence rates for the conventional methods of treating CIN are given in Table 4.19.

4.13.2. Laser Conization versus Cold Knife Conization and Hysterectomy

Since indications for these procedures can be the same in certain circumstances, it is possible to compare the different advantages for each one. In fact, the endocervical extension of the cervical preneoplastic lesions after a colposcopic biopsy for excluding invasive disease requires a specimen for histologic confirmation,[119–121] hence conization or hysterectomy. Following the modern trend of not overtreating the preneoplastic lesion and of conserving the functional integrity by removing a minimum of normal and pathologic tissue, the CO_2 laser conization, if used with proper cutting angles, insures very precise control over the tissue excised. It incorporates the reduction of the operative morbidity correlated with classic cervical conization, which requires hospitalization and general anesthesia, as does hysterectomy.

The CO_2 laser cone resection can be performed on an outpatient basis and intra- and postoperative hemorrhagic complications are also markedly reduced if the hemostatic precautions[80] are used. The classic conization results in significant intraoperative and postoperative risk of complications such as infections and hemorrhage.[122–124]

The healing process is relatively rapid with the CO_2 laser and one of the most important advantages is the visibility of the new squamocolumnar junction and transformation zone, which has the advantage of allowing cytologic and colposcopic follow-up examination.

The cervical surgical Sturmdorf's reconstruction, frequently performed after cold knife treatment, conceals this important zone (which bears the introflection of the resected borders), so that a recurrence can eventually be observed only in a later stage of evolution. By reviewing those cases which had cold knife conization and were subsequently treated by total hysterectomy, residual in situ neoplastic disease was noted in 21% of cases in one series[125] and 51% of cases in another series.[126] Although cervical conization is certainly a more conservative procedure, there is still a relatively high morbidity associated with the traditional techniques of *cold knife conization.*[127] Intraoperative bleeding, delayed hemorrhage, and other late complications such as infertility and high-risk pregnancy have led to cold knife conization being regarded as a minor operation with a major morbidity rate.[128–130] It is therefore logical that gynecologic surgeons seek improved techniques for this operation. Additionally, the incidence of stenosis of the cervical orifice resulting from cold knife conization is 5–25%.[122,129–134] This can lead to impairment of fertility because of menstrual cycle changes, dysmenorrhea, dyspareunia, or dystocia and often requires dilatation. Since the women treated are generally young and are concerned about preserving their ability to bear children, these are important considerations.

Lee[135] examined the reproductive outcome of 97 patients following cold knife conization, and reported a 27% spontaneous abortion rate and a 22% Cesarean section rate in some of the patients because the fibrotic cervices failed to dilate, while 14.5% of these patients had premature deliveries due to cervical incompetence.

Scarring and cervical stenosis have not been demonstrated nor has impairment of reproductive capability been reported as a result of using the CO_2 laser for cone resection.

Finally, the tissue sections obtained by CO_2 laser procedure are no less adequate for pathologic interpretation than those obtained using the cold knife or scissors for cutting the last few millimeters in order to prevent ther-

Table 4.20. Synopsis of Alternative Treatment Modalities for CIN with Endocervical Extension

Variable	Cold knife conization	CO_2 laser conization	Hysterectomy
Operative risk	+	−	+ +
Complications	+ +	±	+
Anatomic and functional conservation	±	+	−
Histologic specimen	+	+	+

mal damage artifact, and the laser procedure allows adequate histologic evaluation of the apex margins.

More experience and clinical trials are needed, however, in order to evaluate the long-term results when compared to the classic methods[136,137] since the reported series[80,98,99] of cases available to date in the literature have not had sufficient follow-up for estimating compared average recurrence rates. Toaff[138] has used the laser conization technique but without hemostatic procedures and concluded that there was no advantage to this application.

It must be remembered that if invasive disease is found, the laser cone resection is still safe. In fact, previous reports[139] have demonstrated the destruction of tumor cells by CO_2 laser without dispersing the cells into deeper tissues; furthermore, the lymphatic and blood vessels are sealed as well. Further treatment could proceed as if the patient had undergone classic conization.

The hysterectomy, as a first choice of treatment for preneoplastic and in situ neoplastic cervical lesions, can be considered an overtreatment for the young reproductive female if no other indication supports this decision. In fact, operative risks, general anesthesia, hospitalization cost, and sterility should be considered excessive treatment when compared to the disease entity.

In conclusion, the serious drawbacks related to classic conization and hysterectomy have to be considered since sufficient elements support the observation that, in a high percentage of cases, cold knife conization can be avoided[140] and that CO_2 laser conization can replace this conventional method as the treatment of choice for endocervical extension of cervical preneoplastic disease (Table 4.20).

4.14. Other Indications for Laser Surgery

Several benign conditions can be successfully treated with CO_2 laser, such as stenosis of the external uterine orifice, chronic cervicitis (even during pregnancy), cervical endometriosis, cervicovaginal adenosis, ectopy, and cervical polyps. Condylomatous lesions and warty atypia have been advantageously treated, especially in multicentric localization of the disease.

Capillary hemangioma of the cervix has been treated with minimal blood loss. The reported case[72] of a large cervical lesion demonstrated the problem of preserving the structural and physiological integrity of the organ in a young girl, who could have required surgical excision or perhaps hysterectomy.

Ectopia or ectropions can be considered as indications for laser vaporization. The relationships among ectopia–dysplasia–carcinoma, age at first intercourse, and use of hormonal contraception have been studied.[56] The treatment of this ectopic disease frequently represents an effective prevention of carcinoma[73,74] and removes the troublesome symptoms of leukorrhea.[75] In the fertile period (25–45 years) it can always be treated, especially in pluriparous women. In the nulliparous woman who wishes to bear children, it is considered advantageous to perform the treatment after conception and delivery.[56] In the postmenopausal period there is little indication because of the end of the metaplastic phenomena. The ectopic area can be vaporized with the CO_2 laser.

Finally, malignant lesions of the cervix can be treated. Palliative bulky lesion reduction can be performed by vaporization. If complete tumor vaporization is technically impossible, partial volume reduction might render the tumor size more responsive to radiation therapy. Chronic cervical disease and other anomalies can lead to reduced fertility or reproductive failures due to mechanical weakness. The CO_2 laser can be used to manage many of these problems.

4.14.1. Stenosis

Stenosis can be congenital with reduced outflow, resulting in retrograde menstruation. Sampson's hypothesis of endometriosis is proposed by this mechanism.

The more common problem of postsurgical stenosis is usually detected. Again, retrograde menstruation with endometriosis, chronic pelvic pain, and reduced fertility may be detected. In addition, certain ablative procedures, such as cryoconization, may result in reduced cervical mucus with impaired sperm transport. The laser can be used to manage the stenosis, with power densities of approximately 1000 W/cm^2, using a laser-integrated colposcope. The entire transform zone is vaporized in a conical geometry. The endocervical canal is vaporized for 1–1.5 cm in depth. During the procedure, bleeding is rarely encountered and generally no anesthesia is required. Incidentally, this is basically the same plan of management for cervical intraepithelial neoplasias. It is important to perform this surgery in the early proliferative phase of the menstrual cycle.

Postoperatively a discharge is expected for 1–3 days. Healing is rapid and usually complete by the 21st–30th day. The new squamocolumnar junction is usually easily detected, and the new external os and canal are patent without stenosis. During the postoperative healing phase no tampons, douching, or intercourse is permitted.

4.14.2. Lacerations

Cervical lacerations can occasionally result in reduced sperm transport and/or weakening cervical support, thereby reducing fertility or promoting fetal wastage. The laser is used to correct this defect under direct vision of the colposcope. The defect is vaporized to a depth of 2 mm along its entire surface. This technique reduces the amount of time usually needed when removing the tissue with a cold knife. Next, 2/0 coated Vicryl suture is used to approximate the defect using interrupted figure-of-eight sutures. The mucosa is closed with 2/0 interrupted coated Vicryl suture.

Coitus is permitted after 4 weeks, but no tampons, douching, or creams are allowed during the healing phase.

4.14.3. Bicollis Configuration

Should a unification procedure be undertaken and the surgeon elects to unify the external cervical canal, we recommend the following: using the laser-integrated colposcope at the time of uterine unification, the septum is vaporized. This double approach allows intrauterine evaluation from the uterine side while the second surgeon vaporizes the septum transvaginally. Again, as with other cervical vaginal procedures, coitus and use of vaginal cream must be avoided for a minimum of 3 weeks.

The major problem with this procedure is the possibility of weakening the cervical canal. However, we do not recommend a concomitant cerclage because the uterine incision may compromise the integrity of the myometrium, and uterine rupture could result in pregnancy. Should the patient, after conception, demonstrate cervical incompetence, a cerclage could be advised if the uterine integrity has been evaluated by hysteroscopy, hysterosalpingogram, and even possible laparoscopy. One must warn the patient of the possible consequences of such surgery.

4.14.4. Adenosis and Cervical Changes Associated with Diethylstilbestrol Exposure in Utero

Today, we no longer believe that vaginal adenosis is a deterrent to conception. In recent studies, fecundation rates showed no statistical differences when compared with a control group of matched females. However, in some females the cervical mucus excess may, though rarely, reduce or hamper sperm transport. In such cases the laser can be used to vaporize the adenotic tissue and promote metaplastic regeneration. In these cases the laser is used to deliver a power density of 500–800 W/cm^2, and the surface is ablated using a raster approach as in cervical intraepithelial ablation. The depth of vaporization will depend upon the glandular extent. Occasionally these glands extend to 5 mm in cervical tissue and up to 3 mm in vaginal tissue.

In preparing the vagina for surgery, make certain the bladder is empty. This will significantly increase the interior vaginal wall thickness. Anesthesia is usually not required. Postoperatively the patient follows recommendations as set forth under the vaginal and cervical procedures described previously.

4.14.5. Polyps

Should a polyp(s) be detrimental to conception, the laser can be used to remove the lesion. If the polyp is pedunculated, set the laser colposcope to deliver power densities of 800 W/cm^2 and vaporize the base of the polyp. The polyp should always be subjected to histopathologic analysis. If the lesion is broad-based, first remove a cold biopsy specimen for histopathologic confirmation, then vaporize the base using the same power density of 800 W/cm^2.

It is most important always to obtain a specimen(s) when dealing with neoplastic growth of the cervix or cervical canal. One case in our practice thought to be a simple adenotic polyp was found to be adenocarcinoma. Therefore, never assume that you can make a definitive histopathologic diagnosis visually or grossly.

4.14.6. Leiomyoma

Cervical leiomyoma are rare but do occur. When encountered, their true relationship to fertility must be carefully weighed against the surgical approach and possible complications at the time of removal. In our experience, we have not yet found a cervical leiomyoma to be the true and only cause of infertility, and, in addition, it is usually associated with other leiomyomata, and removal attempts are fraught with danger.

If one must remove the lesions, then our approach would utilize the laser colposcope to vaporize the tumor until it could be enucleated by blunt dissection. The defect should be carefully closed with 2/0 coated Vicryl suture, and preoperative and postoperative hysterosalpingograms and ultrasonography should be performed to assure patency and complete removal.

4.14.7. Cervicitis

When cervical mucus factors in conjunction with chronic infected mucus glands reduce fertility, the laser can be used. The procedure of eradicating these glands is identical to that described in Section 4.14.4. In addition, we recommend intraoperative aerobic and anaerobic cultures. In the healing phase, repeated cultures assure success. In the postoperative phase, specific parenteral antibiotics are administered in accordance with the antibiotogram. The schedule for resumption of sexual activity is the same as for other cervical or vaginal procedures.

One word of caution: in patients with problems of chronic unresponsive cervicitis, check the coital partner. Obtain a prostatic culture and do a careful penile examination. A high percentage of females have recurrent cervicitis as the result of a "ping-pong" infection with their coital partner.

References

1. Minton JP, Zelen M: A method for predicting malignant tumor destruction by laser radiation. J Natl Cancer Inst *34*:291–296, 1965.
2. Dorsey JH: Excisional and reconstructive surgery with the CO_2 laser, in Bellina JH (ed): Gynecologic Laser Surgery. Proceedings of an International Congress on Gynecologic Laser Surgery and Related Works, New Orleans, 1980. New York, Plenum Press, 1980, pp 197–208.
3. Oosterhuis JW: Lymphatic migration after laser surgery. Lancet *1*:446–447, 1978.
4. Goldman L: Laser surgery for skin cancer. NY State J Med 77:1897–1900, 1977.
5. Fidler JP, Law E, MacMillan GB, et al: Comparison of CO_2 laser excision of burns with other thermal knives. Ann NY Acad Sci *267*:254–261, 1977.
6. Stellar S, Mejer R, Waliass H, et al: Carbon dioxide laser debridement of decubitus ulcers. Ann Surg *179*:230–237, 1974.
7. Madden JE, Edlich RF, Custer JR, et al: Studies in the management of the contaminated wound. IV. Resistance to infection of surgical wounds made by knife, electrosurgery and laser. Am J Surg *119*:222–224, 1970.

8. Fruhmorgen F, Bodem F, Reidenbach HD, et al: Long-term observation in endoscopic laser coagulation in gastrointestinal tract. Endoscopy 7:189–196, 1975.
9. Nath G, Gorish W, Kiefhaber P: First laser endoscopy via fiberoptic transmission system. Endoscopy 5:208–213, 1973.
10. Nath G, Gorish W, Kiefhaber P, Kreitmair A: Transmission of a powerful argon laser beam through a fiberoptic flexible gastroscope for operative gastroscopy. Endoscopy 5:213–215, 1973.
11. Pinnow DA: Polycrystalline fiber optical waveguides for infrared transmission. Appl Phys Lett 33:28–29, 1978.
12. Sakurai Y, Nimsakul N, Tanino R, et al: Japanese fiber-optic induced CO_2 laser in clinical application, preliminary report, in Atsumi K, Nimsakul N (eds): Proceedings, IV Congress of the International Society for Laser Surgery, Tokyo, Nov 1981. Inter Group Corp, 1982, pp 1/30–1/33.
13. Seidman H, Silverberg E, Holleb AI: Cancer statistics 1976: a comparison of white and black populations. CA 26:2–30, 1976.
14. Koss L: Epidemiology of carcinoma of the uterine cervix. Excerpta Med Int Congr Series No. 351, 3:307–313, 1974.
15. Stern E: Epidemiology of dysplasia. Obstet Gynecol Surv 24:711–723, 1969.
16. Christopherson WM: Concepts of genesis and development in early cervical neoplasia. Obstet Gynecol Surv 24:842–850, 1969.
17. Navratil E, Burghardt E, Bajardi F, Nash W: Simultaneous colposcopy and cytology used in screening for carcinoma of the cervix. Am J Obstet Gynecol 75:1292–1297, 1958.
18. Fidler HK, Boyes DA, Worth AJ: Cervical cancer detection in British Columbia. J Obstet Gynaecol Br Commonw 75:392–404, 1968.
19. Feldman JJ, Kent DR, Pennington RL: Intraepithelial neoplasia of the uterine cervix in the teenagers. Cancer 41:1405–1408, 1978.
20. Lindberg LG, Ahlgren M, Nordquist SRB: Cytologic screening and rescreening in detection and prevention of preclinical cervical cancer. Gynecol Oncol 5:121–133, 1977.
21. Bendich A, Borenfreund E, Witkin SS, et al: Information transfer and sperm uptake by mammalian somatic cells. Progr Nucl Acid Res Mol Biol 17:43–73, 1976.
22. Witkin S, Korngold GC, Bendich A: Ribonuclease-sensitive DNA-synthesizing complex in human sperm heads and seminal fluid. Proc Natl Acad Sci USA 72:3295–3299, 1975.
23. Martin EM: Marital and coital factors in cervical cancer. Am J Public Health 57:841–847, 1967.
24. Meisels A, Fortin R, Roy M: Condylomatous lesions of the cervix. II. Cytologic, colposcopic and histopathologic study. Acta Cytol 21:379–390, 1979.
25. Wentz WB, Reagan JW, Heggie AD: Cervical carcinogenesis with herpes simplex virus, Type 2. Obstet Gynecol 46:117–121, 1975.
26. zur Hausen H: Condylomata acuminata and human genital cancer. Cancer Res 36:794, 1976.
27. Pilotti S, Rilke F, Depalo G, et al: Condyloma of the uterine cervix and koilocytosis of cervical intraepithelial neoplasia. J Clin Pathol 34:532–541, 1981.
28. Feldman M, Linzey ME, Srebnik E, et al: Abnormal cervical cytology in the teenager. Am J Obstet Gynecol 126:418–421, 1976.

29. Rotkin D: A comparison of key epidemiological studies in cervical cancer related to current searches for transmissible agents. Cancer Res *33*:1353–1357, 1973.

30. Rotkin D: Adolescent coitus and cervical cancer. Association of related events with increased risk. Cancer Res *27*:603–617, 1967.

31. Hamperl H, Kaufmann C: The cervix uteri at different ages. Obstet Gynecol *14*:621–631, 1959.

32. Langley FA, Crompton AC: Epithelial Abnormalities of the Cervix Uteri. Berlin, Springer Verlag, 1973.

33. Howard L, Jr, Erickson CC, Stoddard LD: A study of the incidence and histogenesis of endocervical metaplasia and intraepithelial carcinoma. Cancer *4*:1210–1223, 1951.

34. Holzer E, Burghardt E: Die lokalisation des pathologischen cervixepithels. II. Aufsteigende Vberhauntung, plattenepithelmetaplasia und basale hyperplasia. Arch Gynecol *210*:395–415, 1971.

35. Coppleson M: The origin and nature of premalignant lesions of the cervix uteri. Int J Gynecol Obstet *8*:539–550, 1970.

36. Reid BL, Garrett WJ: Two types of squamous epithelium of the human ectocervix. A histological and colposcopic study. Austr NZ J Obstet Gynaecol *3*:1–8, 1963.

37. Coppleson M, Reid BL: Preclinical Carcinoma of the Cervix Uteri. Oxford, Pergamon Press, 1967.

38. Fluhmann CF: The Cervix Uteri and its Diseases. Philadelphia, WB Saunders, 1961.

39. Ferenczy A, Richart RM: Scanning electron microscopy of the cervical transformation zone. Am J Obstet Gynecol *115*:151–157, 1973.

40. Jordan JA, Williams AE: Scanning electron microscopy in the study of cervical neoplasia. J Obstet Gynaecol Br Commonw *78*:940–946, 1971.

41. Williams AE, Jordan JA, Allen JM, Murphy JF: The surface ultrastructure of normal and metaplastic cervical epithelia and of carcinoma in situ. Cancer Res *33*:504–513, 1973.

42. Christopherson WM, Parker JE: Microinvasive carcinoma of the cervix, in Gray LA (ed): Dysplasia, Carcinoma *in Situ* and Microinvasive Carcinoma of the Cervix Uteri. Springfield, Charles C. Thomas, 1964.

43. Jordan MJ, Bader GM, Day E: Carcinoma *in situ* of the cervix and related lesions. An 11 year prospective study. Am J Obstet Gynecol *89*:160–182, 1964.

44. Richart RM: Natural history of the cervical intraepithelial neoplasia. Clin Obstet Gynecol *10*:748–784, 1967.

45. Varga A: The relationship of cervical dysplasia to *in situ* and invasive carcinoma of the cervix. Am J Obstet Gynecol *95*:759–762, 1966.

46. Barron BA, Richart RM: A statistical model of the natural history of cervical carcinoma based on a prospective study of 557 cases. J Natl Cancer Inst *41*:1343–1353, 1968.

47. Burghardt E: Besondere Epithelbilder als Ausgangspunkt beginnend invasiven Krebswachstums an der Portio. Geburtshiffe Frauenheilkd *27*:1170–1180, 1967.

48. Barren BA, Richart RM: Statistical model of the natural history of cervical carcinoma. II. Estimates of the transition time from dysplasia to carcinoma *in situ*. J Natl Cancer Inst *45*:1025–1030, 1970.

49. Richart RM, Barron BA: A follow-up study of patients with cervical dysplasia. Am J Obstet Gynecol *105*:386–393, 1969.

159

50. Stern E, Neely PM: Dysplasia of the uterine cervix—incidence of regression, recurrence and cancer. Cancer *17*:508–512, 1964.
51. Richart RM: Cervical intraepithelial neoplasia and the cervicologist. Can J Med Tech *38*:177–180, 1980.
52. Przybora LA, Plutowa A: Histological topography of carcinoma *in situ* of the cervix uteri. Cancer *12*:268–277, 1959.
53. De Virgiliis G, Remotti G, Balzarini MP, et al: Relazione tra eta e localizzazione del carcinoma *in situ* del collo dell'utero. Ann Ostet Ginecol Med Perinat *100*:384–398, 1979.
54. Thompson BH, Woodruff DJ, Davis JH, et al: Cytopathology, histopathology, and colposcopy in the management of cervical neoplasia. Am J Obstet Gynecol *114*:329–338, 1972.
55. Coppleson M, Pixley E, Reid E: Colposcopy: A Scientific and Practical Approach to the Cervix in Health and Disease. Springfield, Charles C. Thomas, 1971.
56. Remotti G, DeVirgiliis G: La cervice uterina nelle varie eta della donna, in: La patologia della cervice uterina. Ann Ostet Ginecol Med Perinat *3*:36–45,1980.
57. Coppleson M, Reid BL: A colposcopic study of the cervix during pregnancy and the puerperium. Br J Obstet Gynaecol *73*:575–585, 1966.
58. Takeuchi A, McKay DG: Area of the cervix involved by carcinoma *in situ* and anaplasia (atypical hyperplasia). Obstet Gynecol *15*:134–145, 1960.
59. Richart MR: Colpomicroscopic studies of the distribution of dysplasia and carcinoma *in situ* on the exposed portion of the human uterine cervix. Cancer *18*:950–954, 1965.
60. Wielenga G, Old JW, Von Haam E: Squamous carcinoma *in situ* of the uterine cervix. II. Topography and clinical correlations. Cancer *18*:1612–1621, 1965.
61. Anderson MC, Hargley RB: Cervical crypt involvement by intraepithelial neoplasia. Obstet Gynecol *55*:546–550, 1980.
62. Thornton WN, Fox CH: Relationship of squamocolumnar function and endocervical gland to the site or origin of CIS of the cervix. Am J Obstet Gynecol *138*:838–839, 1980.
63. Burke L, Covell L, Antonioli D: Carbon dioxide laser therapy of cervical intraepithelial neoplasia: factor determining success rate. Lasers Surg Med *1*:113–122, 1980.
64. Bellina JH, Dunlap WP, Riopelle MA: Reliability of histopathologic diagnosis of cervical intraepithelial neoplasia. South Med J *75*:608, 1982.
65. Casteno-Almendral A, Muller H, Naujoks H, Casteno-Almendral JL: Topographical and histological localization of dysplasia, carcinoma *in situ,* microinvasion and microcarcinomata. Gynecol Oncol *1*:320–329, 1973.
66. Townsend DE, Richard RM, Marks E, Nielsen J: Invasive cancer following outpatient evaluation and therapy for cervical disease. Obstet Gynecol *57*:145–149, 1981.
67. Baggish MS: CO_2 laser for CIN, in Bellina JH (ed): Gynecologic Laser Surgery, Proceedings of the International Congress on Gynecologic Laser Surgery and Related Works, New Orleans, LA, Jan 1980. New York, Plenum Press, 1980. pp 173–196.
68. Sevin BU, Ford JH, Gurtanner RD, et al: Invasive cancer of the cervix after cryosurgery. Pitfalls of conservative management. Obstet Gynecol *53*:465–471, 1979.
69. Griffiths CT, Austin JH, Younge PA: Punch biopsy of the cervix. Am J Obstet Gynecol *88*:695–703, 1964.
70. Townsend DE, Ostergard DR, Mishell DR, Hirose FM: Abnormal papanicolaou smears. Evaluation by colposcopy, biopsies, and endocervical curettage. Am J Obstet Gynecol *108*:429–434, 1970.

71. Ostegard DR: Cryosurgery treatment of cervical intraepithelial neoplasia. Obstet Gynecol *56*:231–233, 1980.

72. Bellina JH, Gyer DR, Voros JI, Raviotta JJ: Capillary hemangioma managed by the CO_2 laser. Obstet Gynecol *55*:129, 1980.

73. Cashman BZ: The role of deep cauterization in the prevention of cancer of the cervix. Am J Obstet Gynecol *41*:216–224, 1941.

74. Peyton FW, Peyton RR, Anderson VL, et al: The importance of cauterization to maintain a healthy cervix. Am J Obstet Gynecol *131*:374–380, 1978.

75. Payne FL: The treatment of leukorrhea. Am J Obstet Gynecol *17*:841–848, 1929.

76. Krantz KE: Discussion of Stafl's laser treatment of cervical and vaginal neoplasia. Am J Obstet Gynecol *128*:134–136, 1977.

77. Sharp F, MacLean AB, More A, Murray EL: Quantitated laser-tissue destruction and the development of a technique for treating cervical intraepithelial neoplasia, in Bellina JH (ed): Gynecologic Laser Surgery, Proceedings of the International Congress on Gynecologic Laser Surgery and Related Works, New Orleans, LA, Jan 1980. New York, Plenum Press, 1980, pp 231–244.

78. Bellina JH, Seto YJ: Pathological and physical investigations into CO_2 laser tissue interactions with specific emphasis on cervical intraepithelial neoplasm. Lasers Surg Med *1*:47–69, 1980.

79. Lisfrac J: Memoire sur une nouvelle methode de practique l' operation de la taille chez des femmes. Gaz Med France *2*:835, 1815.

80. Dorsey JH, Diggs ES: Microsurgical conization of the cervix by carbon dioxide laser. Obstet Gynecol *54*:565–570, 1979.

81. Carter R, Krantz KE, Hara G, et al: Treatment of cervical intraepithelial neoplasia with the carbon dioxide laser beam. Am J Obstet Gynecol *131*:831–836, 1978.

82. Mihashi S, Jako CJ, Incze J, et al: Laser surgery in otolaryngology: interaction of CO_2 laser and soft tissue. Ann NY Acad Sci *267*:263–294, 1974.

83. Verschueren R: The CO_2 Laser in Tumor Surgery. Assen, Amsterdam, Van Gorcum 1976, pp 38–47.

84. Dorsey JH: Excisional biopsy and conization of the cervix, in CR Wheeless (ed): An Atlas of Pelvic Surgery. Philadelphia, Lea and Febiger, 1981, pp 157–159.

85. Baggish MS, Dorsey JH: CO_2 laser for the treatment of vulvar carcinoma *in situ*. Obstet Gynecol *57*:371–375, 1981.

86. Dorsey JH, Diggs ES, Baggish MS: Cytourethroscopy with the direct view contac endoscope. Obstet Gynecol *57*:115–118, 1981.

87. Bellina JH, Voros JI, Kurpel J: Carbon dioxide laser microsurgery in gynecology, in Kaplan I (ed): Proceedings, II International Symposium on Laser Surgery, Dallas, TX, Oct 1977. Jerusalem, Jerusalem Academic Press, 1978.

88. Holmquist N, Bellina J, Danos M: Vaginal and cervical cytological changes following laser treatment. Acta Cytol *20*:290–294, 1976.

89. Baggish MS: High power density carbon dioxide laser therapy for early cervical neoplasia. Am J Obstet Gynecol *136*:117–125, 1980.

90. Jordan JA, Mylotte MS: The treatment of cervical intraepithelial neoplasia by CO_2 laser vaporization, in Bellina JH (ed): Gynecologic Laser Surgery, Proceedings of the International Congress on Gynecologic Laser Surgery and Related Works, New Orleans, LA, Jan 1980. New York, Plenum Press, 1980, pp 245–252.

91. Bellina JH, Wright VC, Voros JI, et al: CO_2 laser management of intraepithelial neoplasia. Am J Obstet Gynecol *141*:828–832, 1981.

161

92. Baggish MS: Carbon dioxide laser treatment for condyloma acuminata venereal infections. Obstet Gynecol *55*:711–715, 1980.
93. Stafl A, Wilkinson EJ, Mattingly RT: Laser treatment of cervical and vaginal neoplasia. Am J Obstet Gynecol *128*:128–136, 1977.
94. Masterson BJ, Krantz KE, Calkins JW, et al: The carbon dioxide laser in cervical intraepithelial neoplasia. Am J Obstet Gynecol *139*:565–567, 1981.
95. Popkin DR: The CO_2 laser in the treatment of CIN, in Bellina JH (ed): Gynecologic Laser Surgery, Proceedings of the International Congress on Gynecologic Laser Surgery and Related Works, New Orleans, LA, January 1980. New York, Plenum Press, 1980, pp 119–130.
96. Benedet JL, Nickerson KG, White GW: Laser therapy for cervical intraepithelial neoplasia. Obstet Gynecol *58*:188–191, 1981.
97. Dorsey J: Cervical healing after laser conization, in Bellina JH (ed): Gynecologic Laser Surgery, New York, Plenum Press, 1981, pp 131–143.
98. Grundsell H, Alm P, Larsson G: Laser conization versus cold knife conization. A prospective, randomized study, in Atsumi K, Nimsakul N (eds): Proceedings IV International Congress, Society for Laser Surgery, Tokyo, Japan, November 1981, Inter Group Corp, 1982, pp 13/15–13/16.
99. Sadoul G, Beuret T: About 40 conizations with the CO_2 laser, in Atsumi K, Nimsakul N (eds): Proceedings IV International Congress, Society for Laser Surgery, Tokyo, Japan, November 23–27, 1981, Inter Group Corp, 1982, pp 13/17–13/20.
100. Baggish MS: Complications associated with carbon dioxide laser surgery in gynecology. Am J Obstet Gynecol *139*:568–574, 1981.
101. Coupez F, Legros R: Traitment des lesions du col uterin par le laser. Un experience de 18 mois. Gynecologie *32*:57–61, 1981.
102. Mazur P: Cryobiology: the freezing biological systems. Science *168*:939–949, 1970.
103. Creasman WT, Need JC, Curry SL, et al: Efficacy of cryosurgical treatment of severe cervical intraepithelial neoplasia. Obstet Gynecol *41*:501–506, 1973.
104. Tredway DR, Townsend DE, Howland DN, Upton RT: Colposcopy and cryosurgery in cervical intraepithelial neoplasia. Am J Obstet Gynecol *114*:1020–1024, 1972.
105. Townsend DE, Ostergard DR: Cryocauterization for preinvasive cervical neoplasia. J Reprod Med *6*:171–176, 1971.
106. Kaufman RM, Irwin JF: The cryosurgical therapy of cervical intraepithelial neoplasia. III. Continuing followup. J Obstet Gynecol *131*:381–388, 1978.
107. Popkin DR, Scali V, Ahmed MN: Cryosurgery for the treatment of cervical intraepithelial neoplasia. Am J Obstet Gynecol *130*:551–554, 1978.
108. Wright VC: Observations regarding patients diagnosed with CIN. The use of cryosurgery and CO_2 laser, in Bellina JH (ed): Gynecologic Laser Surgery, Proceedings of the International Congress on Gynecologic Laser Surgery and Related Works, New Orleans, LA, January 1980. New York, Plenum Press, 1980, pp 217–230.
109. Ostergard DR: Cryosurgery treatment of cervical intraepithelial neoplasia. Obstet Gynecol *56*:231–233, 1980.
110. MacVicar J, Willocks J: The effect of diathermy conization of the cervix on subsequent fertility, pregnancy and delivery. J Obstet Gynaecol Br Commonw *75*:355–356, 1968.
111. Chanen W, Hollyock VE: Colposcopy and the conservative management of cervical dysplasias and carcinoma *in situ*. Obstet Gynecol *43*:527–534, 1974.
112. Hollyock VE, Chanen W: Electrocoagulation diathermy for the treatment of cervical dysplasia and carcinoma *in situ*. Obstet Gynecol *47*:196–199, 1976.

113. Beard RW: Diathermy coning and cautery in the treatment of the eroded cervix. J Obstet Gynaecol Br Commonw *71*:287–292, 1964.

114. Peyton FW, Rosen NA: Cervical cauterization and carcinoma of the cervix. Am J Obstet Gynecol *86*:111–119, 1963.

115. Kolstad P: Diagnosis and management of precancerous lesions of the cervix uteri. Int J Gynecol Obstet *8*:551–560, 1970.

116. Creasman WT, Rutledge F: Carcinoma *in situ* of the cervix. Obstet Gynecol *40*:373–380, 1972.

117. Kolstad P, Klein V: Long term followup of 1121 cases of carcinoma *in situ*. Am J Obstet Gynecol *48*:125–129, 1976.

118. Ostergard DR, Morton DG: Multifocal carcinoma of the female genitals. Am J Obstet Gynecol *99*:1006–1015, 1965.

119. Ostergard DR, Gondos B: Outpatient therapy of preinvasive cervical neoplasia; selection of patients with the use of colposcopy. Am J Obstet Gynecol *115*:783–788, 1973.

120. Hollyock VE, Chanen W: The use of the colposcope in the selection of patients for cervical cone biopsy. Am J Obstet Gynecol *114*: 185–189, 1972.

121. Krumholz BA, Knapp RC: Colposcopic selection of biopsy sites. Obstet Gynecol *39*:22–26, 1972.

122. Holzer E: Conservative treatment of carcinoma *in situ:* a clinical report concerning 866 cases after conization. Obstet Gynecol Surv *34*:870–871, 1979.

123. Phillips JC: Public health aspects of critical care medicine and anesthesiology, Anesth Mortal Clin Anesth *10*:220, 1974.

124. Special Committee Investigating Deaths Under Anesthesia: Report on 745 classified cases, 1960–1968. Med J Aust *1*:573, 1970.

125. Silbar EL, Woodruff JD: Evaluation of biopsy, cone and hysterectomy sequence in intraepithelial carcinoma of the cervix. Obstet Gynecol *27*:89–97, 1966.

126. Garcia RL, Bigelow B, Demoupoulos RI, Beckman EM: Evaluation of cone biopsy in management of carcinoma *in situ* of the cervix. Gynecol Oncol *3*:32–39, 1975.

127. Hester LL, Reed RA: An evaluation of cervical conization. Obstet Gynecol *80*:715–721, 1960.

128. Jones JM, Sweetman P, Hibbard BM: The outcome of pregnancy after cone biopsy of the cervix. A case–control study. Br J Obstet Gynaecol *86*:913–916, 1979.

129. Leimen G, Harrison NA, Rubin A: Pregnancy following conization of the cervix. Complications related to cone size. Am J Obstet Gynecol *136*:14–18, 1980.

130. Onroos J, Keukko P, Kilkku P, Punnonen R: Pregnancy and delivery after conization of the cervix. Acta Obstet Gynecol Scand *5*:477–480, 1979.

131. Davis RM, Cooke JK, Kirk RF: Cervical conization. Obstet Gynecol *40*:23–27, 1972.

132. Villasanta U, Durkin JP: Indications and complications of cold knife conization of the cervix. Obstet Gynecol *27*:717–723, 1966.

133. Attili A, DePalo G: La conizzazione non e un trattamento che assicuri la conservazione della fertilita, in Catanna VC (ed): Proceedings, II Congress of the Society for Italian Surgical Oncology, Florence, Nov 9–10, 1978. Milan, National Cancer Institute, 1978, pp 323–326.

134. Kullander S, Sjoberg NO: Treatment of carcinoma *in situ* of the cervix by conization. A five year followup. Acta Obstet Gynecol Scand *50*:153–157, 1971.

135. Lee NH: The effect of cone biopsy on subsequent pregnancy outcome. Gynecol Oncol *6*:1–6, 1978.

136. Boyes DA, Worth AJ, Fidler HK: The results of treatment of 4389 cases of preclinical cervical squamous carcinoma. J Obstet Gynaecol Br Commonw *77*:769–780, 1970.
137. Bjerre B, Eliasson G, Linell F, et al: Conization as only treatment of carcinoma *in situ* of the uterine cervix. Am J Obstet Gynecol *125*: 143–152, 1976.
138. Toaff R: Use of carbon dioxide laser in gynecological surgery, in Kaplan I, Ascher PW (eds): Proceedings III International Congress Laser Surgery, Graz Sept 1979. Tel Aviv, OT, PAZ, 1979, pp 235–238.
139. Shafir R, Zweig A, Slutzki S, Bornstein L: A use of the carbon dioxide laser in an abdominoperineal resection for epidermoid anal carcinoma: a case report. Br J Surg *65*:565–566, 1978.
140. Heinzl S: Cervical intraepithelial neoplasia degree III: laser therapy yes or no? in: Bellina JH (ed): Gynecologic Laser Surgery, Proceedings of the International Congress on Gynecologic Laser Surgery and Related Works, New Orleans, LA, Jan 1980. New York, Plenum Press, 1980, pp 145–150.

5

Laser Surgery of the Vagina, Vulva, and Extragenital Areas

5.1. Introduction

Carbon dioxide laser therapy has clearly demonstrated its superiority when compared to other conventional methods of therapy for treating vaginal lesions. Lesions in the vagina, which were often overlooked by the gynecologist, are now receiving the attention they warrant. The vagina, with its many rugae, makes close scrutiny a task for the colposcope; however, careful manipulation and spreading of the rugae with a vaginal speculum allow for an easier and more thorough examination. Since the cervix and upper 80% of the vagina originate from the mullerian ducts, lesions affecting the cervix may also appear in the vaginal vault. Conventional surgical methods used for treatment of such lesions have proved to be difficult and less effective because of the limited operating space and obscured areas. The rigidity of the scalpel hinders the surgeon's technique and often produces unwanted effects. Laser treatment has drastically reduced the incidence of complications associated with conventional surgical methods in this complex surgical field (i.e., urethral vesical or rectovaginal fistulae, hematomas, hemorrhage, sloughing of grafts, and/or stenosis with impaired sexual activity).

Dysplasias, carcinoma in situ, condylomatous warts, and vaginal adenosis have been effectively treated with CO_2 vaporization procedures. Viral papillomas, which can be associated with dysplasia, can be identified histologically by biopsy. Lesions which border on carcinoma in situ are difficult

165

to cure and tend to recur. The recurrence rates are similar when one compares conventional surgery with CO_2 laser surgery. However, the CO_2 laser surgery allows retreatment, as often as is necessary to cure the disease, without the morbidity associated with scarring or deformity. Neither stenosis, vesical or rectal fistulae, nor dyspareunia have been noted[1] following CO_2 laser treatment for benign or malignant vaginal tumors. The precision of CO_2 laser treatment allows for ablation of the entire lesion to the desired depth and width, under constant visual microscopic control. This requires careful observation through the colposcope and recognition of the intervening tissue planes.

The areas which can be most advantageously treated with the laser are the fornices and the vaginal vault, because these areas are difficult to treat with conventional methods. Cytologic and histologic examinations prior to therapy are always required. By using 3–4% acetic acid and then Lugol's solution, the borders of the lesion are definitively outlined, allowing for accurate excision.

Either laser microsurgical vaporization or excisional modes can be used for treatment of vaginal lesions. Power output between 10 and 20 W and a power density of 600–900 W/cm^2 are recommended. Transverse electromagnetic mode 00 (TEM$_{00}$) and TEM$_{10}$ of the laser beam have been used to treat vaginal and vulvar lesions.

Adequate tension of the vaginal walls is obtained by using a vaginal speculum. In this way one obtains a smooth surface and better control of beam–tissue interaction; this also prevents the burning of unnecessary areas. A small mirror, such as a laryngeal mirror, is used to deflect the beam laterally; this is especially useful when treating narrow vaginal anatomy, so that one may avoid tangential heating by the laser beam.

Varicose veins in the vagina are not uncommon and must be approached with care. Hemorrhage may occur from a varices, but it can be managed by engaging the usual methods of hemostasis: suture or electrocautery.

5.2. Vaginal Applications

5.2.1. Adenosis

Adenosis was the first gynecologic disease to be treated with the laser. It is frequently found as a mucosal abnormality in adolescents who were exposed to synthetic estrogens during fetal life[2] and represents a theoretical risk for malignant degeneration into clear cell adenocarcinoma.[3,4] This type of lesion is usually symptomatic and is often accompanied by a serosanguinous discharge. The treatment of this disease is the same as for vaginal dysplasia and requires repeated colposcopic examinations in the follow-up period. The expenses involved with hospitalization; postoperative sequelae, such as dyspareunia and dilatation; and to the psychological trauma are among the problems frequently encountered following conventional therapy.

Laser CO_2 vaporization may be indicated when the lesion involves the posterior fornix and/or cervicovaginal junction. These areas are very difficult to treat with traditional methods. Actually the case reports[1,5,6] clearly demonstrate that the colposcopically directed application of the CO_2 laser beam is better controlled and superior to other thermal methods such as electrosurgery and cryosurgery, and it is also superior to excision with the cold knife. The area can be easily ablated by the CO_2 laser and adenosis may be removed with little difficulty and almost no bleeding. Furthermore, hospitalization is unnecessary.

Local or general anesthesia or, in many cases, no palliative may be used, but this depends upon the extent and location of the lesion. Lesions in the upper 80% of the vagina usually do not require anesthesia, while lesions in the lower 20% of the vagina usually do. The patient's threshold for pain tolerance is, however, the final deciding factor.

The vaginal mucosa heals without mutilating scar formation following laser destruction. This important property of laser CO_2 surgery was first reported by Strong and Jako with their experience in vocal cord surgery.[7] Actually neither stenosis, synechia, obstetrical dystocia, nor dyspareunia has been noted. In the previous series no histologically confirmed recurrences were found.[1,8] However, the lack of a means of histologic examination of the entire lesion requires thorough and expert presurgical cytologic and colposcopic evaluation in the obtaining of a representative tissue biopsy specimen. Careful follow-up allows one to easily recognize and retreat small areas that were missed in the initial treatment.

5.2.2. Dystrophy and Neoplasia

Vaginal granulation, following lacerations and accompanied by dyspareunia and postcoital bleeding, as well as dysplasia, carcinoma in situ, and warty dysplasias of the vagina, can be treated with the same technique. Depth of tissue penetration can be controlled without causing injury to the bladder or rectum.[9] The depth of destruction and power density depend on the histologic type of lesion.

Superficial lesions such as granulation tissues can be treated at a relatively low power density (300–400 W/cm^2), while intermediate power output of 600–800 W/cm^2 and 2–3 mm depth is considered sufficient for ablation of condylomata and dysplasias. When the diagnosis is carcinoma in situ, it is advisable to submit the entire lesion for histologic study. This kind of lesion, as well as the dysplastic lesion, requires deeper destruction (3 mm) and higher power densities (1000–1200 W/cm^2). Palliative treatment can be carried out for invasive, primary, or metastatic vaginal carcinoma, with the elimination of bleeding or malodorous discharge.

Hahn[10] reported a case of a 73-year-old patient with chronic bleeding and vaginal telangiectasia. Treatment with the CO_2 laser achieved coagulation of the superficial vaginal vessels and complete remission of symptoms.

Previous reports demonstrated[8] a high recurrence rate (28%) after a 3-mm-deep vaporization for vaginal intraepithelial neoplasia. Careful attention must be given to treating older women with atrophic vaginal walls. Deeper destruction can be approached only in young women with estrogenized mucosa, where the risk of fistula is somewhat reduced.

Better results have been recently reported[11] in the treatment of a group of patients with vaginal intraepithelial neoplasia. The treatment was successful in 1 of 10 patients with the CO_2 laser, while the results from a comparative group treated with topical 5-fluorouracil were not as favorable. Carbon dioxide laser treatment was performed at 3–4 mm of estimated depth, and no local complications were reported.

Finally, CO_2 laser techniques have a number of advantages when one compares them to conventional surgery for procedures such as partial or total vaginectomy.

5.2.3. Postoperative Care and Follow-up

During the postoperative period only minimal analgesics may be required. There can be a serosanguineous discharge which may be odorous. The use of an antiseptic vaginal cream is sometimes prescribed to reduce the possibility of secondary infections.

Vaginal dilation is contraindicated because of the trauma that would be imposed on delicate, healing tissues. However, when extensive lasing must be performed, a vaginal dilator may be necessary. Granulation tissue has been observed on occasion and can be removed with chemical cautery or a repeat of the lasering treatment. Healing time varies from 4 to 6 weeks. Vaginal douching, intercourse, and the use of tampons should be avoided for at least

2–3 weeks. Intravaginal manipulation should be performed only by the surgeon, preferably 10–14 days after laser treatment.

Follow-up Pap smears and colposcopy should be performed at 2–6 weeks to evaluate the healing process. During the first year, the patient should be evaluated cytologically and colposcopically every 3 months. Persistent disease can then be identified and retreated if necessary. Thereafter, the patient should be seen every 6 months until healing is complete and no abnormal pathology is present.

5.2.4. Reconstruction

5.2.4.a. Longitudinal Vaginal Septum In defects resulting from unfused mullerian ducts, the laser is used to cut and vaporize the vaginal septum. To perform this dissection we use the operating microscope with micromanipulator with power densities of up to 10,000 W/cm^2. The magnification allows for precise dissection and rapid identification of microbleeders and, if bleeding results, a monopolar high-frequency current is used.

Postoperatively no vaginal packing, tampons, creams, or douches are allowed for the first 3 weeks. The patient is seen in 10 days and gently examined. By the third to fourth week healing is complete and coitus may be resumed.

To date, we have performed this procedure on three women with no complications.

5.2.4.b. Transverse Vaginal Septum We have seen two cases of transverse vaginal septum. As this septum acts as a barrier to sperm transport, we use the laser to resect the tissue. Transverse vaginal phenomenal septum occurs in approximately 1 of 80,000 females. The procedure is carried out by placing a No. 5 Foley catheter through the septum aperture and distending it. General anesthesia is used. Traction on the catheter allows for septal-vaginal junction identification. We prefer to use the microscope with the micromanipulator as described in Section 5.2.4.a. Bleeding is not usually encountered but can be easily controlled by monopolar high-frequency current. The vaginal mucosa does not need to be sutured unless a large defect remains.

Postoperative patients should refrain from intercourse for 6 weeks. As with other vaginal procedures, no tampons or intravaginal creams are recommended. However, douching with warm water after the third week is permitted.

5.2.4.c. Gartner's Duct Cyst and Other Vaginal Inclusion Cysts The cyst is exposed using nonreflective instruments. If the cyst is small it can be totally vaporized. However, when large cystic structures are treated we prefer the following technique.

Anesthesia is not generally required. First, set the power density to 800–1000 W/cm^2. Next, incise the cyst wall to create an oval or circular window. Complete the excision and submit the specimen for histopathologic analysis. Culture the cystic fluid using aerobic and anaerobic media. Occasionally we have detected gonococcal organisms in benign-appearing vaginal wall cysts. The cysts should now look like hard-boiled eggs with the ends cut off. To complete the procedure, change the power density to 100–300 W/cm^2 and irradiate the inner aspect of the cyst wall. This irradiation will photocoagulate the remaining secretory cells.

Postoperative instructions include abstinence from intercourse for 21 days. Warm water douche can be used after the first examination indicates that healing is adequate. We prefer to perform this examination approximately 7–10 days after surgery. The healing phase is rapid and does not result in vaginal narrowing or scar formation. We do not recommend vaginal dilatation. To date, we have had no complications or complaints from patients treated in such a fashion.

5.3. Vulvar Applications

5.3.1. Introduction

Vulvar tissues are subject to a number of diseases, which can be due to infections, irritants, injury, cellular changes, or venereal diseases. Lesions of the vulva and the perineum can be treated with the CO_2 laser with equal effectiveness (Table 5.1). Unfortunately, patients, for many reasons, fail to seek medical assistance until the disease is in advanced stages. When disease is treated in the early stages, most patients experience little or no surgical discomfort, and minimal postsurgical problems (i.e., scarring or disfigurement). Viral diseases, which have been present for some time, do cause problems for the gynecologist, both in effecting a cure and with regard to extent of the surgery involved. The general principles that apply to disease of the cervical epithelium also apply to the epidermis of the vulva. The terminology of the International Society for the Study of Vulvar Disease has been used in this text.

The CO_2 laser is the instrument of choice for treatment of several kinds of lesions. The method of CO_2 laser treatment for exophytic and nonexophy-

Table 5.1. CO₂ Laser Applications for Disease of the Vulva

Dystrophy
    Hypoplastic (formerly lichen sclerosus, atrophic vulvitis, kraurosis, etc.)
    Hyperplastic (formerly hypertrophic vulvitis, neurodermatitis, leukoplakia, etc.)
        Without atypia
        With atypia: mild, moderate, severe
    Mixed (lesions that contain both hypoplastic and hyperplastic areas)
        Without atypia
        With atypia: mild, moderate, severe
Intraepithelial neoplasia
    Carcinoma in situ (formerly Bowen's disease, erythroplasia of Queyrat,
        carcinoma simplex)
    Paget's disease (a distinct clinicopathologic entity)
Condyloma acuminatum
Inclusion cyst
Papillomata
Herpes simplex virus type II
Hemangioma
Hyperplastic labia minora

tic condylomata acuminata viral lesions and other sexually transmitted diseases, such as herpes simplex virus, type II, and molluscum contagiosum, is described in the following section. Complete ablation of the lesions eliminates the disease, but the patient must be made aware of the venereal nature of the disease and cautioned against reinfection by her partner.

5.3.2. Preoperative Analysis

As with any intraepidermal pathology, the precise histologic cell type, extent of surface involvement, and depth of penetration are critical in the preoperative work-up. All vulvar lesions are thoroughly examined under magnification and by palpation. Appropriate biopsy specimens are taken. Toludine blue stain is used to help increase diagnostic efficiency.

Anesthesia is used as needed: general, conduction, or local. The extent of the lesion governs the selection of anesthesia. Small discrete lesions can be managed with a local anesthetic, while a superficial "skinning" vulvectomy requires either general or regional anesthesia. The steps necessary for accurate prelaser evaluation of vulvar lesions include:

1. Identification of lesion
2. Colposcopy and photography
3. Toludine blue test
4. Histologic confirmation

5.3.3. Dystrophic and Neoplastic Lesions

Premalignant in situ lesions of the vulva[12-14] and invasive neoplasia or dystrophic lesions can require treatment of a small area or the entire vulva by CO_2 laser ablation. The results have been low recurrence rates, relief of symptoms, and progressive rehealing, with conservation of the anatomy and normal function.[12,15,16]

Bowen's disease is frequently multicentric and radical surgery usually results in severe deformity. Laser surgery, however, can preserve the normal contours of the vulva, while the diseased area can be radically vaporized or excised. The necessity for histologic confirmation must be emphasized in order to rule out tumor invasion before laser vaporization can be undertaken.

Hyperplastic dystrophy, lichen sclerosus, and mixed dystrophy are characterized by alterations of the epithelial surface growth with or without atypia and can be considered precancerous lesions.[17] Although the matter remains controversial, only 1–2% of these lesions have been shown to develop into carcinoma in situ over long periods of time. Intractable pruritus and tissue breakdown, however, often cause great discomfort to the patient.

Vulvar dystrophy, with or without atypia, is best treated by deepithelializing the entire labial surfaces. The technique employed is most important. Many authors have written and discussed their experiences with vulvar disease and the laser. The management is based on the biophysics of the laser and its tissue interaction. If patients are followed up carefully, the postoperative discomfort which has been reported often, can be considerably reduced. After accurate diagnostic evaluation, including specific stains and biopsy for histologic confirmation, even where conventional therapeutic attempts[18,19] have failed, CO_2 laser ablation of the dystrophic tissue can achieve a successful result and can be used repeatedly, under a local anesthetic if necessary.

Should a more advanced disease be suspected, the method given for carcinoma in situ of the vulva should be used. If it is required, definitive therapy for microinvasive or frank invasive carcinoma can be scheduled.

5.3.4. Premalignant Disease and Degenerative Dystrophia

The patient is placed in the dorsal lithotomy position. Aqueous solution may be used to prep the perineum. Next, outline the outer limits of the zone to be deepithelialized using 500 W/cm^2. Then outline the inner limits of the resection. It may be helpful to divide the area of excision into quadrants. Power output of 10–15 W is required for vulvar excision or vaporization relative to the desired depth. Adjust the power density to 500–800 W/cm^2. These power settings with 2-mm spot size are suggested for precise technique through the operating microscope.

Begin the raster approach to deepithelialization as outlined in the cervix (x-y-z). A deepithelialization of 2–3 mm should be performed with rapid sweeps of the laser beam. A uniform depth of ablation of 3 mm and 4 mm beyond the margins of the lesions is recommended to remove the lesion effectively to its base. Do not create a carbonized field. If excessive carbonization begins to develop, increase your power density, sweep the beam at a more rapid rate, and clean the area with a wet sponge or use irrigation. Do not continue to raster the same areas without allowing sufficient time for tissue cooling. The perineal lesions can be treated at the same time; this includes the perirectal areas. In a two-stage operation (i.e., hemivulvectomy is not performed) the entire vulva can be treated. This is very important in ensuring that diseased areas are not missed.

5.3.5. Carcinoma in Situ

The diagnosis of carcinoma in situ of the vulva, like that of so many diseases of the female genitalia, is increasing. Whether the increase is due to a better educated public and a more acute awareness of health and hygiene, or to more advanced, sophisticated diagnostic techniques is not certain. It is probably a combination of these and the fact that society has become more sexually permissive. Nevertheless, the rates of such disorders continue to climb.

The CO_2 laser can be used to manage carcinoma in situ of the vulva, as this is a slowly developing tumor. Conservatism and caution are the key words. Repeated treatments can be performed without the untoward effects of conventional surgery.

5.3.6. Primary or Secondary Invasive Neoplastic Lesions

Successful radical vulvectomy resection and vaporization of recurrent lesions have been reported[20] for primary or secondary invasive neoplastic lesions. Carbon dioxide laser surgery is especially useful in treating patients of advanced age, patients with severe medical problems, such as diabetes, or patients who require anticoagulant therapy. These are poor candidates for traditional surgery because of delayed healing time; they are subject to secondary infections and, therefore, septicemia is a threat.

In spite of the extended surgical time, the hemostatic properties of the CO_2 laser, the lack of wound infection during healing, and the ease of application indicate the choice of this method of treatment. When a radical vulvectomy is performed (with histologic confirmation) healing after laser treatment has been reported, in some cases, in 6 weeks.[21] Furthermore, the treated areas are tender but have minimal to no scarring without obvious damage to the structure. The original anatomic configuration has been preserved; intercourse can be resumed without difficulty, while other surgical methods result in sexual dysfunction and stenosis.

5.3.7. Procedure

First the lesion is preoperatively evaluated by the techniques presented for vulvar dystrophy. When the diagnosis is definitive for carcinoma in situ, it is advisable to have the entire lesion available for histologic study. To accomplish this, each lesion and a margin of excision 5 mm beyond its periphery is undercut with the laser to a depth of 4–5 mm. This tissue is excised with the laser beam using a power density of 800–1200 W/cm^2, lifted off with Allis forceps, and submitted for microscopic evaluation. Higher power densities of 1400 W/cm^2 are required for deeper resection procedure. The edges of the resection are smoothed using the laser. The depth of tissue destruction or removal determines the success of the surgery, and adequate depth is important for cure. It must be recognized also that, in the vulva, excess depth of destruction produces complications, lengthens healing time, and increases scarring. Should bleeding occur, then high frequency is used for coagulation. The specimen is then submitted for histologic confirmation of in situ carcinoma. Should the specimen contain an invasive carcinoma, appropriate management should then be undertaken.

The lateral extent of tissue destruction accomplished at one operation depends upon the condition of the patient and the judgement of the surgeon. The labia majora and minora, clitoral area, perineum, and perianal region can be treated in one surgical procedure. However, this may be too extensive for some patients' tolerance. Removing the lesion in stages with either a local or general anesthetic may be preferable for most patients.

5.3.8. Tissue Reaction

The immediate appearance of the vulva at the operative site is one of desiccated tissue with charring. Induration, exudation, and edema follow after 24 hr. On the third day a gray necrotic membrane forms over the operative field. Some investigators have reported that when both sides of the introitus have been lased at the same time the tissue may agglutinate with fine adhesions. This complication is probably a reflection of excessive depth of destruction, and scarring may occur in addition to agglutination. Digital separation facilitates proper healing and drainage of exudate retained in the vagina. Topical estrogen can be applied to the adhesions, and gentle traction will separate the tissue.

5.3.9. Postoperative Management

The lased site should be considered as a thermal burn even though the heat coagulum zone may only extend 600 μm below the impact site. Various medications have been employed to encourage primary healing, but isotonic saline soaks in a whirlpool or pulsator apparatus are now recommended. Patients may experience moderate discomfort for the first 24 hr. In cases of extensive dissection for severe vulvar disease, micturition may become difficult. Occasionally, catheterization has been required to alleviate the dysuria.

With complete reepithelialization there is restoration of the normal anatomic architecture. Strictures, when they do occur, are minimal. When this technique is properly executed, scarring is not a problem. Edema and induration subside in 10–12 days. Sloughing of the eschar with complete healing takes 4–6 weeks. As with cervical and vaginal lesions, recurrence of disease depends on adequate eradication of all foci of the principal and associated lesions. Rates of persistent disease following laser therapy vary with the type and extent of the disease, but the effectiveness of treatment with the modality is in each instance comparable or superior to conventional treatment. Additionally, the preservation of normal anatomic configuration and the absence of disfigurement and scarring are important benefits of laser therapy for vulvar disease.

A preoperative explanation of the postoperative care is optimal as it will probably promote greater adherence to the care. Patients should be told of the possibility of minor discomfort or a burning sensation. Mild oral analgesics are usually ordered, or Xerofom® may be applied topically. A Foley or suprapubic catheter may be inserted to eliminate pain when voiding. Today, as well as in the past, a urinary catheter is not recommended unless voiding becomes impossible. Again, if the surgeon adheres to the principle of rapid beam movement and tissue cooling, pain and urinary retention can be kept at a minimum.

Prior to discharge, patients must receive printed instructions for self-care at home, including a list of abnormalities in healing which warrant contacting the physician. The need for inpatient care is directly proportional to the extensiveness of the surgery.

Since the healing course after treatment of small lesions is rapid, the patient can be discharged within 24 hr. In most cases, by day 13 complete reepithelialization of the vulvar treated area is noted and all discomfort has ceased. But recovery may vary considerably from patient to patient.

A total cutaneous vulvectomy will usually require a 1- to 3-day hospital stay. It is usually advantageous to begin these instructions before and after admission so that areas of confusion may be resolved. The instructions include:

No intercourse until healed
Cornstarch for itching
Cotton panties, only if necessary
Sitz bath two or three times daily
Irrigation of the perineum with povidone–iodine solution
Hair dryer used to dry perineum
Water bottle for voiding
Stool softeners
Tucks® or witchhazel pads
Perineal lamps

On the first postoperative day we begin whirlpool baths. These are administered three times a day. They not only wash away dead tissue and promote healing, but also relieve the stricture of healing tissue. Perineal lamps aid in keeping the vulvar surface dry. Patients are advised to bring a hair dryer to the hospital and are then taught to use the dryer, set on cool, to dry the perineal area, while standing with one leg up on a chair. The hair dryer will reduce moisture and should be used after bathing or voiding. (Caution: all electrical equipment brought into the hospital must be checked by the Biomedical Engineering Department prior to use.) Perineal irrigation and cool air drying are used after micturition and defecation. Witchhazel-impregnated cotton swabs are used after defecation. In some cases, oral analgesics are prescribed, and may be required for up to 3 weeks following surgery.

Patients are advised not to wear underwear during the initial postoperative period. Once they have been discharged, if they feel it is necessary to wear panties, only cotton panties may be used. Labial fusion is not a problem and digital separation may be sufficient. The patient may complain of minor itching associated with the healing process, or that her panties stick to the healing. Cornstarch and normal saline may be used for this complaint, but the patient must be cautioned against using any scented talcums. Providing a mirror for the patient to visualize the postoperative site usually helps allay her anxiety, as she can see the progressive healing.

Laser surgery has been noted to produce excellent healing and return of normal organ function. Patients experience a minimum of discharge and very few patients have delayed bleeding, pain, or other adverse reactions. Persistent disease is rare, but can easily be retreated. As for carcinoma in situ, since these lesions are relatively small, the use of lasers has proven to be effective. The treatment and care are the same as those described in Section 5.3.3.

5.3.10. Complications, Results, and Follow-up

After the vaporization procedure the postoperative courses are free of complications and patients receive only mild oral analgesics. Fever can develop within the second day, but will respond to antibiotics; on the third day, edema and a subtle necrotic membrane form in the treated area. The white exudate is usually sterile.

We have now found that in extensive perineal deepithelialization immediate intraoperative treatment with Decadron® (dexamethasone; 4 mg intravenously, 4 mg intramuscularly) followed by 5 g methylprednisolone given orally three times a day, will prevent the excessive postoperative edema and the rare pyrexic response. The pyrexic phenomenon can be quite alarming to the physician if it has not been previously encountered. It usually develops 1–3 hr postoperatively with temperature elevation to 102°F. We believe this is probably due to the surface destruction and release of histamines or histaminelike substances. It has not been found to be a bacterial response. More investigations are needed to determine its exact etiology.

Lobraico[16] reports a series of 27 cases of vulvar dystrophy treated with the CO_2 laser. The end results were encouraging and advantageous when compared to the failure rate of conventional techniques. Since the premalignant and neoplastic lesions, even multicentric lesions,[23] tend to recur after treatment, the patient must be examined every 3 months for the first year, and thereafter every 6 months.

In a case of invasive vulvar carcinoma managed by the carbon dioxide laser, the reporting physician stated that a hemivulvectomy (cutaneous type) was performed for a carcinoma in situ on the posterior fourchette. The patient was instructed to return in 6 weeks to complete the other side. However, due to an extremely harsh winter, the patient did not return for 6 months, at which time the other side was treated. Later a lesion was noted in the posterior fourchette and diagnosed as invasive carcinoma. This case illustrates the need for completing the management in a single stage and appropriate follow-up examinations.

Recurrent lesions of vulvar dysplasia, carcinoma in situ, or invasive carcinoma can be diagnosed by cytologic, colposcopic, or histologic examination[25] and can be retreated repeatedly with the CO_2 laser as they appear. This kind of treatment can be considered as elective for vulvar lesions, especially in young women.

5.4. Lower Genital Tract Multicentric Viral Lesions

5.4.1. Condyloma Acuminatum Lesions

Condylomatous lesions are occurring with increasing frequency in young women in the industrialized western world.[26] The lesions are mostly located in the prickle cell layer of squamous epithelium. The epithelial thickening below the proliferating prickle and basal cell layers determines acanthosis. The papilloma papovavirus infection causes lesions in the cervix, vagina, vulva, and perineal regions, singularly or in clumps.

Cervical condylomatouslike lesions have been recently recognized to appear frequently as nonexophitic lesions or inverted condylomata, with mosaic punctuation or a leukoplastic appearance.[27] Since cytologic and histologic changes are similar to dysplastic processes[27] and are frequently associated,[28,29] their preneoplastic significance is considered common knowledge.

As is well known, topical application of podophyllin[30] and 5-fluorouracil, and electrosurgical and cold knife ablation, have had unsatisfying results.[31] Moreover, in pregnancy, when the above-mentioned drugs are contraindicated, it is still necessary to eradicate these lesions in order to prevent infectious contact and to prevent the risk of laryngeal papilloma in the newborn during the labor.[32] In these cases, CO_2 laser treatment can be used with confidence.

5.4.2. Preoperative Analysis

Follow the guidelines for cervical intraepithelial neoplasia (CIN). In addition, the gynecologist must examine all suspected areas, as with any CIN lesion (Table 5.2). This includes the anus and rectum, and careful scrutiny of the vaginal walls, hymenal ring, and urethral orifices. In addition, the patient should probably be screened using a 3 hr glucose tolerance test and

Table 5.2. Preoperative Evaluation for Condyloma Acuminatum

Identify all lesions with colposcope
  Cervix
  Vagina
  Urethra
  Vulva
  Rectum
Obtain histologic confirmation

serum immunoelectrophoresis. A significant number of prediabetics or undetected diabetics have been found in our condyloma acuminatum population. Furthermore, if the immunoelectrophoresis reveals low IgG, we pretreat with gamma globulin (0.1 mg/kg body weight) and repeat this dose in 60 days.

Finally, and of greatest importance, is the complete "colposcopic" evaluation of the consort(s). A urologic examination without magnification is *not* sufficient. Careful viewing (under magnification) of the penile glans, shaft, and scrotum is mandatory, and these lesions should be biopsied routinely for confirmation. If the urologist is unwilling to diagnose in a similar fashion, then the male partner can be managed by vaporizing the penile lesion with the CO_2 laser. A local anesthesia may or may not be required. If a small discrete lesion or a few discrete lesions are found, short-duration (0.1-sec) impacts at 500 W/cm^2 will thermally inactivate the DNA of the condyloma acuminatum. The lesion should be vaporized to the same plane as its surrounding penile tissue.

If the male evaluation is omitted, a 35–50% recurrence in the female can probably be expected. Should the male refuse treatment, the primary patient must be informed that she cannot be efficiently treated unless she abstains from coital activity with the suspected male.

5.4.3. Sequence of Therapy

When dealing with cervical condylomata, follow the technical approach outlined in the discussion of CIN management. However, additional safeguards are required if one is to effect a complete cure.

When dealing with lesions of the external and internal genitalia, the following treatment sequence is recommended: cervix, vagina, rectum, urethra, vulva. This order has been chosen to reduce bacterial contamination. It also prevents mechanical trauma to tissues previously treated with the laser.

5.4.4. Technique of Management

Local infiltration of xylocaine (1%) (Lidocaine®) or Carbocaine® (mepivacaine) is suggested for vulvar CO_2 laser treatment, while vaginal warts do not require anesthesia.

First and foremost the perirectal and anal canal should be evaluated. All lesions should be vaporized at power densities of 300–500 W/cm^2. Next, visualize the cervix and vaporize the entire transformation zone to a depth of 2–4 mm. Similar power densities are employed. All vaginal lesions are treated to a depth of 1–2 mm. Finally the perineal condylomata acuminata are vaporized to a depth of 1 mm.

The precision of CO_2 surgery allows the destruction of the lesion and the preservation of healthy tissues. The high thermal effect that results in cellular evaporation may also destroy the local viral particles that could perpetuate the disease; therefore it could have clinical significance. In fact, residual disease due to viral particles may be responsible for the so-called multiple primary squamoid neoplasia,[33] while the special properties of the CO_2 laser can avoid the possibility of recurrent disease.[15] Moreover, the proper laser action causes alteration of the nerve ending, which results in an immediate relief of pain.

5.4.5. Postoperative Management

The immediate postoperative phase consists of nonintervention. This means that for the first 3 weeks following therapy, no douching, use of tampons, intercourse, or examination should be undertaken. The patient is informed to expect slight to moderate discharge (bloody to serous in type) for the first 1–3 days. Thereafter, she may experience a mild leukorrhea for an additional 1–3 days. Abstinence from intercourse should last 4–6 weeks. In addition, if coitus is undertaken during the third to sixth week, it is strongly recommended that condoms be used.

The first postoperative visit should be performed in the latter part of the third week or early in the fourth week. A moistened speculum should be gently inserted to visualize the cervical area. Do not attempt to apply acetic acid or clean the surface. The new epithelial surface tensile strength does not return to its maximum until after the 40th day. This phenomenon can be readily appreciated by applying a wet cotton-tip applicator to the cervical epithelial covering before the third week after surgery. A sheet of cells can be easily torn free from its underlying stroma.

After the 40th day, the patient should be colposcoped to determine the extent of the healing and detect any abnormal pathology that may exist. If the surface appears healed and the patient is insistent, coitus may be resumed but condoms should be used. The next visit should be 90 days following therapy. Again colposcopic examination is undertaken and a cytologic sample is taken. The second examination should be performed in the ninth month following therapy. We have observed that 95% of all residual disease will be detected on or before this examination. Thus, if one must conserve visits, then the third- and ninth-month examinations are considered mandatory. If both examinations, cytologic and colposcopic, are normal, the patient can be considered "cured" and returned to your routine examination schedule. The semiannual approach is suggested.

5.4.6. Complications and Results

Healing is rapid and infection is minimal because the laser beam should only come into contact with diseased tissue. There is virtually no scarring with this treatment because the depth of destruction is well controlled by the operator. Epithelial continuity is established within 3 weeks. The minimal damage of the underlying structure allows minimal alteration of anatomic structure.

Baggish[5] and Schellhas[20] have demonstrated excellent results by CO_2 laser vaporization or resection of any size of vulvar exophitic condylomatous lesions in a large series of cases. Also for the patients treated during pregnancy[10] despite vascular hyperemia and even in inaccessible areas, the procedure has been successful and is virtually bloodless.

Baggish[5] reports an overall recurrence rate of 5% in a selected series of 110 patients previously treated with other methods (5-fluorouracil, cryosurgery, podophyllin); in 23% of those cases a second CO_2 laser treatment was planned in order to eradicate the extensive disease. Periurethral edema and pain were reported in one case and were cured with 2 days of catheterization. No recurrence or major complications were reported with other treated series.[10,22,23,34]

Thus successful treatment with the CO_2 laser appears to be related to the selective destruction of the pathologic tissue to sufficient depth, with conservation of the healthy surrounding tissue. Nevertheless, CO_2 laser treatment can fail if the appropriate depth (the prickle cell epidermic layer for condylomatous lesions) is not reached.

The technique and results are valid for other viral sexually transmitted lesions such as herpes genitalis and molluscum contagiosum.

5.4.7. Herpes Simplex Virus Type 2

Herpes simplex virus type 2 is a cutaneously induced viral infection that can present as vesicular and genital ulcerative lesions of the vulva, vagina, or cervix. The causative agent is a DNA core virus, usually sexually transmitted. Today, with the change in social norms, this disease is approaching epidemic proportions in all socioeconomic classes.

The major problem facing the gynecologist is the natural history of this virus. Once the virus is transplanted into a mucous membrane, replication begins. Some of the viral particles are thought to migrate up the dendritic processes to the dorsal root ganglion. Here in the ganglion nuclei the virus may become dormant. Under stress, or other exciting factors, the nuclear viral DNA is activated and descends the dendritic process to recreate a vesicular cutaneous eruption.

The CO_2 laser has been used[36,37] to irradiate the vesicular eruptions and reduce the total number of cutaneous viral particles. By applying the appropriate power densities, the DNA core of the virus is thermally inactivated. The virus has a DNA core; its codons can be interrupted by heat. The adenine–thymine bond breaks at 65°C while the guanine–cytosine bond will dissociate at 100°C. The major advantage in this energy application is the reduction of the total number of viral particles at the epidermal level, thereby reducing the probability of neuron ascent. This reduction appears to alter the natural history of the disease. In our patient population, we have noted a resolution in the symptoms of the patients treated. By using laser surgery in the vesicular and ulcerative phase, the recurrence rates appear to be reduced.

We have noted three populations based on therapeutic response:

Group A. Primary disease
Group B. Recurrent disease with long intervals between recurrence
Group C. Chronic recurrence with regular intervals between recurrence.

The most effective management occurs in Group A and the least effective in Group C. This therapeutic effectiveness is probably related to the natural history of the disease. In the primary lesions, the number of viral particles is limited and, if exposed to the laser, is reduced to immunologically manageable levels. In the chronic and recurrent group, the dorsal root ganglion continues to supply the viral particles.

In using the laser for herpes management, the most important facts to keep in mind are that the virus is inactivated at 100°C and that the viral pathology is in the superficial layers of the epidermis. Once the virus has become associated with the dendritic process, the laser is not effective. Thus the irradiation should be ≤ 100 W/cm^2 using a beam focus of 2–3 mm. The vesicles should be vaporized and their bases and the adjacent tissue irradiated. The depth of coagulation should be limited to the superficial layers. If the energy penetrates to a great depth, the heat necrosis may create a new problem. This management usually gives subjective relief in most, if not all, cases. A drainage catheter may be required in severe cases, as periurethral ulceration can cause acute urine retention.

Postoperative management is identical to that outlined for the vulva, vagina, and cervix. We strongly recommend that condoms be used for 3 months following treatment to prevent sexual transmission. If there is no recurrence after 3 months, the couple can resume coitus without using barrier methods.

5.5. Other Sites

5.5.1. Peritoneal Labial Fusion

Labial fusion may result from previous surgical ablative procedures for diseases such as condyloma acuminatum. Rarely, we have seen persistent but incomplete labial fusion causing dyspareunia. To remove the fusion, one simply uses local anesthetic to reduce operative pain. A glass probe is placed through and behind the fusion, to absorb the energy once the fusion has been cut. The handpiece laser, PD $\sim 1 \times 10^5$ W/cm^2, is used as a scalpel. Bleeding is rare and can be easily controlled by pressure or high-frequency current.

Postoperatively, we recommend peritoneal irrigation twice a day, genital digital separation of the opposing surfaces at least three times daily for 1 week, and loose-fitting undergarments. Healing is usually complete by the third week.

5.5.2. Hymenotomy

Using the laser for a hymenotomy is what we would consider overkill. However, if one does have a laser it can be used to cut a circular aperture in the hymenal membrane. Occasionally we have used the laser to vaporize hymenal tags which have resulted in dyspareunia. One should place a wet gauze on the vagina to act as a backstop for the incident laser energy that may escape into the vaginal vault.

5.5.3. Anal Lesions

Care must be exercised when using the laser for management of peri-rectal and anal canal lesions. The lesions should be removed to a depth of no greater than 2 mm. The CO_2 laser has been reported to be successful when used to excise epidermoid anal and perianal carcinoma in an abdominal perineal resection.[35]

5.5.4. Periurethral Lesions and Skene's Ducts

The laser can be used to remove, excise, or vaporize urethral meatal lesions. A catheter is not generally required in the postoperative period.

5.5.5. Bartholin's Gland Abscess and Cyst Management

The CO_2 laser can be used to incise and drain an infected Bartholin's gland. Under appropriate anesthesia, the gland surface along the squamo-mucosal junction is elliptically incised. Cultures for aerobic and anaerobic bacteria are obtained. The cavity is then irrigated with normal saline. The edges of the cavity are separated and a defocused beam of 50–100 W/cm^2 is used to photocoagulate the inner abscess wall. This technique will reduce the bacterial flora and improve the healing phase. Appropriate antibiotics are administered. A small drain can be inserted, but is not required. Healing is usually complete in 10–15 days.

A Bartholin's gland cyst can be managed in a similar fashion. An elliptical cutaneous incision is made and submitted for histologic evaluation. Occasionally a benign-appearing cyst is found to contain a papillary or glandular carcinoma. The inner cavity is then irradiated with power densities of 50–100 W/cm^2. Healing is usually complete in 12–15 days.

5.5.6. Other Cutaneous Lesions

The gynecologist may be called upon to treat other cutaneous lesions and may elect to use the CO_2 laser. Following the principles of having the diagnosis confirmed by histology, correct identification of all lesion boundaries, complete removal, and proper follow-up will limit the probability of error. To avoid or shortcut any one of the above practices is to invite trouble.

References

1. Bellina JH, Polanyi TG: Management of vaginal adenosis and related cervico-vaginal disorders in DES-exposed progeny by means of carbon dioxide laser surgery. J Reprod Med *16*:295–296, 1976.
2. Adduci J: Gynecological surgery using the CO_2 laser. Intern Surg *63*:72–74, 1978.
3. Herbst AL: Exogenous hormones in pregnancy. Clin Obstet Gynecol *16*:37–50, 1973.
4. Scott JW, Seckinger D, Puente Duany W: Colposcopic aspects of vaginal adenosis in DES children. J Reprod Med *12*:187–193, 1974.
5. Baggish MS: Carbon dioxide laser treatment for condylomata acuminata venereal infections. Obstet Gynecol *55*:711–715, 1980.
6. Stafl A, Wilkinson EJ, Mattingly RT: Laser treatment of cervical and vaginal neoplasia. Am J Obstet Gynecol *128*:128–136, 1977.
7. Strong MS, Jako GJ: Laser surgery in the larynx. Ann Otol *81*:791–798, 1972.
8. Baggish MS: CO_2 laser surgery for benign and malignant lesions of the vagina, in Bellina JH et al (eds): Gynecologic Laser Surgery, Proceedings of an International Congress on Gynecologic Laser Surgery and Related Works, New Orleans, LA, Jan 1980. New York, Plenum Press, 1980, pp 73–94.
9. Upton J: Discussion of Stafl's laser treatment of cervical and vaginal neoplasia. Am J Obstet Gynecol *128*:134–136, 1977.
10. Hahn GA: The carbon dioxide laser in gynecology. Phila Med *74*:344–347, 1978.
11. Petrilli ES, Townsend DE, Morrow CP, Nakao CY: Vaginal intraepithelial neoplasia: biological aspects and treatment with topical 5-fluorouracil and the CO_2 laser. Am J Obstet Gynecol *138*:321–328, 1980.
12. Baggish MS, Dorsey JH: CO_2 laser for the treatment of vulvar carcinoma *in situ*. Obstet Gynecol *57*(3):371–375, 1981.
13. Neyens H: Laser therapy: How well does it work. Contemp Ob/Gyn *13*:199–202, 1979.
14. Schellhas HF, Fidler JM, Rockwell MJ: The carbon dioxide laser scalpel in the management of vulvar lesions, in Kaplan I (ed): Proceedings I International Symposium on Laser Surg, Israel, Nov 5–6, 1975. Jerusalem, Academic Press, 1976, pp 133–135.
15. Krantz KE: Discussion of Stafl's laser treatment of cervical and vaginal neoplasia. Am J Obstet Gynecol *128*:134–136, 1977.
16. Lobraico RV: The use of CO_2 laser in vulvar dystrophy, in Bellina JH (ed): Gynecologic Laser Surgery, New York, Plenum Press, 1981, p 291.
17. Di Saia PJ: Intraepithelial neoplasia of the vulva. Female Patient *2*:55–57, 1977.
18. Mering JH: A surgical approach to intractable pruritus vulvae. Am J Obstet Gynecol *64*:619–627, 1952.
19. Friedrich EG: Lichen sclerosus. J Reprod Med *17*:147–153, 1976.
20. Schellhas HF, Fidler JP, Rockwell RJ, et al: Resecting vulvar lesions with the CO_2 laser. Contemp Ob/Gyn *6*:35–39, 1975.
21. Bellina JH: Carbon dioxide laser in gynecology. Obstet Gynecol Annu *6*:371–391, 1977.
22. Forney JP, Morron OP, Townsend DE, DiSaia JP: Management of carcinoma of the vulva. Am J Obstet Gynecol *127*:801–806, 1977.
23. Lobraico RV, Townsend DER: CO_2 laser surgery for vulvar lesions, in Bellina JH et al (eds): Gynecologic Laser Surgery, Proceedings of an International Congress on Gynecologic Laser Surgery and Related Works, New Orleans, LA, Jan 1980. New York, Plenum Press, 1980, pp 279–290.

24. Invasive vulvar cancer—treated with CO_2. Personal communication, Dr. Pierre Martin-beau, Cleveland Clinic.
25. Di Re F, Lupi G. Bandieramonte G: Terapia chirurgica delle recidive del carcinoma vulvare, in Veronesi U, Di Re F, et al (eds): Le Neoplasia dell'Apparato Genitale Femminile. Milano, CEA, 1978.
26. Oriel D: Genital warts in sexually transmitted disease, in Caterall RD, Nicol CS eds: Sexually Transmitted Diseases. Academic, London, 1976, p 186.
27. Meisels A, Fortin R, Roy M: Condylomatous lesions of the cervix. II. Cytologic, colposcopic and histopathologic study. Acta Cytol *21*:379–390, 1977.
28. Meisels A, Fortin R: Condylomatous lesions of the cervix and vagina. I. Cytologic patterns. Acta Cytol *20*:505–509, 1976.
29. Yabe Y, Koyama H: Virus and carcinogenesis in epidermodysplasia verruciformis. Gan *64*:167–172, 1973.
30. Slater GE, Rumack BH, Peterson RG: Podophyllin poisoning. Obstet Gynecol *52*:94–96, 1978.
31. Graber EA, Barber H, O'Rourke J: Simple surgical treatment for condylomata acuminata of the vulva. Obstet Gynecol *29*:247–250, 1967.
32. Wilson J: Extensive vulvar condylomata acuminata, necessitating Caesarean section. Austr NZ J Obstet Gynaecol *13*:121–124, 1973.
33. Woodruff JD, Williams TJ: Multiple sites of anaplasia in the lower genital tract. Am J Obstet Gynecol *85*:724–743, 1963.
34. Bellina JH: Gynecology and the laser. Contemp Ob/Gyn *4*:24–34, 1974.
35. Shafir R, Zweig A, Slutzki S, Bornstein LA: Use of the carbon dioxide laser in an abdominoperineal resection for epidermoid anal carcinoma: a case report. Br J Surg *65*:565–566, 1978.
36. Bellina JH: The carbon dioxide laser in gynecology, Part II. Curr Probl Obstet Gynecol JM Leventhal (ed), 1:26–31, 1–35, 1981.
37. Baggish M: CO_2 laser treatment of viral venereal disease, in Atsumi K, Nimsakul N (eds): Proceedings, IV International Congress on Laser Surgery. Tokyo, Japan, November 1981, Jnter Group Corp, 1982, pp 13/10–13/11.

6

Intra-abdominal Applications

6.1. Introduction

In 1974 the CO_2 laser was adapted to the operating microscope for reconstructive pelvic surgery. Early experimental research demonstrated that this new energy transfer system had many potential advantages for surgery involving the fallopian tubes.[1,2]

Microsurgery is the technique of performing surgery wherein the operative field is viewed by the surgeon through a dissection microscope. The microscope expands the range of the surgeon's vision and, by allowing him to see more, facilitates very intricate repair procedures on extremely delicate and small structures. Microsurgery requires not only specially designed instruments but also an understanding of microstructural physiology, the ability to execute delicate movements with minimal trauma to tissue, and perfect hemostasis, yet it can potentially be performed by specialists in every area of surgery (Table 6.1).

The CO_2 laser adaptation to the operating microscope for reconstructive surgery of the female reproductive tract has been tested and used with substantial success. The advantages of this adaptation include:

1. Precision of application
2. The ability to reach otherwise inaccessible areas
3. The ability to vaporize dense adhesions
4. Reduced to absent bleeding
5. Reduced to absent postoperative adhesion formation
6. Significant reduction in operative time

**Table 6.1. Gynecologic Procedures Well-
Adapted to CO_2 Microsurgery**

Salpingolysis
Ovariolysis
Adhesiolysis
Cornual reimplantation
Tubal reanastomosis
Fimbrioplasty
Salpingostomy
Metroplasty
Myomectomy
Endometrioma excision and ablation
Vaginal reconstruction(s)
Cervical reconstruction(s)
Vulvar reconstruction

In order to use the CO_2 laser effectively in microsurgery, one must adhere to strict principles of application. First and foremost, the surgeon must be confident in microsurgical techniques and adhere rigidly to those principles set down concerning tissue handling, suturing, and a septic technique. Once these are mastered, a definite knowledge of the relevant biophysics is necessary in order to predict the effects of the CO_2 laser and utilize it to its maximum. This includes a thorough working knowledge of laser–tissue interaction, the mechanisms of heat transfer and decay, power density concepts, and the utilization of TEM in tissue vaporization, coagulation, and cutting.[3] Finally, and of similar importance, is the acquisition of the proper equipment. Today many types of lasers are for sale, each claiming its own advantage. The laser microsurgeon must be knowledgeable, lest he buy a system that is not optimum for his needs.

In utilizing the CO_2 laser in endometriosis, the ability of the surgeon to reflect the beam off a specialized mirror is of paramount importance. The mirror must have a highly reflective metallic coating. Infrared energy of 10.6 μm can be effectively reflected (95%) by polished silver surfaces. In ablating endometrial implants of the retrouterine surfaces, interior ovarian surfaces, or fossa recesses, the mirror technique has major advantages. In addition, the microsurgical micromanipulation of the integrated operating microscope allows the surgeon to operate in confined recesses without instruments obstructing his visual field. The modification of the OPM 6 Zeiss microscope with laser micromanipulation allows the surgeon to visualize constantly while simultaneously incising and vaporizing the diseased tissue (Fig. 6.1). Currently no other surgical technique has this advantage.

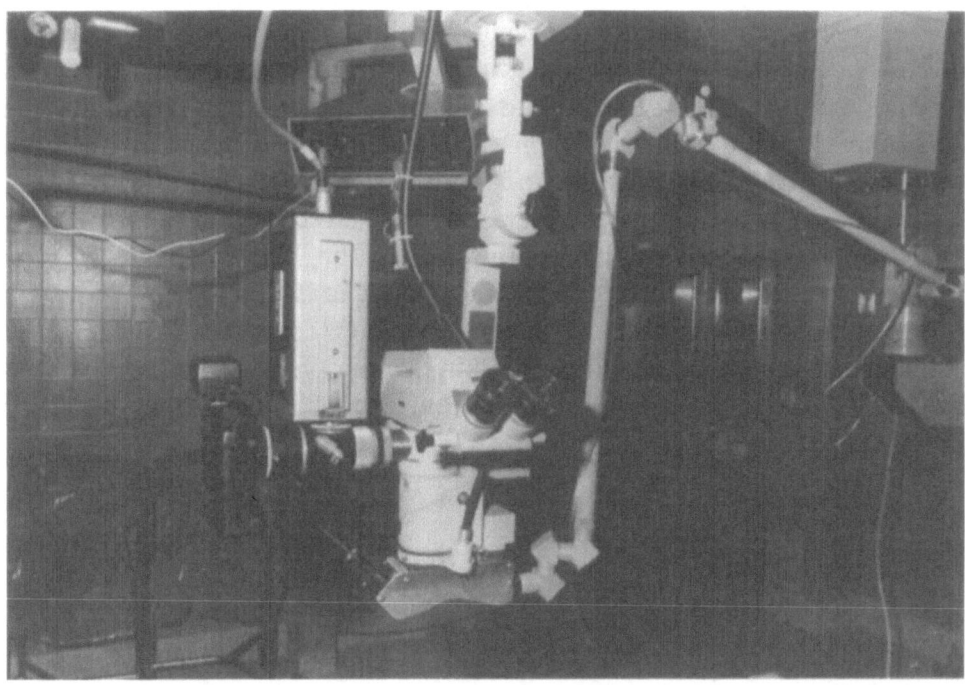

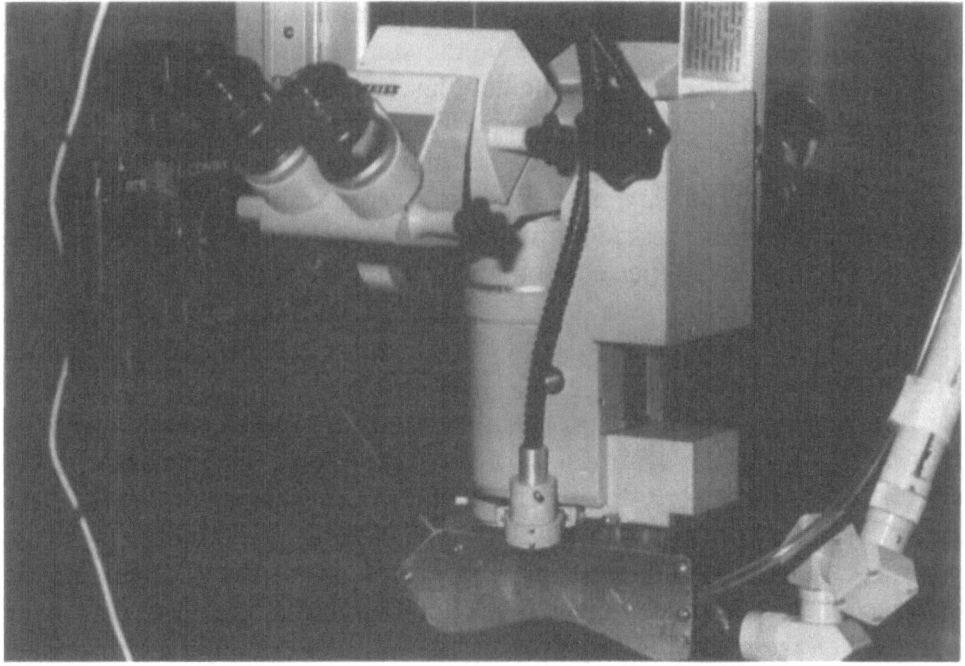

Figure 6.1. (Top) Broad view of the OPM 6 Zeiss microscope that has been fitted with a modified micromanipulator. (Bottom) The laser-articulated delivery assembly is shown to the right of the microscope.

Today we open the abdomen using a high-frequency current generator. The power output is 250 W in the cutting wave form. Once the skin is incised we switch to the "blend" wave form to cut and coagulate simultaneously. The fascia is incised in a similar fashion. The peritoneum is opened with sharp dissection. In the past, we used the 50-mm focal length CO_2 laser to incise the skin but found the high-frequency current as effective, but much quicker. The major difference is in the healing phase. The high-frequency current produces greater tensile strength in less time. This is due to the increase in tissue destruction and fibroblast and macrophage response. The increased collagen deposition is of benefit in the skin healing phase but not in the peritoneal work. The increase in collagen can lead to synechia and adhesion formation.

6.2. Instrumentation

For microsurgery, the colposcope or operating microscope is attached to both the laser manipulator and a special gimbaled mirror. The narrow laser beam entering from above strikes a gimbal-mounted mirror which is located between the monocular optical axes of the stero microscope. The mirror is positioned at 45° to the primary incident laser beam and deflects the energy along the viewing axis of the microscope. This arrangement must be modified (see Section 6.2.2) if a biheaded steroscopic microscope with recording system is to be substituted. Apertures in the mirror permit normal viewing with the microscope. A lens located in the primary incident laser beam focuses the energy to a spot at a distance equal to the working distance of the microscope objective. By appropriate lens selection (i.e., germanium, gallium arsenide, or zinc sebenide), this distance can be made anything from 10 to 50 cm or more.

The gimbal-mounted mirror permits the beam to be steered to any location within ±3° of the central axis of the microscope. The diameter of the working area is, therefore, about 10% of the working distance. To move the mirror about the gimbal axis, a joystick type of control is provided in a convenient location a few inches to the right or middle of the microscope. The mechanical linkage between the joystick and the gimbal is arranged to make the motion of the beam directly proportional to the same joystick movement with a demagnification of 7:1. The sensitivity and naturalness of this adjustment allow the surgeon to position the beam with confidence and precision to any preselected location.

One additional feature is necessary: to predict with accuracy, prior to exposure, where the focused energy will make contact with the work site. This ability is provided by a marker system which projects a visible image of a light source into the focal plane of the microscope eyepiece. Reflection of the marker light from a beam splitter attached to and located in the same plane as the metal mirror which directs the laser beam results in the image of the visible marker appearing on the work surface and moving in a one-to-one relationship with the impact point of the laser beam. A similar arrangement, but using a helium–neon laser, is coupled to the other laser systems. The markers coincide with the CO_2 laser impact point.

6.2.1. Current Laser System for Microsurgery

Below are listed the current models available in the United States for microsurgery adaptation. Each system has its own advantages and disadvantages. A microsurgeon contemplating a purchase should test each system and decide for himself which is best.

1. Sharplan 733, 791
2. Merrimack
3. Coherent 450
4. Biophysics Medica
5. Xanar

We believe that the major points to consider in a laser acquisition are as follows:

1. Power output of >30 W at the final exit port, *not* at the laser head.
2. Articulation system to allow placement at foot of operating table or other location, as desired
3. Smoothly articulating handpiece assembly
4. Variable focal lengths
5. Micromanipulator assembly
6. Service and maintenance contract
7. Inservice training for operating room personnel

6.2.2. Laser Micromanipulator

Currently, micromanipulators are produced by most manufacturers (Fig. 6.2). The micromanipulator is an optical platform containing an articulated mirror at 45° to the incident laser beam. Most micromanipulators

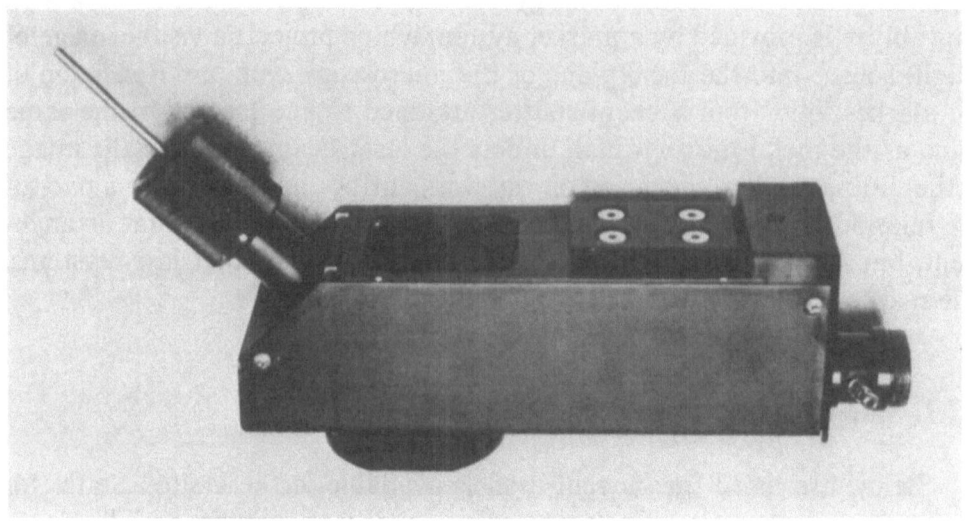

Figure 6.2. Micromanipulator to adapt CO_2 laser to operating miscroscope.

contain a set of fixed-focus lenses which allow the surgeon to change his working distance and focal spot size. The major disadvantage of current models is that the articulated mirror obstructs 30% of the surgeon's viewing field when attached to a binocular steroscopic microscope. In order to over-come this problem, one must modify the current models by extending the optical platform and changing the articulated mirror from 45° to 49°. This eccentric placement results in a beam–tissue interaction that is 85° rather than 90°. This slight deviation from the perpendicular results in a very small and not significant alteration in tissue heat flow. The major gain in this new arrangement is that the surgeon can videotape or record while operating without loss of image to the recording devices or his own visual field.

Additionally, the surgeon should require the manufacturer to modify the system, or modify the system himself, to yield a working distance of 300 mm with a laser focus of $<500~\mu$m. All manufacturers today can accomplish this at a nominal additional expense.

Once the micromanipulator has been properly modified, it must be cus-tom fitted to the surgical microscope. This fitting is mandatory to allow fine adjustments in the system so as to have all planes parafocal. If the visual field does not correspond to that of the recording system, then the final pictures or videotape images will be out of focus. Also, certain microscopes have objective lenses that protrude or retract in the zoom mode; allowances must be made. When dealing with a double-objective steroscopic system, the micromanipulator must be fitted to one side and modified so as not to obstruct the second objective system.

Once mounted, the micromanipulator should be marked so as to be easily removed or replaced to the exact location on the microscope suspension. This allows for cleaning of the manipulator. The reflective articulated mirror should be cleaned with acetone and lens paper only. Never use an abrasive object that could scratch the highly polished surface. The gallium arsenide lenses should be cleaned in a similar fashion. Do not gas-sterilize the system, as the ethylene oxide will remove or damage the infrared coating on the lens surface.

Alcohol or Cidex® can be used to cleanse the outside of the manipulator, but soaking will begin a leeching process from the lens-mounting surface into the metallic lens. This leeching will reduce the focal properties of the system and eventually necessitate complete and expensive lens replacement.

6.2.3. Omega Modification of Laser Micromanipulator

In this modification the optical platform was lengthened sufficiently to allow the articulated mirror to be placed beyond the 300-mm objective lens of the OPM 6 microscope. The mirror articulated assembly was repositioned to 85° to replace the infrared focal point within the viewing field of the surgeon. A spacer was added to the dovetail to allow for rapid on/off assembly. In addition, care was taken to mill the spacer so that it always returned to the exact loci on the microscope attachment assembly. This exact fit design prevents the necessity for realignment each time the micromanipulator is removed for cleaning (Fig. 6.3).

The lens assembly was fitted with three lenses to allow the choice of variable focal points of the infrared energy. We selected 500-μm, 1-mm, and 3-mm focal points at 300-mm working distance. We can vary this system by changing the Zeiss objective lens to 400 mm and thereby obtain three additional focal points. This arrangement gives six discrete focal points of infrared energy for microsurgery.

Finally, the protective side walls of the micromanipulator were sculptured to allow for maximum lumination from the bifid light pipes of the OPM 6 microscope (Fig. 6.4).

Once completed the assembly was mounted and checked to assure proper alignment of the HeNe pointer to the surgeon's viewing field via the OPM 6 microscope.

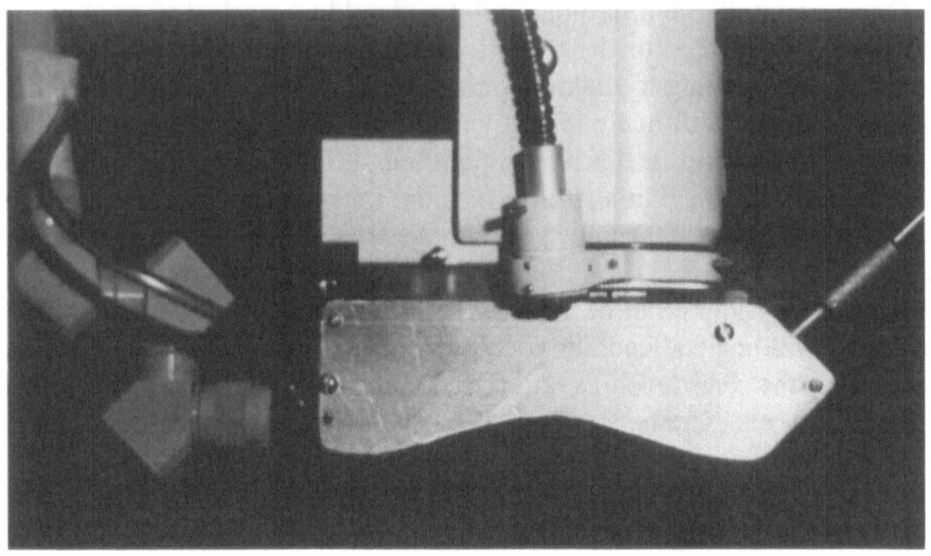

Figure 6.3. Modified laser micromanipulator designed to fit the OPM 6 microscope.

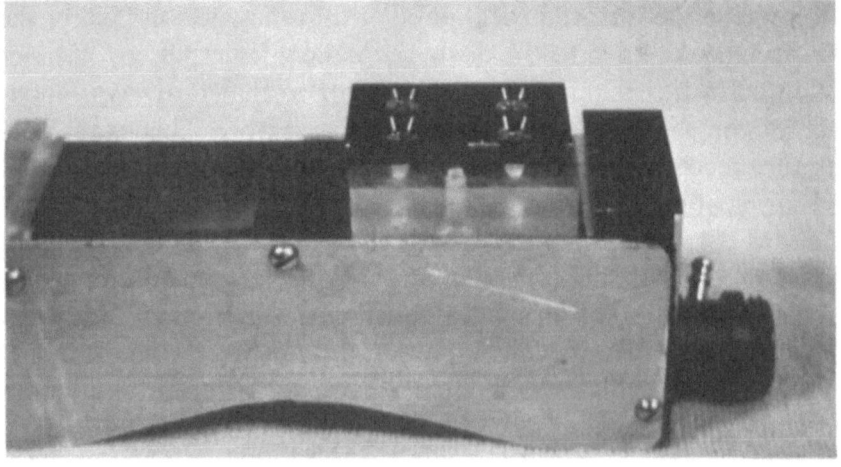

Figure 6.4. Side view of modified micromanipulator with sculptured walls to allow for proper illumination.

6.2.4. Laser Scalpel

The laser can be used with a fixed-focus hand-held assembly. There are usually three focal lengths available: f:50 mm, f:125 mm, and f:150 mm. Each has a fixed focus but the focal point can be varied by moving the hand. These lenses can generate power densities of up to a million W/cm^2 depending upon the laser input and final focus diameter. Great care must be used in handling these laser scalpels. All laser scalpels have a nitrogen input port for laminar flow across the lenses. This gas flow across the lens prevents back splatter from the tissue, which could damage the coated lens surface. The laser scalpel is used as a scalpel but has the added advantage of limited tissue interaction. However, when one cuts across a large vessel it will bleed and could require cauterization or suture.

6.2.5. Laser Accessory Instruments

The major tool used by the laser microsurgeon is the quartz glass rod, which will absorb the incident energy of the laser. These rods can be shaped into any desired configuration by the surgeon. We use them as elevators and manipulators. The laser is then fired onto the surfaces and the tissue is severed. We prefer to use a new rod if the glass shows pitting or fatigue. They are inexpensive and can be fashioned on site by the operating room personnel. A propane torch will heat the glass rod to its melting point, allowing for shaping or bending.

We have developed a glass-rod holder which allows a light pipe to be attached to the glass rod. This assembly allows for excellent transillumination of pelvic structures.

6.2.6. Laser Laparoscopy

Because of the coherent properties of a laser, its energy can be channeled through a laparoscope. An operating laparoscope (OD = 10 mm) has been modified to allow for passage of the 10.6-μm beam (Fig. 6.5). Specialized modification of the operating channel allows the focusing lens and gas to flow through the same channel. The gallium arsenide lenses focus the laser to a 1-mm spot size 2 cm beyond the end of the laparoscope. This exact prefocused beam can be used to cut fine adhesions or vaporize endometriomas. The laparoscope has a channel for plume evacuation. A newer mod-

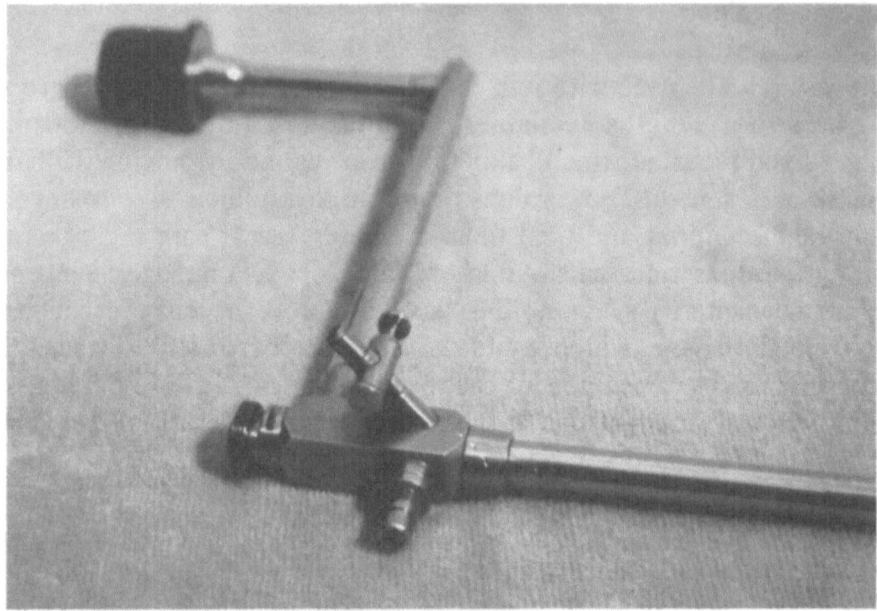

Figure 6.5. Laser operating microscope: phototype.

ification has been developed which allows a second puncture to carry the laser energy. Again the lens systems focus the laser to a 1-mm spot size 2 cm beyond the probe tip.

In both systems a HeNe laser is used as a target light. In the combined operating laser laparoscope the HeNe beam does not always correspond exactly with the infrared focus. The manufacturers have placed a crossed hair arrangement in the surgeon's viewing window. This arrangement allows the surgeon to test fire the system and correct the crossed hairs for exact beam alignment.

This laser laparoscope is a rigid system and still needs many refinements. However, with the advent of the flexible CO_2 fibers, many of the difficulties in this system will be overcome. In addition, specialized probes are needed to absorb the 10.6-μm energy, lest it be reflected to another surface. Ceramic-coated probes are being developed which will solve this problem.

6.2.7. Operating Room Modification

A laser operating room should be large, 25 $\times$ 30 if possible. The location of the operating table should allow one access to either side of the table without becoming entangled in electrical cords, suction tubing, or gas lines. We prefer for the surgeon to stand on the left side of the patient. The laser is placed at the foot of the operating table and the articulating arm elevated to allow for maximum clearance. This elevation allows a Mayo stand to be placed at the foot of the table. An additional Mayo stand is placed to the right of the surgeon which serves as a private tray containing the instruments he uses most. The microscope is ceiling-mounted and attached to the laser via the articulating arm from the foot of the table. A micro-high-frequency cauterization system is suspended over the right shoulder of the surgeon.

The anesthesiologist can provide his services at the head of the table and is kept out of harm's way. (N.B.: The anesthesiologist must wear protective glasses at all times during the laser procedure. In the sitting position, the anesthesiologist's eyes are usually in direct line with the exit port of the laser–micromanipulator assembly. If a defect exists in the alignment, theoretically a packet of photons could hit the eye of the anesthesiologist and result in corneal damage.)

The suction for laser surgery should be piped with an inline filter to remove tars or other substances which tend to foul the vacuum pumps. We have found that the disposable inline filter, together with a semipermanent filter and the vacuum system, is most effective. This system is extremely cost-effective and prevents vacuum pump failures.

In addition, we have found that mandatory presurgical checking of equipment ensures success.

Daily checklist:
1. CO_2/N_2/He gas bottle pressure
2. Visual inspection of lens and reflective mirrors
3. Wall suction semipermanent filter
4. Ground system alarms
5. Test firing of laser to assure proper alignment
6. Video alignment and system parafocal check
7. Luminescence of light pipes

Weekly checklist:
1. Power output of laser
2. Vacuum (torr) pressure

We have a chart in the operating room which records the diopter correction(s) for each surgeon. In addition, the chart records the diopter correction for the assistant. Because we use a steroscopic microscope the surgeon's right lens system can and usually does vary from the surgeon's left lens system. Thus each eyepiece must be individually corrected to the surgeon's eyes. This is done in conjunction with focusing the recording system.

In order to align the system properly, the following operations must be performed:

1. Place the proper objective lens in the microscope (e.g., f:300).
2. Place a f:300 focusing radicule in one eyepiece (e.g., left).
3. Focus the radicule until two distant crosses appear.
4. Without using the eyepieces focus the video system using the monitor. Adjust the microscope assembly up or down until the (left) eye is in focus.
5. Check the 16-mm focus camera system and video system.
6. Lock all systems in place.
7. Correct right eyepiece by rotating the diopter correcting lens until proper focus is noted for right eye.
8. Record the diopter correction next to the surgeon's name and the date. (N.B.: with time every diopter correction will change.) Repeat with all personnel until all diopter corrections are recorded.

Your visual system is now parafocal and corrected to your eyes.

6.2.8. Recording System: General

The OPM 6 microscope used by our surgical team contains a 50/50 beam splitter with a single exit port. This exit port can receive a teach arm adaptor, 16-mm camera attachment, video adaptor, or 35-mm camera adapter. Currently Urban produces a 16-mm/35-mm dual adaptor and a video/35-mm adaptor, but not a 16-mm/video adaptor. However, at the senior author's request a 16-mm/video adaptor of his design is now available from Zeiss.

We prefer to use the Bieleau 16-mm camera and a Circon* video tube for recording. Cine recording is done with tungsten ASA 400 positive film. If a movie is contemplated then negative film is substituted; a negative results in a better-quality 16-mm movie. A word of caution: a movie is very expensive to produce; it is currently estimated to cost between $500 and $1000 per minute of edited and titled sound film.

---

*Circon, 749 Ward Drive, Santa Barbara, California 93111.

6.2.9. Recording System: Specialized Video–Cine Modification

Our operating room has been modified to allow continual viewing by the family while simultaneously recording the procedure on ¾-in. video and 16-mm cine photography.

One monitor is viewed by operating room personnel, the second by the video technicians, and the third by the family. A closed-circuit audio system allows the surgeon to communicate with the family and discuss his or her findings while operating. It also allows the surgeon to activate the 16-mm camera and record when specialized or noteworthy events occur. Should publications require illustrations, the 16-mm frames are analyzed and reproduced as black and white or 35-mm color slides. The flexibility of this recording system can be appreciated when one attempts to video record and later create a 16-mm movie of the same sequences.

6.3. Microsurgical Procedures

The patient is taken to the surgical suite and a general anesthetic is given. A culture (aerobic and anaerobic) of the cervical canal is taken. The vagina is prepped with an antiseptic solution. A Humi®* cannula is inserted into the endometrial cavity and distended. A catheter is inserted into the urinary bladder. The vaginal pack is inserted to help elevate the corpus uteri. An intraoperative hysterosalpingogram may be performed. Methylene blue dye is added to the water-soluble radiopaque medium to determine intra-abdominal spillage. The surgeon performs a standard laparoscopic examination. Findings are noted and filmed. At this point the procedure can be aborted or advanced to the microsurgery phase. Should the surgeon desire consultation with a family member, an audio/video relay allows for direct communication, through closed-circuit television, to a private consultation room. A permanent audio and visual record is made of this discussion, including the surgeon's recommendations and the additional consent of the appropriate family member.

This phase concludes the intraoperative evaluation. The abdomen is reprepped and draped, and the skin incision is made. An O'Conner–O'Sullivan self-retracting retractor is placed in the abdominal cavity and intra-

*United Marketing Resources, UNIMAR.

abdominal packing is placed. The operating microscope with laser micro-manipulator is draped with a sterile polyethylene bag and positioned over the incision. Depending upon the pathology of the case, the laser microsurgeon and attending microsurgeon may perform one or a combination of the procedures described below.

During microsurgical procedures, all patients receive methylprednisolone sodium succinate at a rate of 100 mg/hr. The same medication and dosage is continued for the first 24 hr, then replaced by methylprednisolone 15 mg/24 hr for 5 days with declining dosage over the next 5 days. Doxycycline hyclate 100 mg/12 hr is administered intravenously then orally for 10 days. Adjustment in antimicrobial therapy is based upon cultures taken at surgery. At the termination of all surgical procedures, the abdomen is irrigated with 1500–2000 ml of normal saline, then 100 ml of 70,000-mol.-wt. dextran (32%) is added and the peritoneum is closed. Postoperatively, the patients are usually ambulatory the first day and are placed on a regular diet.

Hysterosalpingographic studies are done cinefluorographically using atraumatic techniques prior to discharge (5th–7th day) in some cases. Hysterosalpingograms are performed using water-soluble contrast media mixed with 100 mg of hydrocortisone succinate and 25 mg of 1% xylocaine. The total mixture is 20 ml. Instillation rate is dependent upon the fluoroscopy picture. Cinefluorography is used in all hysterosalpingograms in an attempt to prevent needless pressure upon suture lines. X rays are taken according to standard procedures, labelled and kept for future follow-up. The video record is similarly processed.

At 1, 3, and 6 months, patients complete a follow-up questionnaire concerning complications, menses and general health, and personal gynecologist's evaluations. If the patient has not conceived within the expected time interval based on the type of procedure done, a repeat of the hysterosalpingogram and second-look laparoscopy are recommended.

Should conception be suspected, patients are instructed to obtain confirmation via a serum beta subunit pregnancy test. If possible, echograms are immediately ordered to document conception and to determine placement of the conceptus. This serves as an early detection for ectopic pregnancy.

6.3.1. Adhesiolysis

Adhesive processes are removed using a micromanipulated laser beam with PD from 2×10^3 W/cm^2 to 1×10^4 W/cm^2. Each adhesion should be removed from its origin and insertion. Because laser energy dissipation is finite and limited, adjacent tissue injury is minimal particularly at high power densities. Therefore, adhesions arising from the bowel can be removed on the serosal surface. A glass probe is used to absorb excess energy. The adhesions separate cleanly if gentle traction is applied.

All serosal surfaces giving rise to an adhesive process are relasered with PD ~800–1000 W/cm^2. We believe this reduces postoperative adhesion formation. This belief has been confirmed on second-look procedures and by other investigators.

Because the laser beam is electromagnetic energy, it behaves according to the laws of physics. This conformity allows the surgeon to utilize mirrors in the abdominal cavity to direct the beam. Thus the surgeon can operate under structures such as the ovary and around corners. A front-silver-surfaced mirror with an integrated light bundle (Narco Pilling Company) can be used to remove adhesive processes inferior and lateral to the ovary by reflected energy. The utilization of energy in this fashion is a major advance in surgical technique and is particularly useful for this type of anatomically complex situation.

6.3.2. Fimbrioplasty and Salpingostomy

The diseased fimbria are examined and placed on saline-soaked Telfa® pads. Adhesive processes are removed using the micromanipulated laser with PD ~2 × 10^3 W/cm^2 to 1 × 10^4 W/cm^2. The tubal ostia are identified by direct observation and/or transillumination. If required, a neo-ostia can be created by exposing the dependent "dimple" to 1 × 10^5 W/cm^2 for 0.5 sec. The neo-ostia is then cannulated with a tapered glass probe and transilluminated. Vascular radiations are identified and radial incisions made in the serosal surface. The geometric configuration of the radial incisions is a function of tubal distortion, tubal neovascularization, and ovarian location. The preferred geometry places the fimbrial ostia in juxtaposition to the ovarian surface.

The radial incisions are made with PD 5–8 × 10^3 W/cm^2. This power density range creates precise lines of tissue separation with minimal thermal injury. The zone of thermal necrosis is usually sufficient to seal microcapillaries. Arterioles greater than 1 mm in diameter may require high-frequency microcoagulation. The incised surfaces are liberally irrigated with isotonic saline to remove loose debris and carbonized tissue.

The serosal surfaces adjacent to the radial incisions are then irradiated at 100–300 W/cm^2. The surface heating causes linear protein contraction and tubal mucosal eversion. Usually 3 to 4 No. 8/0 coated Vicryl sutures are placed (serosa to serosa) to assure eversion.

Mucosal surfaces are carefully evaluated for microadhesions. If noted, they can be removed using PD $\sim$1–5 $\times$ 10^3 W/cm^2. Glass probes are used to absorb excess and deflected energies. Normal saline is used to remove loose debris and carbonized matter. Tubal patency is evaluated by chromopertubation.

6.3.3. Tubal Reanastomosis

Reanastomosis preparation begins with the tubal segments. The proximal and distal segments are prepared in similar fashion. The serosal layer is vaporized with PD $\sim$800–100 W/cm^2 thereby exposing the muscular coat. The muscular coat is then incised to the mucosa with PD $\sim$5 $\times$ 10^3 W/cm^2. Mucosal division is performed with cold instruments. Each segment is washed free of debris and carbonized matter with isotonic saline. Patency is assured by anterograde chromopertubation and retrograde chromopertubation. Retrograde chromopertubation is performed by cannulating the fimbria using a No. 18 gauge Jelco® Sialistic Catheter.

Closure of the tubal defect is accomplished by microsuturing, not laser welding. The mesosalpinx is approximated with No. 6/0 coated Vicryl® sutures. Four No. 8/0 coated Vicryl® sutures are placed at 6, 9, 3, and 12 o'clock positions in the muscular coat. Care is exercised to avoid mucosal suturing. A final layer of No. 8/0 coated Vicryl® is placed at 4, 8, 10, and 2 o'clock positions in the serosal layer. No guides or stints are used. Gentle chromopertubation is used to assess luminal apposition.

In certain sterilization procedures, the ampullary segments have been severed, leaving a terminal fimbrial cul-de-sac arrangement. In these specialized cases, a glass probe is placed in the fimbrial cul-de-sac, and pressure applied with transillumination. Under direct microscopic view the avascular fibrotic site is vaporized in a drill fashion. This aperture is enlarged to accommodate the proximal ampullary segment. Suturing is then performed in the muscular and serosal layers.

6.3.4. Cornual Reimplantation

This procedure is technically the most difficult of all fallopian tube microsurgical procedures, and therefore must be performed with extreme care. After appropriate abdominal preparation the fundus is exposed. The site for reimplantation is chosen to avoid venous and arterial plexus if possible. The myometrium is then infiltrated with vasopressin (1 ml of 1:2000

Pitressin® in 5 ml normal saline). A No. 30 gauge needle is preferred for cornual infiltration. The uterine cavity is distended with hypertonic solution ($>$150 mm Hg). This solution is used to compress the endometrium and absorb the exit laser energy. A cornual neo-ostia is created using the f:50 mm hand-held laser with PD $\sim$5 $\times$ 10^5 W/cm^2. A cylindrical incision is completed and the excised myometrium submitted for histopathology. Cultures (aerobic and anaerobic) are now taken of the neo-ostia. Intrauterine fluid pressure is reduced to stop transabdominal flow. The diameter of the neo-ostia is enlarged to accommodate the distal tubal segment. A microruler is used to assure proper calibration.

The distal tubal site is prepared by vaporizing the serosal surface with PD $\sim$800 W/cm^2. This process exposes the tubal muscularis. The terminal tubal fimbriotic cap is incised with PD $\sim$1 $\times$ 10^5 W/cm^2 to the mucosal level. The muscosa is incised using cold instruments.

The distal tubal segment is now transfixed into the cornual neo-ostia with No. 6/0 and No. 8/0 coated Vicryl® sutures. Prior to final fixation the lasered sites are irrigated free of all debris and carbonized matter. This technique assures mucosa–mucosa, muscularis–muscle, and serosal–serosa closures. A water-tight seal is not necessary. No splinting is used. Final aerobic and anaerobic cultures are taken at the fimbrial segment. At the termination of the surgical reconstruction, patency is tested by pressurizing the intra-uterine hypertonic solution.

6.3.5. Ectopic Pregnancy: Linear Salpingostomy

After appropriate abdominal entry, usually via a Pfannenstiel's incision, the tube containing the ectopic pregnancy is placed on a wet Telfa® pad with protective moistened laps separating the adjacent vital structures. All peritubal adhesions are incised using the carbon dioxide laser as the primary cutting tool. The antimesenteric surface, over the gestational site, is then incised with the laser. Usually the gestational products appear as a blood clot containing the gestational sac. The sac and blood clot are carefully, under microscopic vision, teased free from the tubal mucosa. In this phase the operating microscope is invaluable in isolating small venous and arteriolar bleeding points allowing for microbipolar cauterization. The tubal mucosa is then irrigated with physiological saline to insure that all bleeding points have been identified. A number 5 umbilical catheter (Sherwood Medicallo) is then gently inserted into the distal segment of the tube and advanced into the incision area. The proximal portion of the fallopian tube is cannulated in a similar fashion completing the tubal splint insertion. The tubal muscularis layer is then approximated with interrupted number 8/0 coated Vicryl® sutures. Care must be taken not to produce tension of the suture line. The serosal layer is closed in a similar fashion. Once the sutures are properly placed, the intraluminal umbilical catheter is gently withdrawn. Just before one withdraws the intraluminal catheter, 25 ml of heparinized saline is used as an irrigant and the catheter is then gently withdrawn during the final 5 ml of irrigation. The pelvic cavity is irrigated with sufficient quantities of normal saline to remove all fibrinous clot products. During closure, 200 ml of 70,000-mol.-wt. dextran (32%) is placed in the pelvic cavity. Postoperatively, the patient receives methylprednisolone 15 mg daily for 5 days. In addition, we empirically administer doxycycline hyclate 200 mg daily, in divided dosage, for 10 days.

During the recovery phase, barrier contraception is suggested for a minimum of 3 months. When a menstrual cycle is missed, a beta human chorionic gonadotropin pregnancy test is ordered. Ultrasonography is then performed to detect the exact location of the gestation.

To date, we have performed six procedures using this technique. In all cases, the blood loss was minimal. Three intrauterine pregnancies have resulted in this approach and to date no repeated tubal pregnancies have occurred. The major advantage the CO_2 laser has added to the corrective approach is the ease of excising or incising tubal tissues in a relatively bloodless fashion.

6.3.6. Endometriosis

Two complementary methods exist for the management of endometriosis. Danocrine or other drug suppression and reconstructive surgery can control pelvic endometriosis in a significant number of females. Prior to management, all cases of suspected endometriosis should be classified in accordance with the American Fertility Society Classification.

6.3.6.a. Endometrial Implants Implants along the uterosacral ligaments or other serosal surfaces are vaporized with low PD ~150–300 W/cm^2. Rapid beam raster movement are used to "erase" the implant until stromal tissue is identified. This technique can be used on bowel surfaces, vessel surfaces (with care), or other vital structure surfaces.

Occasionally the beam is used in the pulse mode ($t = 0.05–0.1$ sec). If a vessel or surface structure seems extremely thin, use traction to elevate the endometrioma away from the underlying stroma and then vaporize. If one is very concerned, simply inject, with a 25 gauge needle, a small wheal of saline under the lesion and then vaporize. The saline barrier will completely absorb the CO_2 laser.

We prefer to use the micromanipulator and sweep the beam rapidly over all endometrial implants. The silver-surfaced mirror is extremely beneficial in giving access to the ovarian fossa, uterine ligaments, and other areas usually inaccessible to direct microscopic vision.

6.3.6.b. Endometrioma: Ovarian Type

Ovarian endometriomas that are small (<2 cm) are decapitated by cutting around the ovarian–endometriomal junction. The cap removed is submitted for pathology. The base is thoroughly washed free of all debris. The laser is then used to photocoagulate the internal walls PD ~300 W/cm^2. We do not close the resulting defect. Second-look laparoscopy has revealed the defect to close spontaneously and rarely, if ever, to adhere to adjacent structures.

The larger endometriomas are approached in a similar fashion, resecting the cap with PD ~1 $\times$ 10^4 W/cm^2 and photocoagulating the internal surfaces. The deeper ovarian surface defect is approximated using No. 4/0 coated Vicryl® sutures, and No. 5/0 coated Vicryl® is used to close the surface defect.

Implants on the ovaries are vaporized by the technique described in Section 6.3.6.a. All carbonization should be thoroughly washed free prior to abdominal closure.

6.3.6.c. Bowel Endometrioma

To date, we have performed seven primary large bowel endometriosis resections with the CO_2 laser in the cutting mode (PD ~1 $\times$ 10^4 W/cm^2). The sigmoid colon was the site in all cases. We excised the tumor through the mucosal surface and performed a primary bowel closure. In none of the cases was the bowel completely transected. The largest defect was 3 cm in diameter and was closed primarily without a diverting colostomy. In all cases no apparent fecal contamination was noted. We believe that the laser sterilized the resection site, thus increasing our success. In addition, the limited tissue injury probably resulted in a stronger closure plane.

All patients were placed on nasogastric suction until bowel sound returned. Thereafter, a progressive diet was administered. No postoperative complications have resulted to date. None of the patients developed a mechanical ileus. All had a bowel movement by the third postoperative day, and none developed a febrile response. This afebrile response must be viewed in light of our protocol of administering antibiotics for 10 days postoperatively and our steroid management.

We do not believe that our technique should be attempted or selected over other managements unless the surgeon feels confident in his ability to repair bowel. In addition, he should be prepared to accept the risk of bowel perforation and possess the ability to cope with such a complication if it occurs.

6.3.7. Uterine Anomalies

6.3.7.a. Septal Defects   When an intrauterine anomaly is detected, the CO_2 laser system can be used in place of the conventional scalpel. We prefer first to inject the serosal and muscular layers with 1:2000 pitocin diluted in 10 cc normal saline. A 25 gauge needle is preferred for the injection. The handpiece with 10-cm focal length is chosen. This configuration yields a focal diameter of 125 μm generating PD $\simeq 1 \times 10^5$ W/cm^2.

The procedure begins with the outlining of the fundal area to be excised. Then the laser is used to cut down to the septum. A glass probe is inserted under the septum, which is then excised or vaporized depending upon the thickness and location. Because of the laser hemostasis the procedure can be accomplished in short order. Should the septum extend toward the internal os, the laser is used to vaporize this septum. We prefer to place a Humi® cannula prior to surgery to facilitate anatomy identification. No intrauterine device (IUD) is inserted postoperatively. The myometrium is closed in three layers. The first muscular layer is closed with No. 3/0 coated Vicryl® running sutures, the second with No. 3/0 coated Vicryl interrupted sutures. The serosal layer is then closed using a subserosal running suture. This technique results in suture lines which are not exposed, thereby theoretically reducing adhesions.

Postoperatively, we recommend estrogen supplement for 6 weeks, (conjugated equine estrogen 2.5 mg orally daily). In addition, we request that contraception be practiced, preferably barrier technique for 3 months. In the third month a hysterosalpingogram and ultrasound sector scan of the uterine cavity is used to detect weakness or deficient uterine healing. Should a defect be identified, it should be repaired prior to the patient attempting pregnancy. To date, of the four patients treated by this technique, none have been noted to have a defective scar. One patient has conceived, but was delivered by caesarean section at the 39th week of gestation. We do not believe that the laser will create a stronger healing in muscle when compared to other modalities. However, we do find that the reduced operative time, blood loss, and technical ease of procedure give the CO_2 laser major advantages.

6.3.7.b. Bicornuate Uterus Fetal wastage resulting from a failed mullerian unification can be corrected by the CO_2 laser. We prepare the patient in the same fashion as for intrauterine septal defects. The serosa and myometrium are injected with a dilute Pitressin® solution (1 cc of 1:2000 in 10 cc normal saline). The line of excision is traced over the serosal surface with the hand laser PD $\simeq$ 1000 W/cm^2. The muscular dissection is carried out with PD $\simeq$ 1 $\times$ 10^5 W/cm^2. We also employ high-frequency monopolar current to cauterize larger vessels. Once the excision is complete, the defect is closed in three layers. Again we employ the subserosal closure to limit peritoneal exposure of the coated Vicryl® suture.

Postoperative care and pregnancy recommendations are identical to those described in Section 6.3.7.a.

6.3.7.c. Uterine Leiomyomata Today, with reconstructive advances, we are attempting to excise large intramural leiomyomata. Small leiomyomata present little difficulty, but tumors in excess of 3 cm may present serious technical problems, particularly when adjacent to tubular anatomy or great vessel structures. The procedure begins by testing for tubal patency. Next, palpation of the tumor is used to select the best surgical plane. The serosa is injected with a dilute Pitressin® solution (see Section 6.3.7.a.). A semilunar incision is made. We do not remove this flap, as it will be used in repairing the defect at the termination of the leiomyomata removal. The flap is carefully dissected from the superior portion of the tumor. Next, by blunt dissection, most leiomyomata will be enucleated. However, we prefer to do laser excision in areas where the capsule is densely adherent to myometrial stroma. We use power densities of 1 $\times$ 10^5 W/cm^2 for this dissection. Again, we employ high-frequency monopolar current for large-vessel hemostasis. Once the tumor is removed from its encapsulation, the base is irrigated and all bleeding sites coagulated using monopolar current under direct microscopic vision. Again, tubular patency is checked to detect if the intramural portion of the fallopian tube has been disrupted. If it has, careful microsurgical repair with No. 8/0 coated Vicryl® is recommended.

Once hemostasis has been achieved, the myometrial defect is closed with No. 4/0 coated Vicryl® in interrupted figure-eight sutures. The serosal flap is placed over the defect and sculptured to fit the defect. The laser is used at PD 1 $\times$ 10^5 W/cm^2. The flap is placed on a wet Telfa® pad to prevent the laser from injuring additional myometrial tissue. The final closure of the flap is accomplished with No. 5/0 coated Vicryl® using a running subserosal technique.

We have found that very large leiomyomata, 8–10 cm in diameter, can be effectively removed by the above procedure. Using the microscope and laser, the utero-ovarian arcuate system can be identified and dissected from the capsule wall.

As with all procedures that weaken the inherent myometrial structure, we recommend a minimal healing phase of 4–6 months. Barrier technique for contraception is our preference. Again, after the healing period, evaluation of intrauterine anatomy by hysterosalpingogram and ultrasound is undertaken. When these results are questionable, a hysteroscopic examination will usually resolve the issue. If a defect is present, a second but much less extensive procedure is performed to correct the defect. We excise the defect and close the layers as described in Section 6.3.7.a.

6.3.8. Tubal Anomalies

6.3.8.a. Intraluminal Polyps With newer and more sophisticated diagnostic procedures, polyps or defects in the intramural or isthmic portion of the fallopian tube are being detected. In order to remove these, our approach is to incise the antimesentery surface of the tube using the 125-μm beam at PD 1×10^5 W/cm^2. Care in dissection must be exercised so as not to cause contralateral mucosal damage. We prefer to cannulate the fimbria with a number 5 umbilical catheter, and irrigate the site in an anterograde fashion. The liquid phase prevents contralateral mucosal surface damage. Once the lumen is exposed, the polyp is carefully elevated and excised with the laser. The tissue is sent for pathologic identification. The base of the polyp is vaporized. The tubal incision is then closed using interrupted No. 8/0 coated Vicryl® sutures on the muscular layer. The serosal surface is enclosed with a running No. 7/0 coated Vicryl® suture. At the termination of the suturing the tubal mucosa is flushed with hypertonic solution to remove tissue fragments and other substances that could promote intraluminal blockage.

6.3.8.b. Bifid Fallopian Tubes We have encountered two fallopian tubes which we believed were truly bifid in nature (reduplication). One case was detected during reconstructive surgery after ectopic pregnancy rupture. The two channels originated at the ampullary portion and ended in what appeared to be two separate fimbrial ostia (a greater ostia and a lesser ostia). We thought that the ectopic pregnancy originated at the junction of the two internal channels. We excised the lesser channel and repaired the ampullary segment. The repair resulted in a single channel. A small glass probe was inserted in the distal minor fimbrial ostia and then threaded to the junction of the ampullary portion. The tract was incised over the glass rod and then totally excised with the CO_2 laser. The lesser ampullary ostia was identified and closed with No. 8/0 coated Vicryl®. Anterograde chromopertubation assured closure of the accessory channel. The serosa was then closed over the primary channel using No. 8/0 coated Vicryl® in two layers. Both patients have achieved pregnancy and delivered without complications.

6.3.8.c. Defective Fimbria Ovarica   In certain cases, occasionally congenital but usually iatrogenic, the fimbria is found to be unattached to the ovarian surface. In this arrangement, fimbrial ovum pickup is difficult if not impossible. We have begun to correct these defective fimbrial ovarica by the following technique.

First, the fimbrial segment is placed adjacent to the ovarian surface, making absolutely certain that all anatomical planes are obeyed. Next, the laser at power density ~ 300 W/cm^2 is used to create a transplant channel in the surface of the ovary and the corresponding channel in the meso-ovarian surface onto the inferior portion of the fimbria. Then No. 8/0 coated Vicryl® is used to attach the tube to the ovary using the channel vaporized by the laser as the transplant site. Once complete, the architectural arrangement increases ovum pickup as the fimbria is adjacent to the ovarian surface. The procedure is easy to perform, and if all other factors have been excluded in the fertility dysfunction, it can result in pregnancy in less than 6 months.

Of the five patients on whom we have operated, all have conceived. Analysis of our cases revealed four to be iatrogenic in nature and only one thought to be congenital. One must be extremely careful in fimbrial dissections lest an iatrogenic fimbria ovarica defect result.

6.3.9. Ovarian Procedures

6.3.9.a. Cystectomy   Preservation of ovarian function in the young reproductive woman is directly dependent upon ovarian tissues. Surgical procedures should attempt to:

1. Preserve the maximum ovarian tissue
2. Prevent, if possible, secondary infections resulting in adhesions
3. Avoid secondary pelvic surgical infections

In order to achieve these goals, the surgeon must plan his surgical approach. The vascular anatomy and tubal and fimbrial architectural geometry must be considered. For example, the primary ovarian incision should be placed, if possible, 180° away from the fimbrial ovarian area. An incision in the fimbrial ovarian area could result in tubal agglutination, omental or bowel adhesion formation, and secondary sterility. If, in the same case, the incision could be along the antimesosalpinx area and the cyst enucleated or excised, theoretically the possibility of secondary infertility is lessened.

6.3.9.b. Incisional and Excisional Approach   Cystic ovarian structure in young reproductive ovaries can be first incised using a power density of 800–1000 W/cm^2. The serosal surface, if possible, should be incised at the junction of the cyst wall and ovarian surface. This area has the maximum serosal cooling and will limit iatrogenic rupture. Next, attempt to use a knife handle or Metzenbaum scissors to shell out the cyst. If successful, the ovarian defect is then photocoagulated with 100–300 W/cm^2 to reduce bleeding and assure a sterile cavity. The ovarian wound edges are closed with No. 6/0–4/0 Vicryl® using either an operating microscope or loupe. Ovarian surface blood clots and tissue debris are washed with saline and the procedure is terminated.

We prefer to place 7000-mol.-wt. dextran in the pelvic cavity prior to abdominal closure.

6.3.9.c. Wedge Resection   Today, a wedge resection is reserved for very special cases. Should it become necessary to remove a wedge of ovarian tissue then care must be undertaken to reduce secondary tubal damage.

First, the ovary must be completely exposed. The excisional lines of dissection should be on the antimesosalpinx surface and should not encroach upon the fimbrial ovarium.

The power density should be at the maximum, 5×10^5 W/cm^2. An elliptical incision is preferred using traction on the wedge. Care must be exercised to avoid damaging the deep ovarian medullary tissue.

Closure of the ovarian defect is very important. Use a microsurgical approach. Place interrupted sutures in the deeper ovarian stroma using No. 6/0 Vicryl®. Hemostasis is critical. All vessel oozing, no matter how slight, must be reserved. Use the microcoagulation if necessary. Finally, the ovarian surface is closed with No. 6/0 or 7/0 Vicryl® sutures. A running suture is preferred. All ovarian blood clots are removed with saline. Again, we prefer to place 100 cc of 70,000-mol.-wt. dextran in the pelvic cavity prior to abdominal closure.

6.3.10. Rectovaginal Repair

This repair technique is reserved for small apical fistulae. Large defects need more extensive dissection and tissue plane separation.

The repair begins with a preoperative bowel cleaning. We do not find that a complete bowel preparation is necessary. A thorough cleaning enema should be performed the morning of surgery. A low-residue diet is given for 24 hr preceding surgery. A pHisoHex® douche is given the night before surgery and repeated the morning of surgery. Prophylactic antibiotics are not administered preoperatively.

The patient receives a general or regional block. Preoperative vaginal cleansing is performed with povidone/iodine solution. The dorsal lithotomy position is used. A weighted vaginal speculum and Haney retractor are first wrapped with a wet Curlex to prevent laser beam reflection. The fistula site is exposed.

We prefer a vaginal dissection following the classical Lasko technique. The mucosa is completely denuded. Then, using No. 3/0 Vicryl®, a three-layer closure, ending with the vaginal mucosa, is performed.

Postoperatively the patient receives a low-residue diet for 3–5 days and then is placed on a regular diet. Flatulent food products should be avoided for 21–30 days. Should constipation become a problem, use mild bowel stimulants (i.e., Dialose® Plus).

Intercourse should definitely be postponed for 40 days or until complete healing is evident.

6.4. Conclusion

Increased demand for sterilization reversal and surgical treatment for tubal occlusion has resulted in a developing and explosive interest in microsurgery. Results of microsurgical repair of the fallopian tube are far greater than with gross surgical techniques. There remains, however, substantial room for improvement. The need for a more perfect hemostasis, reduced operating time, and theoretical reduction of postoperative adhesions and tubal occlusion from scarring prompted the experimental use of the CO_2 laser by the senior author in reconstructive microsurgery from 1974 to 1979.[4] The results of the first 14 cases were encouraging: 9 conceptions and 5 viable infants. Two ectopic pregnancies occurred. Unfortunately, results of the other pregnancies are unknown, and some of the original 14 patients preferred not to attempt pregnancy.

Subsequently, other investigators, notably in France and West Germany, began utilizing the laser in microsurgery.[5–7] Animal models, used abroad and in the United States, confirmed increased postoperative tubal patency, and demonstrated that limited laser tissue injury reduced adhesion formation. All investigators confirmed the intraoperative hemostasis and reported reduced operating time in these studies.

To date, we have performed over 1000 microsurgical procedures with the CO_2 laser microsurgical system. We have not had any complications. No wound separations or infections have been noted. Patients' recovery was complete by the fifth postoperative day and they were allowed to return home, sometimes traveling as many as 18,000 miles to their homeland.[8]

Analysis of our operative time revealed a significant reduction in our operative time. This reduction in operating room time will translate into financial savings for the patient.

The CO_2 laser is another step into the future, and we hope that it is not the final step.

References

1. Klink F, Brosspietzsh R, Klinzing LV, et al: Animal *in vivo* studies and *in vitro* experiments with human tubes for end to end anastomotic operation by a CO_2 laser technique. Fertil Steril *30*:100–102, 1978.
2. Von Klinzing, Grosspietzsch R, Klink F, et al: Zur operativen refertilirisierung durch laser technique. Fortschr Med *96*:357–359, 1978.
3. Bellina JH, Seto YJ: Pathological and physical investigations into CO_2 laser-tissue interaction with specific emphasis in cervical intraepithelial neoplasia. Lasers Surg Med *1*:47–69, 1980.
4. Bellina JH: Reconstructive microsurgery of the fallopian tube with the carbon dioxide laser—procedures and preliminary results. Reproduccion 5:1–17, 1981.
5. Grobpietzsch R, Inthraphuvasak J, Klink F, Oberheuser F: Experiments on operative treatment of tubular sterility by CO_2 laser technique, in Kaplan I, Ascher PW (eds): Laser Surgery, Vol III, Part 1. Tel Aviv, Israel, OT-PAZ Press, 1979, pp 256–262.
6. Inthraphuvasak J, Grobpietzsch R, Klink F, Oberheuser F: CO_2 laser beam in gynecological microsurgical operations . . . A preliminary report, in Kaplan I, Ascher PW (eds): Laser Surgery, Vol III, Part 1. Tel Aviv, Israel, OT-PAZ Press, 1979, pp 263–268.
7. Bruhat MA, Mage G, Pouly JL: Use of the CO_2 laser in neosalpingostomy, in Kaplan I, Ascher PW: Laser Surgery, Vol III, Part 1. Tel Aviv, Israel, OT-PAZ Press, 1979, pp 271–273.
8. Bellina JH: Microsurgery of the fallopian tube with carbon dioxide laser: eighty-two cases with follow-up. Lasers Surg Med 2:129–136, 1982.

Appendixes

Appendix A. The Zeiss Operating Microscope 215
    I. Optical Principles, Illumination Systems, and
        Support Systems 217
    II. Individual Parts, Handling, Assembling, Focus-
        ing, and Balancing 223
    III. Accessories 233
    IV. Documentation 239
    V. Maintenance and Cleaning 253
Appendix B. Patient Information: Laser Surgery 257
Appendix C. Discharge Instructions 259
Appendix D. Informed Consent............................ 261
Appendix E. Laser Certification 263
Appendix F. Societies 267
Appendix G. Publications 269
Appendix H. Glossary of Laser Terminology 271

A

The Zeiss Operating Microscope

The optical principles of the Zeiss OPMI 1, 6-S, and 7 P/H operating microscopes are discussed, along with standard and fiberoptic illumination
systems and the range of currently available support systems.

JOURNAL OF MICROSURGERY   1:364–369   1980

THE OPERATING MICROSCOPE
I. OPTICAL PRINCIPLES,
ILLUMINATION SYSTEMS,
AND SUPPORT SYSTEMS

PETER HOERENZ, Dipl.-Ing.-Phys.

Editor's Note: This is the first in a series of five articles by Mr. Hoerenz on the basic principles and construction of the operating microscope. Future articles will discuss the individual parts of the microscope, accessories, methods for documentation, and maintenance and cleaning.

Since the invention of the operating microscope and the spread of microsurgical procedures through the various surgical disciplines, a large number of specialized operating microscopes have appeared in the world marketplace. The discussion here will focus on three operating microscopes manufactured by Carl Zeiss, the OPMI 1, 6-S, and 7 P/H, which are designed to meet the needs of otorhinolaryngology, neurosurgery, gynecology, urology, plastic surgery, and the other surgical disciplines (figs. 1–3).

OPTICAL PRINCIPLES

The optical principles of the OPMI 1 instrument are presented in figure 4. At the front end of the microscope, a large-diameter main objective lens receives an image of the object situated at the objective's focal point and projects this image to infinity. This means that the light rays

leaving the front objective are parallel to each other. Behind the front objective there is a miniature telescope system, the magnification changer, which, much like field glasses of the Galilean design, takes the parallel-ray image from the main objective lens and increases or decreases its magnification. The rays that leave the Galilean system are again parallel and are picked up by another telescope system—the binocular tubes. The objectives of the binocular tubes transmit intermediate images of the object to the eyepieces, or oculars, under repeated magnification.

In effect, within each microscope, a multiple-step magnification takes place, and this is expressed in the magnification formula:

$$M_v = \frac{f_T}{f_0} \times M_E \times M_C$$

In order, therefore, to calculate the visual magnification (M_v) of a microscope, it is necessary to have data on the focal length of the binocular tube (f_T), the magnification factor of the magnification changer (M_C), the focal length of the principal objective (f_0), and the magnification power of the eyepieces (M_E). The Zeiss OPMI 1 microscope provides five magnification steps in a range of $1:6$, the Zeiss OPMI 6-S zoom system provides a continuous magnification range of $1:4$, and the OPMI 7 P/H zoom system provides a continuous magnification range of $1:5$. The data for the factor M_C of the magnification changers in these three systems are presented in table 1.

From Carl Zeiss, Inc., New York, NY.

Address reprint requests to Mr. Hoerenz at Carl Zeiss, Inc., 444 Fifth Ave., New York, NY 10018.

Received for publication September 29, 1979; translated revision received January 15, 1980.

0191-3239/0105/0364/$00.00/0

Appendix A: Zeiss Operating Microscope

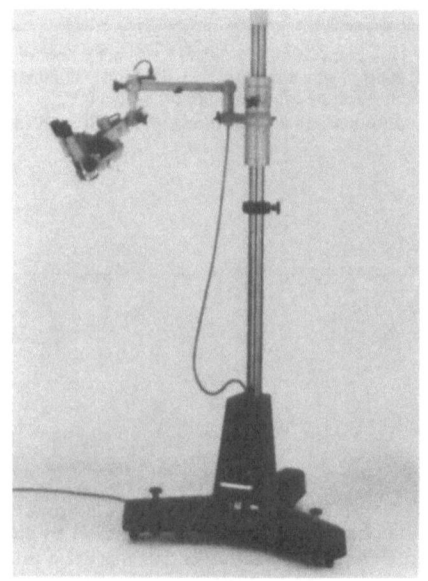

Figure 1. A Zeiss OPMI 1 with moveable floor stand.

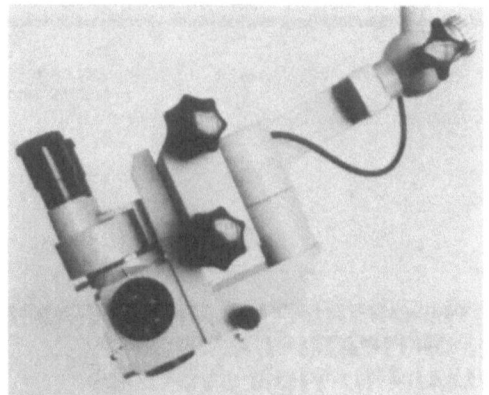

Figure 2. A Zeiss OPMI 1 microscope.

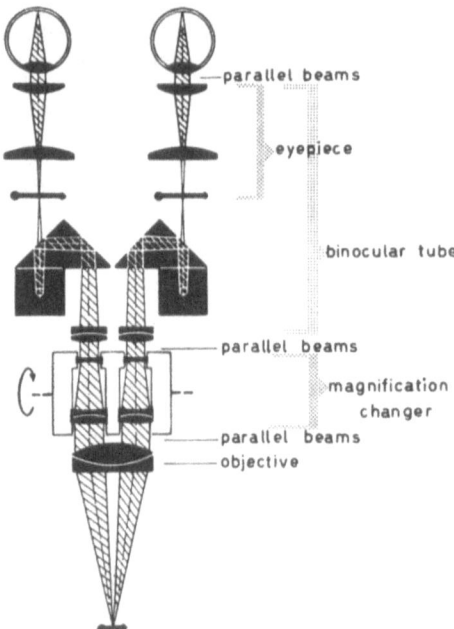

Figure 4. A schematic diagram demonstrating the optical principles of the Zeiss OPMI 1 microscope.

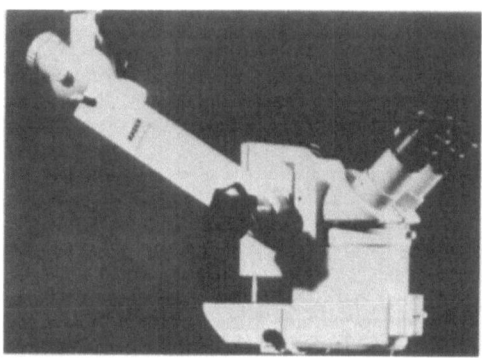

Figure 3. A Zeiss OPMI 6-S with inclined binocular tubes.

Table 1. Magnification factors (M_C) for the OPMI 1, OPMI 6-S, and OPMI 7 P/H magnification changers.

Microscope	Magnification changer dial setting	M_C
OPMI 1	6	0.4
	10	0.6
	16	1.0
	25	1.6
	40	2.5
OPMI 6-S (zoom)	0.5	0.5
		1.0
	2.0	2.0
OPMI 7 P/H	0.5	0.5
	1.0	1.0
	2.5	2.5

218

Table 2. The size of the field of view (mm) and the total magnification power of an OPMI 1 equipped with 125-mm binocular tubes and 20× eyepieces.

Focal length of the main objective	Magnification changer dial setting									
	6 (0.4)[a]		10 (0.6)		16 (1)		25 (1.6)		40 (2.5)	
	Field of view	Magnification	Field of view	Magnification	Field of view	Magnification	Field of view	Magnification	Field of view	Magnification
200 mm	40	5×	27	7.5×	16	12.5×	10	20×	6	31×
225 mm	44	4.5×	30	6.5×	18	11×	11	18×	7	28×
250 mm	50	4×	33	6×	20	10×	12.5	16×	8	25×
275 mm	57	3.5×	36	5.5×	22	9×	14	14.5×	9	23×
300 mm	67	3×	40	5×	25	8×	15	13×	10	21×

[a]*Numbers in parentheses are the factors on the new OPMI 1 magnification changer knobs.*

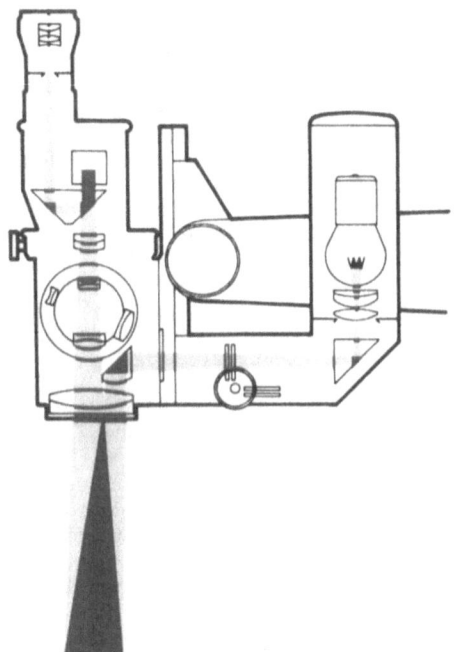

Figure 5. A diagram demonstrating the coaxial illumination system.

The focal lengths of main objectives used in microsurgery are graduated from $f_o = 150$ mm to $f_o = 400$ mm in steps of 25 mm. It should be noted here that the focal length of the objective is equal to its working distance, and it is therefore necessary to bring the object to be viewed to the exact distance of the focal length of the lens (see fig. 4).

Binocular tubes, either straight or inclined, are available in two lengths or focal lengths of $f_T = 125$ mm and $f_T = 160$ mm.

Finally, one needs the magnification power (M_E) of the oculars in order to complete this simple calculation. Four different ocular magnifications are available: 10×, 12.5×, 16×, and 20×.

With this information, it is easy to determine the minimum and maximum magnifications of the most frequently used combination of microscope components. For example, an OPMI 1 equipped with a 300-mm objective, 125-mm binocular tubes, and 20× eyepieces produces a minimum magnification of:

$$M_{v\ min} = \frac{125}{300} \times 0.4 \times 20 = 3.3$$

and an upper-range magnification of:

$$M_{v\ max} = \frac{125}{300} \times 2.5 \times 20 = 20.8$$

Data for other combinations are presented in table 2.

The size of the field of view, which obviously changes as the magnification changes, is equally simple to calculate. The formula for determining the diameter of the field of view is

$$F = \frac{200}{M_v}$$

so that in the example above, the microscope at its lowest magnification has a maximum field of view of about 60 mm (diameter) and, at its highest magnification, a field of view of about 10 mm (table 2).

ILLUMINATION

The illumination of the operating field is supplied by an additional built-in ray path in the microscope (fig. 5). A low-voltage incandescent bulb (6 V 30 W or, formerly, 6 V 50 W) is situated in a precentered lamp socket in the lamp housing on the back side of the microscope. A collecting system and two reflecting prisms transmit the light through the front objective in the immediate vicinity of the ray paths of the image, without, however, in any way interfering with these rays. The illumination finally reaches the surgical wound almost parallel to the viewing axes and, under ideal conditions, produces a bright, uniformly illuminated, circular spot. This spot is concentric with the microscope's field of view. This type of illumination, termed "coaxial," is capable of providing shadow-free illumination even in very deep and narrow wounds. The low-voltage incandescent lamp receives its power through a cable connected to an outlet on the microscope's horizontal arm. A transformer is built into the base of the microscope stand.

In the last few years, glass fiber illumination sources have both supplemented and displaced the incandescent lamp coaxial system. One reason for this is the problem of heat build-up from the incandescent lamp inside the microscope, especially when the microscope is fully draped. In addition, many surgeons find the heat radiating from the lamp housing uncomfortable when they are using the short, straight binocular tubes.

A second and perhaps more important reason is the difficulty of replacing the 6-V bulb if it burns out during an operation. Under such circumstances, replacing the bulb can result in a time-consuming procedure, because it is necessary to redrape the microscope. Because the glass fiber illumination housing is mounted outside the microscope drapery and is designed with a practical drawer system, a bulb change is possible in seconds.

Additional advantages of glass fiber illumination are an increase of the diameter of the illuminated field and a major gain in light intensity. At the moment, a combination of glass fiber illumination and built-in incandescent lamp gives the highest attainable light level. This is especially useful when film and photographic attachments on the microscope are being used. (More details on the subject of fiber illumination will be provided in a future article on accessories.)

An important point to remember when evaluating light sources is not only their brightness but also their life spans. Unfortunately, brightness, also called luminance, and life span have a detrimental relationship to one another. If the surgeon wants to increase the light intensity by overloading the bulb, he sacrifices the life span of the bulb. For example, by doubling the light output—thereby doubling the illumination level in the operating field—the life span of the lamp is reduced by 93%. For this reason, increasing the brightness by raising the voltage is limited by natural boundaries, namely, the point at which the life span of the lamp is reduced to a few hours and falls within the time period required for completing the surgical procedure. Under no circumstances, therefore, should the voltage be raised so high that the life span of the bulb is reduced to less than 10 hours.

Manufacturers of bulbs are very hesitant to give statements on the life span of bulbs. Therefore, the only way to establish absolute clarity on this subject is through a series of tests. This also applies to the adjustment of the primary voltage in the transformer, and naturally, of course, to the use of voltage controls in instruments with voltmeters. It has been established that most of the 6-V incandescent bulbs whose life span at 6 V amounts to 200 hours, will have their life span reduced to zero if the voltage they receive reaches about 10–11 V, i.e., they burn out at those levels. Overloading of these bulbs beyond a 9-V limit should therefore never be allowed. Moreover, the voltage level noted here must be measured at the socket of the lamp. Measurements made at the outlet on the microscope's horizontal arm usually give values that are higher by 0.5 to 1.0 V. The voltage drops before it reaches the lamp socket because of resistance in the connecting cable. For example, readings of 9.5 to 10 V at the outlet will drop to 9 V at the lamp socket.

Regarding illumination of the operating field and observed brightness, it must be mentioned that a change in the working distance resulting from a change to an objective with a different focal length changes the illumination levels attainable in the operating field. As a general rule, the longer the focal length, the less brightness is attainable. Thus, a change in working distance from 200 mm to 300 mm produces a 58% loss in "viewed," i.e., observable brightness. This is caused by two factors: the illumination intensity in the operating field itself is decreased by the increased working distance, and the effective

Table 3. Reduction of brightness with increasing working distance.

Working distance of the main objective lens	Measured light value	% of light lost
200 mm	100%[a]	0
250 mm	64%	36%
300 mm	42%	58%

[a]*The measured light value at 200 mm is set at 100%; the point of measurement is behind the eyepiece.*

aperture of the optical viewing system is also diminished. Table 3 provides a summary of these relationships.

The need for more light with increased working distances is, therefore, widely felt. The human eye is physiologically capable of adapting itself to different light levels, and especially to low light levels, and is consequently able, even under unfavorable light conditions, to make work possible. On the other hand, movie cameras, still cameras, and television cameras record light losses more objectively and register them immediately with underexposures. A knowledge of these illumination-reduction relationships is therefore extremely important to anyone interested in photography through the microscope.

MICROSCOPE SUSPENSION SYSTEMS

There are a variety of support systems available for mounting the operating microscope. Among these are moveable floor stands with internal counterweights and manual up and down movement; motorized floor stands with mechanical up and down movement controlled by foot pedal; ceiling mounts with manual and electromechanical height adjustment; and finally, the microscope stand developed by the firm of Contraves A.G. in Zürich, Switzerland, which is equipped with an electromagnetic clutch system, permitting an absolute equilibrium condition and, consequently, free movement of the balanced microscope with or without accessories (fig. 6). This instrument's position adjustment is controlled by a mouth-operated switch that also serves as the microscope control stick.

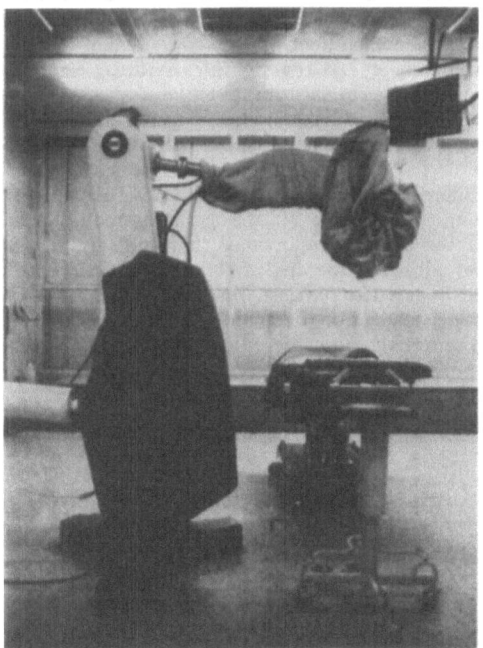
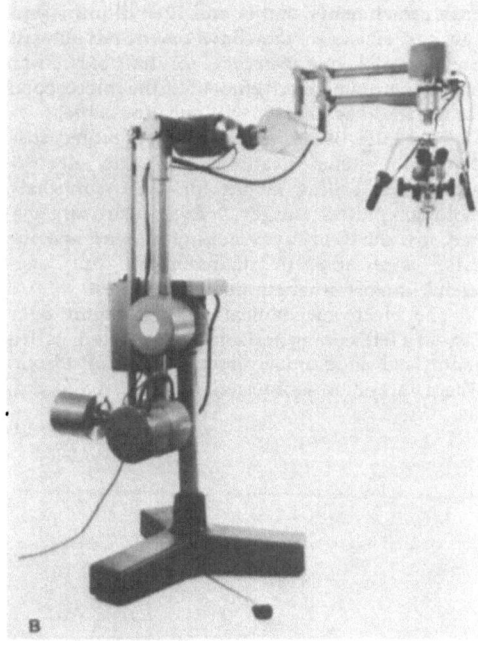

Figure 6. (A) Prototype of the Contraves stand in the operating room of the Kantonsspital Zürich. (Courtesy of Prof. Dr. M.G. Yasargil, Neurochirurgische Universitätsklinik, Kantonsspital Zürich, Switzerland.) (B) The Contraves stand.

221

The special advantage of this microscope support is that it drastically reduces the effective operation time because maneuvers in repositioning the microscope can be carried out easily and swiftly.

All floor stands are moveable and, depending upon the various patient positions for the different microsurgical operations, can be set up in different places around the table so that they interfere as little as possible with the surgeon and the assisting personnel. Once the microscope support is brought into position, it is made stationary through the use of brakes. In the case of the Contraves microscope stand, its massive weight alone provides for a safe stationary position. Furthermore, because of the extensive reach of the Contraves arm system, it is always set up on the upper left end of the operating table when used by right-handed surgeons and on the upper right side for left-handed surgeons.

The latest additions to the line of microscope suspension systems are those that are mounted on operating room ceilings. They allow absolute freedom of movement around the operating table and they come equipped with additional features such as auxiliary outlets for cameras, flash attachments, and 6- and 12-V illumination systems. However, they have one disadvantage: they restrict microsurgery to that particular operating room since removal of the microscope for use in other rooms is no longer possible.

There are two types of ceiling-mounted suspension systems available: (a) the electromechanical ceiling mount for use in ophthalmology, plastic surgery, and neurosurgery; and (b) the Contraves ceiling mount specifically applicable to neurosurgery but also useful in most other surgical disciplines.

The electromechanical ceiling mount consists of a telescoping horizontal arm system with a motorized or manual vertical travel of 48 cm. The arm system is internally counter-balanced, and the microscope can be moved up and down manually, much like the movement on a counter-balanced floor stand. For those who prefer motorized movements, the vertical travel at 3 mm/sec can be controlled by a foot switch. All controls of the fully motorized OPMI 6-S, namely, zooming and focusing, are remotely controlled by means of a foot-control panel.

The ceiling-mounted Contraves suspension system offers exactly the same features as the Contraves floor unit with the addition of extra free space on the floor next to the operating table. All operating microscopes, motorized and manual, can be attached to the Contraves ceiling mount, and, in the case of the motorized microscope, the function of the zoom magnification changer is controlled with a simple two-action foot switch since the internal focusing of the microscope body is no longer needed on the Contraves stand. Naturally, all accessories normally used with microscopes mounted on floor stands can be attached and counter-balanced on the ceiling suspension systems.

Ideally, ceiling mounts are best installed in operating rooms during the construction of the operating suite. They may be installed in existing operating rooms, but finding the appropriate point of attachment may be complicated by the presence of existing lighting fixtures, electric wiring, overhead tubing for anesthesia, air-conditioning ducts, and heavy traffic areas overhead that could cause ceiling vibrations. Therefore, because of the potential for protracted construction problems and the subsequent long-term closing of the operating room, it is of the utmost importance that sufficient time be allowed to analyze the situation with all concerned parties, including the architect, the construction firm, the manufacturer's representative, and the microsurgeons. This detailed and long-range planning should minimize the downtime of the operating room facility.

The major components of the Zeiss OPMI 1, OPMI 6-S, and OPMI 7 P/H are discussed along with details on handling and assembling the components, changing couplings, focusing, and balancing the microscope system prior to use.

JOURNAL OF MICROSURGERY   1:419–427   1980

THE OPERATING MICROSCOPE. II. INDIVIDUAL PARTS, HANDLING, ASSEMBLING, FOCUSING, AND BALANCING

PETER HOERENZ, Dipl.-Ing.-Phys.

Editor's Note: This is the second in a series of five articles by Mr. Hoerenz on the basic principles and handling of the operating microscope. The first article, on optical principles, illumination systems, and support systems, appeared in Journal of Microsurgery *1:364–369, 1980. Future articles will discuss accessories, methods for documenting surgical procedures, and maintenance and cleaning.*

The importance of the optical and illuminating properties of the operating microscope in the successful use of the instrument is often underrated. In order to put these technical properties to full use, however, it is extremely important to have a knowledge of the separate parts of the operating microscope and to be able to handle and assemble these parts, to focus, and to balance the instrument.

Basically, the operating microscope is composed of three major components: the main objective, the microscope body, and the binocular tube system. These three components can be seen clearly in figures 1 and 2.

THE MAIN OBJECTIVE

The main objective is a lens system that is attached to the front or lower end of the microscope body by means of a threaded mount. The focal length of the lens system is engraved on the side, for example, f = 300 mm. This lens number simultaneously gives the focal length of the lens and the free working distance available between the microscope and the surgical field when that lens is used. The objectives are easily interchangeable, and they are available in various focal lengths (and, therefore, various working distances) in graduated steps of 25 mm. It is advisable to begin equipping the microscope with objectives properly selected for the various specific tasks it will encounter. The most commonly used focal lengths are 150, 175, and 200 mm in ophthalmology; 200, 225, 250, 275, and 300 mm in neurosurgery; 200, 300, and 400 mm in otolaryngology; 250, 300, and 320 mm in gynecology; and 200 mm in hand and reconstructive surgery.

Use of the proper working distance can greatly lessen strain, especially in operations of long duration, and a difference of 25 mm often can determine the body comfort or the positioning of the arms and hands of the surgeon. Therefore, tests should be conducted by every user of the instrument to determine exactly which objectives provide the most comfortable working distances.

THE MICROSCOPE BODY

The microscope body, which includes the magnification changer, makes up the middle section of the instrument. The body is attached mechanically to a support yoke that allows the instrument to be tilted. On the outside of the body of the OPMI 1 are knobs for manual focusing.

From Carl Zeiss, Inc., New York, NY.

Address reprint requests to Mr. Hoerenz at Carl Zeiss, Inc., 444 Fifth Ave., New York, NY 10018.

Received for publication February 27, 1980.

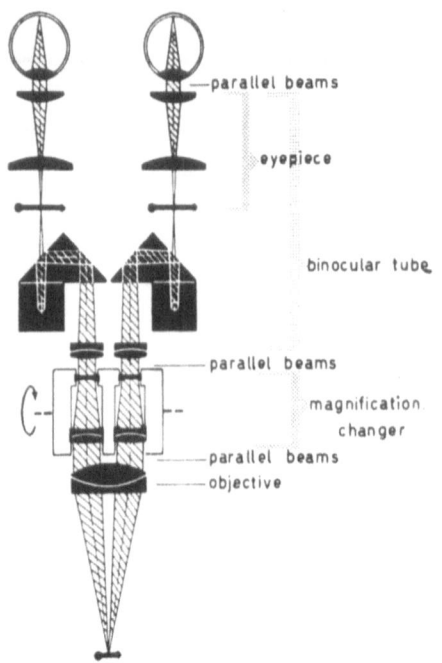

Figure 1. Schematic diagram of the optical principles of the Zeiss OPMI 1. Note the three major components of the microscope: the main objective, the microscope body (housing the magnification changer), and the binocular system.

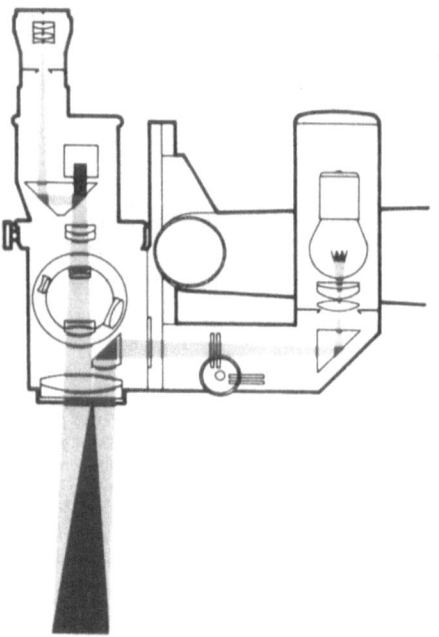

Figure 2. A cross-section diagram of the Zeiss OPMI 1, demonstrating the three components and the coaxial illumination system.

Motorized microscopes, such as the OPMI 6-S and the OPMI 7 P/H, are focused via electric hand or foot switches.

In the center of the microscope body are manual control knobs for changing the magnification; this is stepwise on the OPMI 1, and continuous on the OPMI 6-S. The OPMI 7 P/H (a microscope especially designed for plastic and hand surgeons) has no external manual controls (fig. 3). All focusing and magnification adjustments are made electrically and are controlled by remote switches. By eliminating all external knobs, it was possible to devise a microscope of such slim design that two surgeons working at positions 180° from each other both have unobscured, unhindered access to the surgical field.

On the lower end of the microscope body is the threaded receptacle for the front objective. On the upper end of the microscope body is a dovetail receptacle with a knurled clamping screw, which serves as a receptacle for the attachment of accessories, or in the simplest case, for the attachment of the binocular tube system (fig. 4).

THE BINOCULAR TUBE SYSTEM

The binocular tube system permits stereoscopic viewing. The system is comparable to a telescope; in fact, it is constructed on the same principle and can be used as field glasses. On the lower side of the system, there is a dovetail that is the counterpart of the dovetail receptacle on the microscope body and serves to fasten the system to the microscope and ensure that the optical axes of the binocular tubes align precisely with those of the microscope body when the clamping screw has joined the two parts together. The two objectives of the binocular tubes, visible as two blue-colored lens surfaces 16 mm wide, are built into the system's dovetail (the blue color results from a nonreflective optical coating).

Inside the upper end of the binocular tubes are spring-loaded supports for the eyepieces or oculars. Mechanical clamps ensure that the oculars always sit securely inside the tubes and do not fall out when the microscope body is tilted into a horizontal position (or lower). The

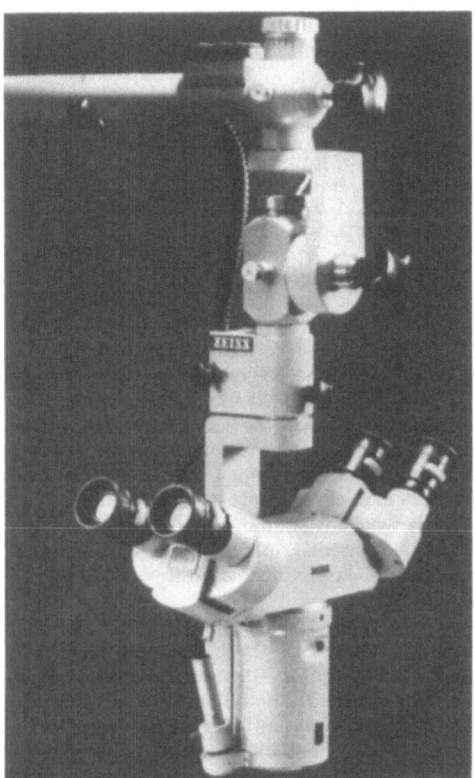

Figure 3. The Zeiss OPMI 7 P/H with no accessories. The OPMI 7 P/H is designed for plastic and hand surgery and allows two surgeons to work simultaneously at positions 180° opposed to each other. Note the lack of external focusing and zoom controls.

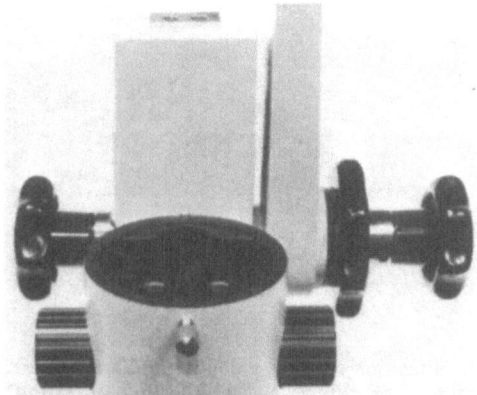

Figure 4. The dovetail receptacle of the microscope body.

HANDLING AND ASSEMBLING THE SEPARATE PARTS OF THE MICROSCOPE

Changing Objectives. The objectives are equipped with a very fine thread that must be very carefully engaged into the threaded receptacle on the microscope body. This task can be simplified by turning the objective first in a counterclockwise direction until a soft "click" is heard, which indicates that the thread is engaged, and then by carefully turning the objective in a clockwise direction until it is completely screwed into the microscope body and comes to its end stop. It is essential that one take care not to leave fingerprints on either the lenses of the magnification changer or the objective itself when changing objectives. In the event a lens is soiled, it can be cleaned (the cleaning of lenses will be discussed in a future article on cleaning and maintenance of the operating microscope).

Magnification Changer. After inserting the objective, one should make certain that the movement of the magnification changer is in order, namely, that it moves between magnification steps with light force and audible engaging clicks on the OPMI 1 and that it zooms smoothly on the OPMI 6-S and OPMI 7 P/H. A sharp rubbing or squeaking sound (or a faulty zoom) indicates that the mechanical guides are dry. In this case, servicing the instrument is immediately necessary.

The magnification changer of the OPMI 1 has the capacity to magnify as well as reduce the image received from the main objective in five different steps. The numbers engraved on the magnification changer (6, 10, 16, 25, and 40) serve only as coefficients and indicate the actual

distance between the binocular tubes can be adjusted inward or outward to allow for differences in the pupillary distance of different users. This is especially important for the basic focusing procedure of the microscope.

The oculars make up the last part of the assembled microscope (fig. 5). They are, as already mentioned, interchangeable and are available in four different magnifying powers: 10×, 12.5×, 16×, and 20×. In procedures with long working distances and small surgical fields (such as in neurosurgery), the 300-mm objective is used with the 20× oculars. With shorter working distances, where one needs lower total magnifications for a relatively large surgical field (such as in ophthalmology), eyepieces with a lower magnification are recommended. In such cases, 12.5× eyepieces will be preferred.

225

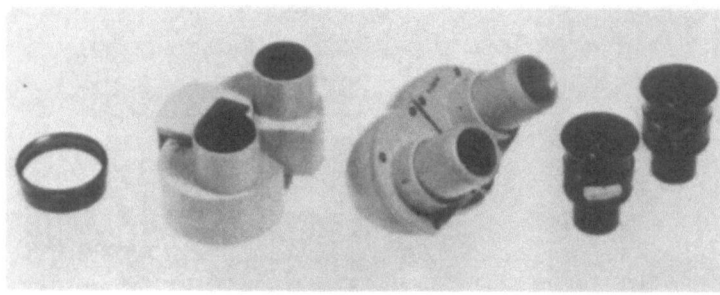

Figure 5. A 300-mm main objective, straight and inclined binocular tube systems, and 20× oculars.

magnification only for a definite optical combination (see table 1). On the magnification changer knob of the newer OPMI 1, the factors 0.4, 0.6, 1, 1.6, and 2.5 have replaced the old numbers and serve for the computation of total magnifications as discussed in the previous article (*J Microsurg* 1:364–369, 1980).

Binocular Tubes. Binocular tubes are available in straight and inclined forms and in two different lengths, short tubes of 125 mm and long tubes of 160 mm (fig. 6). The long tubes produce a slightly higher magnification than the short tubes; the short tubes, on the other hand, have the advantage of reducing the total length of the microscope by 25 mm. How the microscope is to be used, i.e., in the horizontal, inclined, or vertical position, will determine whether straight or inclined binocular tubes should be inserted into the dovetail receptacle. Before attaching the binocular tubes, one must make sure that neither the objectives of the magnification changer nor the exposed lenses of the binocular tubes are soiled by dirt or fingerprints.

The knurled screw in the dovetail of the microscope body must be screwed out quite far in order to allow the insertion of the binocular dovetail. The binocular system should be tilted slightly in order for the small cutout on the binocular dovetail to engage the positioning pin of the dovetail of the microscope body. Then, the binocular system should be inserted until the dovetails are neatly joined. The knurled screw then should be tightened carefully to fasten both parts together.

At this point the working condition of the geared movement of the binocular tubes that permits the pupillary distance to be adjusted should be checked. The adjustment mechanism should be relatively stiff but, at the same time, easily and continuously adjustable with the application of light force. If it is very loose and the gearing on both tubes is shaky—thereby producing uneven and jerky adjustments—the system must be repaired immediately. An unanticipated change in the pupillary distance during an operation can be extremely disturbing and uncomfortable.

The final step in assembling the microscope is the insertion of the oculars. Before inserting

Table 1. The size of the field of view (mm) and the total magnification power of an OPMI 1 equipped with 125-mm binocular tubes and 20× eyepieces.

	Magnification changer dial setting									
	6 (0.4)[a]		10 (0.6)		16 (1)		25 (1.6)		40 (2.5)	
Focal length of the main objective	Field of view	Magnification	Field of view	Magnification	Field of view	Magnification	Field of view	Magnification	Field of view	Magnification
200 mm	40	5×	27	7.5×	16	12.5×	10	20×	6	31×
225 mm	44	4.5×	30	6.5×	18	11×	11	18×	7	28×
250 mm	50	4×	33	6×	20	10×	12.5	16×	8	25×
275 mm	57	3.5×	36	5.5×	22	9×	14	14.5×	9	23×
300 mm	67	3×	40	5×	25	8×	15	13×	10	21×

[a]Numbers in parentheses are the factors on the new OPMI 1 magnification changer knobs.

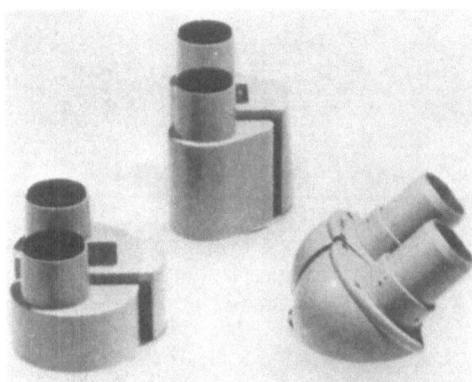

Figure 6. Interchangeable binocular systems: (left) short straight tubes, (center) long straight tubes, and (right) short inclined tubes.

the eyepieces in the binocular tubes, one should check that the lens surfaces are clean. When the oculars are inserted into the binocular tubes, they should be forced down into the sleeves of the tubes as far as possible. If the image quality is poor, a check of proper seating should be made. Often, the surgeon will be unable to achieve a clear and sharp image because one of the oculars is not fully inserted into the tube.

OCULAR FOCUSING

One of the most important steps in the basic focusing of the microscope is the correct adjustment of the oculars. Each ocular permits a spherical diopter adjustment of −9 to +9 dpt. Through these adjustments, it is possible for surgeons who wear glasses with a spherical correction to set the microscope oculars to their individual eyeglass prescription and work without spectacles. In those cases where the surgeon

wears glasses that correct for corneal astigmatism, it is recommended that the oculars be set at zero correction and the surgeon wear his glasses while using the microscope. Under these circumstances, the rubber cups attached to the eyepieces must be curled down and used as supports for the eyeglasses. Surgeons with normal vision likewise set the oculars at zero; however, they would use the rubber eye cups in the normal position. The eye cups shadow the eyes and prevent the influx of disturbing outside illumination (fig. 7).

For those ametropic surgeons who do not know the correction values for their eyes, the following procedure for the basic focusing of the oculars is appropriate:

1. Remove the binocular system from the microscope body.
2. Use the binocular system as field glasses and view a distant object, such as a tree or a house.
3. Rotate both diopter scales counterclockwise to their end stop. To rotate the oculars, depress the locking button (the orange-colored button on the new oculars).
4. Close one eye and, with the open eye, view the target while simultaneously rotating the diopter ring slowly in a clockwise direction until the target appears in sharp focus. Do not go beyond this point.
5. Read and make a note of the diopter value that appears on the ocular index scale. Repeat this procedure three times and select the mean of the three readings. This value represents the individual correction for the eye tested.
6. Repeat the procedure for the other eye. The diopter correction values determined by these procedures are valid for all other oculars and microscopes.

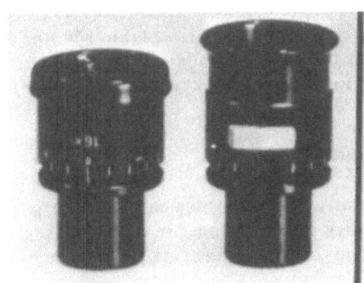
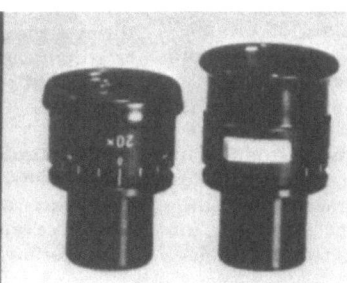

Figure 7. Interchangeable oculars of 16× and 20×. Note the diopter scale and the diopter lock. The rubber eyecups can be curled down and used as rests for glasses.

In the event that the eyepieces are not equipped with locking devices, it is advisable to tape them securely in place to prevent any inadvertent rotation and change of setting.

ADJUSTING THE PUPILLARY DISTANCE

The correct adjustment of the binocular tubes to the pupillary distance of the user is of great importance for stereoscopic viewing and maximum brightness. The most suitable object to view under the microscope for this purpose is a sheet of graph paper.

FOCUSING THE MICROSCOPE

There are several basic rules that underlie the focusing of the microscope which, if followed, will simplify the use of the instrument (especially where frequent changes are made from low to high magnification). After the ocular and pupillary distance adjustments noted above are completed, the microscope is set to its highest magnification level and, descending from above the surgical field, is focused upon an object. Focusing at the highest magnification level is done because the minimal depth of field at this magnification is extremely critical and leads to perfect focus for all other magnification levels. Thereafter, the surgeon only has to switch to another magnification and does not need to refocus the instrument. If the instrument is repositioned, however, the procedure must be repeated.

A microscope adjusted according to the procedures noted above will allow the user to work for long periods without fatigue and will ensure a minimum number of adjustments, optimum brightness, and perfect focus of all accessories attached to the instrument.

ADDITIONAL CHECKS

Before the operating microscope is used, two additional tests should be made.

First, the focusing mechanism of the manual OPMI 1 is controlled by two large hand knobs that protrude from opposite sides of the microscope body. In the event that the tension of the focusing mechanism must be changed, these two knobs must be rotated in opposite directions to one another. In order to loosen the mechanism, the knobs are rotated away from each other, i.e., in a counterclockwise direction. To increase the stiffness of the mechanism, the knobs must be turned toward each other, i.e., in a clockwise direction. The force required to accomplish these adjustments is somewhat large.

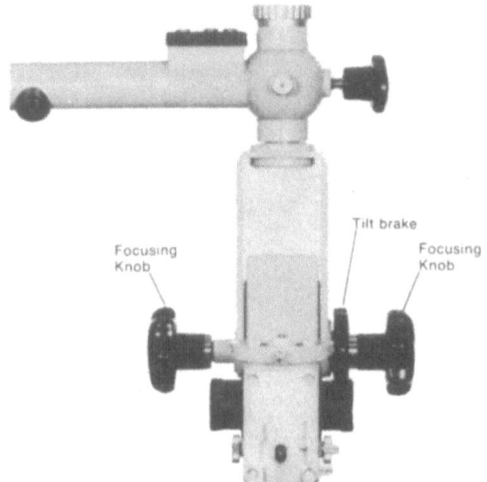

Figure 8. The body of a Zeiss OPMI 1, demonstrating the focusing knobs and tilt brake.

The mobility of the focusing mechanism should be so smooth and exact that the instrument with its attached accessories will focus easily but will not sink under its own weight, especially when it is used in the vertical position (fig. 8).

Second, the tilting of the microscope around the horizontal axis is controlled by a brake knob that can be adjusted for stiffness of movement. This brake knob is situated on the focusing axis between the yoke and the right-hand focusing knob. Turning this wheel clockwise increases the brake friction to the point where movement is prevented, whereas turning the knob in the opposite direction increases the mobility of the yoke to the point where it will swing freely. It is important to adjust the tilting resistance to the point where the microscope with all of its attached accessories is easily moveable, but not to where the microscope is on the verge of tipping over. The OPMI 6-S has a geared friction clutch tilting device that allows free rotation of the microscope when the clutch is unlocked and continuous tilt via a manual knob when the clutch is locked.

DISMANTLING AND CHANGING COUPLINGS

The great variety of microsurgical procedures often necessitates major changes in the outfitting and positioning of the operating microscope.

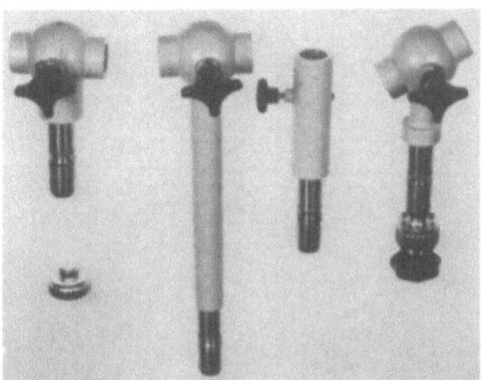

Figure 9. Couplings currently available for use with the Zeiss floor stand.

Changing objectives in order to alter the working distance and removing and replacing the binocular system have already been discussed. It is obvious that in order to use the microscope in the vertical position, inclined binocular tubes of 125 mm are preferred, and it is equally obvious that the straight binocular tubes can be used only when the microscope is used in a horizontal or inclined position. Changing the position of the microscope in many cases, however, is possible only by changing various couplings of the total suspension system.

So many couplings are available to change the position of the microscope that it is advisable to seek the optimal solution to a specific problem through experiments in the laboratory. Figures 9 and 10 illustrate couplings that are used in neu-

rosurgery, otology, ophthalmology, gynecology, and reconstructive surgery.

Changing couplings is very simple. To disconnect a coupling, the silver safety screw should first be removed from the top side of the bolt. Next, the safety pin on the side of the ball-shaped receptacle should be pulled out of the support coupling. The coupling to be removed then can be pulled out. One coupling can be inserted into another by pushing the bolt into the receptacle until the clearly audible click of the spring-loaded safety pin is heard. The safety screw is then tightly screwed into its seat. Some couplings have a set screw instead of a spring-loaded safety pin. This set screw can be loosened or tightened with a small screwdriver.

When removing the microscope from the horizontal support arm of the floor stand, it is important to remember that the microscope has considerable weight. At the moment the safety pin is pulled, the counterweights within the column of the floor stand will pull the horizontal arm violently upward as a result of the abrupt unburdening. This can lead to damage when the heavy counterweights hit the base of the stand. It is necessary, therefore, to make certain that the star knob above the point of rotation of the horizontal arm on the carriage is securely tightened before removing the microscope from the horizontal arm. Once the carriage is locked on the column, all possible coupling combinations may be inserted between the microscope yoke and horizontal arm without the danger of the counterweights falling.

Every time a coupling is changed, one should make sure the coupling bolt in the receptacle moves easily without squeaking. This test can be made only when the star knob is loosened fully.

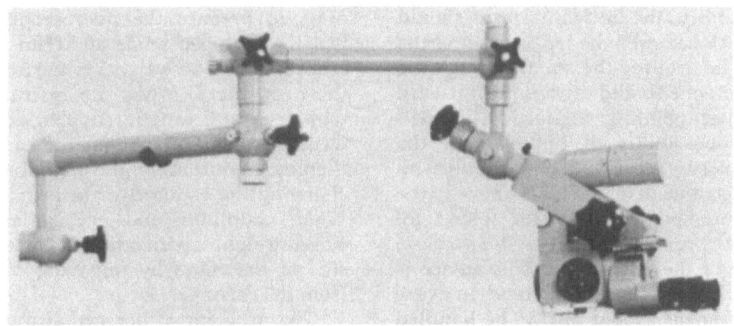

Figure 10. An OPMI 1 and couplings set up for posterior work in neurosurgery.

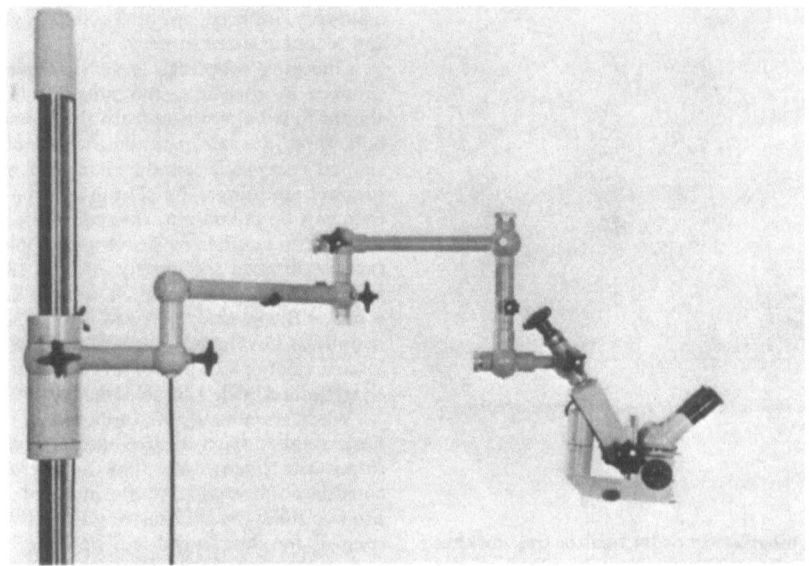

Figure 11. *The motor head attachment on the floor stand column with the microscope suspended for surgery on a supine patient.*

If scratching or squeaking is heard, the coupling should be removed and greased with a light coat of Vaseline.

The rotating joints of the horizontal arm may be damaged if a turning movement is attempted while the star knob is securely tightened. If movement is attempted, the locking bolt of that screw can, in an unfortunate case, mar the internal rotating axis of the coupling. This can make the movement of the coupling difficult or even impossible, even after the star knob is loosened. This type of damage can be repaired only by a service mechanic.

Another point to keep in mind when setting up the microscope is that in order to maintain maximum stability, the horizontal arm should always be positioned over the longest foot of the wheel base. When rolling the stand through the operating room, one should always push it with the longest foot pointing forward. This will minimize the possibility of tipping over the stand when crossing electric cables or bulges in the floor. When the instrument is moved, the horizontal arms should always be folded together so that the center of gravity is drawn close to the column of the floor stand. This advice is also valid for the motorized floor stand. In every case, the instrument should always be handled by two people when it is being moved.

BALANCING THE MICROSCOPE

The equilibrium of the microscope when mounted on the horizontal arm should be calculated in connection with variations in any equipment or accessories. Whenever accessories and couplings are changed, so, naturally, is the total weight of the instrument, which is concentrated at the far end of the horizontal arm. The counterweight within the column, however, remains unchanged. Consequently, when extreme weight changes are made to the instrument, it loses its equilibrium and can no longer be used in a free-moving, unfixed fashion.

It is therefore advisable, from the very beginning, to prepare the microscope in its most heavily equipped mode and then to counterbalance it with lead weights in the inner column of the floor stand. When the instrument is used with less total weight, supplementary counterweights can be placed on top of the carriage, thereby maintaining the equilibrium without changing the counterweight inside the column. When couplings and accessories are added again, weight equalization can be adjusted outside of the stand by removing counterweights from the carriage.

The problem of balance also can be solved through the use of two accessories: the motor

230

head and a balancing device produced by Urban Engineering (Burbank, CA).

The motor head system is based on the principle of the slipping clutch and allows either motorized or manual height adjustments of the microscope (fig. 11). Manual adjustments require a moderate expenditure of force. The friction level of the slipping clutch is adjusted so that it can control unbalanced weight on the microscope of ± 3 kg. In the event, however, that the additional weight on the microscope is greater than 3 kg, the motor is not capable of moving the microscope upward. The 3-kg limit, however, is sufficient to cover most of the commonly used accessories.

The motor head, which is made in two versions with focusing speeds of 2.5 mm/sec and 5 mm/sec, can be mounted on all nonmotorized floor stands. It is especially useful for focusing the microscope in vertical or near vertical positions. The 2.5-mm/sec speed is preferred for use with the OPMI 7 P/H. When the microscope is used in a horizontal position, the motor head can only be used for centering the height of the instrument over the surgical field and not for focusing.

The mechanical device produced by Urban Engineering for assisting in balancing consists of a steel cable that is wound on a spring-loaded drum. The drum is attached to the head of the microscope column. The extreme end of the cable has a loop that is securely attached to the highest star knob on the carriage of the floor stand. The spring tension of the cable is adjustable and can easily assimilate the increased weight of the microscope and accessories. During height adjustments, the cable runs up and down the entire column without in any way being a hindrance. When spring tension is high, however, the range of vertical travel is somewhat limited.

In summary, the trouble-free use of an unhindered, free-moving operating microscope can be achieved by counterbalancing its weight through one of the following methods:

1. Compensating the weight in the inner column.
2. Use of the motor head.
3. Use of the Urban Engineering balance device.
4. Use of the motor head together with the Urban Engineering device.

The Contraves stand may be balanced by adjusting the counterweight through inward rotation if accessories have been removed and through outward rotation if accessories have been added. For extra heavy loads, such as large TV cameras, additional weights can be added to the large standard counterweight.

Proper balance is essential with the Contraves stand in order to enjoy the full advantage of a free, "floating" microscope. It is therefore imperative that the person responsible for setting up the microscope be absolutely familiar with the detailed instructions in the Contraves user manual.

In conclusion, it should be stressed that ease of using the microscope during surgery can only be achieved by properly adjusting, focusing, and balancing the system beforehand. If attention is paid to these matters, the surgeon will be able to forget the optical device altogether in the course of performing an operation.

The beam splitter, observation tubes, and assistant's microscope, available as accessories for the OPMI series of operating microscopes, are discussed.

JOURNAL OF MICROSURGERY   2:22-26   1980

THE OPERATING MICROSCOPE. III. ACCESSORIES

PETER HOERENZ, Dipl.-Ing.-Phys.

Editor's Note: This is the third in a series of five articles by Mr. Hoerenz on the basic principles and handling of the operating microscope. The first article, on optical principles, illumination systems, and support systems, appeared in Journal of Microsurgery 1:364–369, 1980. The second article, on individual parts, handling, assembling, focusing, and balancing, appeared in Journal of Microsurgery 1:419–427, 1980. Future articles will discuss methods for documenting surgical procedures, and maintenance and cleaning.

In all of the disciplines that use microsurgery, there is a great deal of interest in microscope systems that allow direct co-observation during an operation or that allow documentation of the progress of an operation. This interest largely has been satisfied in the OPMI microscopes by a series of accessories.

THE BEAM SPLITTER

The beam splitter is the principal part that makes possible the attachment of other observation and documentation accessories. In the first article on the operating microscope (*Journal of Microsurgery* 1:364–369, 1980), the advantages of the telecentric optical system were explained, and as shown in Figure 1, there are several points in the path of the light traveling through the microscope where parallel rays are available. A unique advantage of parallel rays is that

From Carl Zeiss, Inc., New York, NY

Address reprint requests to Mr. Hoerenz at Carl Zeiss, Inc., 444 Fifth Ave., New York, NY 10018.

Received for publication March 24, 1980.

0191-3239/0201/0022 $01.25/0

they can be manipulated easily without unfavorably influencing the quality of the image. Consequently, it is possible to insert beam-splitting cubes in the path of the parallel rays that allow a portion of the rays to pass unhindered, yet divert another portion of the rays away from the original path to the outside at a 90° angle. Two such cube systems are found in the beam splitter pictured in Figure 2.

The OPMI beam splitter has a beam-splitting ratio of 50:50. This means that 50% of the light coming from the operating field is available to the principal observer through the binocular tubes and the other 50% is diverted for use in the accessory attached to the side of the microscope. It is important to mention that the accessory presents a view of the operating field that is identical to the view through the binocular tubes.

As in Figure 1, Figure 3 schematically shows the path of the light rays through the microscope, but in Figure 3 a beam splitter has been inserted between the binocular tube system and the magnification changer. A photo adapter tube is attached to the right side of the beam splitter. The photo adapter, which will be discussed in detail in a future article, is equipped with an objective ($f = 220$ mm) that focuses the incoming parallel-ray image to the film plane of the camera.

The beam splitter is approximately 50 mm in depth, and, therefore, adds little to the overall length of the entire microscope. The beam splitter is attached to the microscope body in the same manner as the binocular tube system (see *Journal of Microsurgery* 1:419–427, 1980). Again, it is worthwhile to point out that one should ex-

233

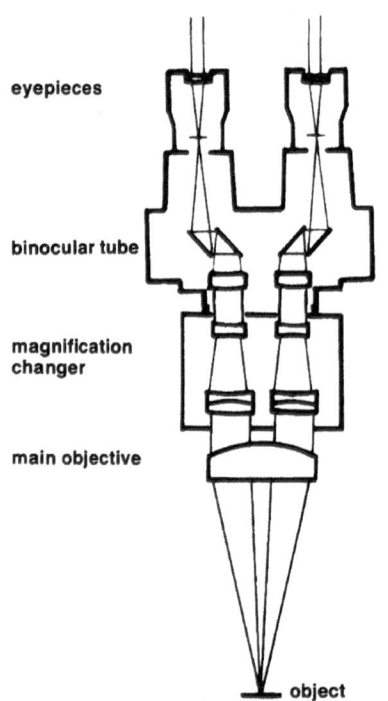

eyepieces

binocular tube

magnification
changer

main objective

object

Figure 1. A schematic diagram demonstrating the optical principles of the Zeiss OPMI microscopes. Note the parallel rays between the main objective and the magnification changer and between the magnification changer and the binocular tubes.

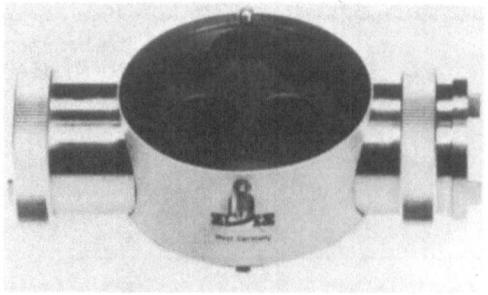

Figure 2. The beam splitter for the Zeiss microscope with two openings for attachment of accessories.

amine all glass surfaces and clean any that are soiled before assembling the components. In the case of the beam splitter, there are six glass surfaces that must be checked.

CO-OBSERVATION WITH THE BEAM SPLITTER

Three different systems are available to make possible direct co-observation during an operation. Two of these systems are monocular, and the third is binocular and stereoscopic.

The monocular tubes are differentiated by their lengths. The shorter tube can be used by an assisting surgeon, while the longer tube is more suitable for a guest observer.

The stereoscopic co-observer tube is ideal for an assisting surgeon in neurosurgical, ophthalmologic, and otologic procedures. It is shown attached to the right side of the beam splitter in

Figures 4 and 5. It makes it possible for an assistant to take an active part in the operation by providing him with a stereoscopic view. The stereoscopic depth perception available to the assistant through the stereo tube is somewhat shallower, however, than that available through the main binocular system. This is because the two viewing axes of the stereo co-observer tube run through only one side of the microscope body. The observer will be able to accustom himself to the given stereopsis in a short time, however, and will begin to see the operating field in three dimensions.

All three of the co-observer systems are constructed in a manner that allows the observer to obtain the same magnification and field of view as the microscope operator by selecting the proper ocular and, in the case of the stereo adapter, the proper binocular tubes. Since the beam splitter is mounted on top of the microscope body, the magnification and the field of view through the co-observer tubes change when the magnification changer is set at a new magnification. In many cases, however, it is desirable and possible to give the observer a wider field of view of the operation with less magnification by choosing eyepieces with a lower power.

The lower portion of the co-observer tube, which is inserted into the beam splitter and secured with a screw ring, has a rotating joint that allows the observer to find a comfortable position and to align the viewing direction accordingly. This viewing position is set by raising the sliding sleeve on top of the joint of the tube, rotating the tube to the desired position, and securing it by releasing the spring-loaded sliding sleeve. This maneuver causes the image being viewed to rotate, but this can be straightened

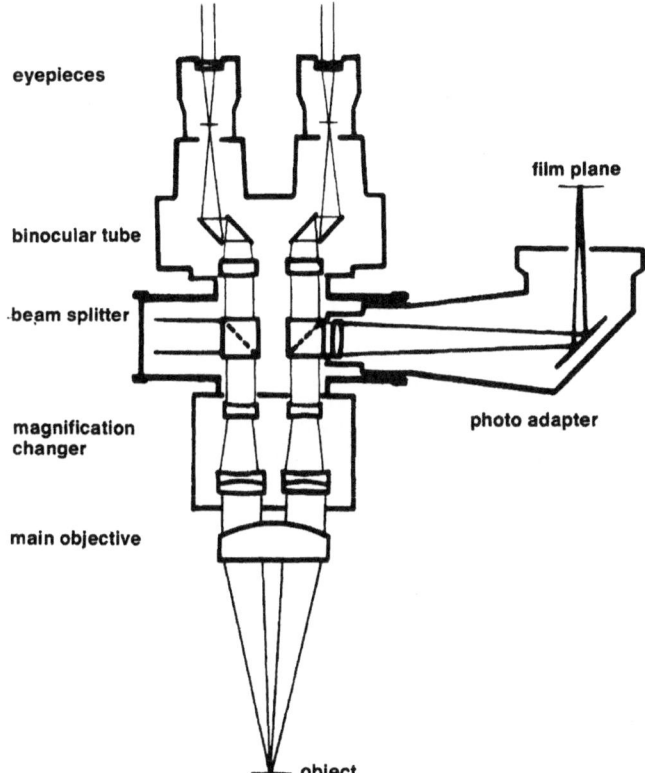

eyepieces

film plane

binocular tube

beam splitter

photo adapter

magnification
changer

main objective

object

*Figure 3. The path of the light rays in an
OPMI microscope with a beam splitter
inserted between the magnification
changer and the binocular tube system.*

again with the aid of the rotation prism system, which is located inside the tube and which is operated by a corrugated metal ring located around the tube. This ring can be turned until the view of the operating field through the co-observer tube is at exactly the same angle as the view without the microscope. Positioning of the image is made easier for the observer if the microscope operator describes the position of an object in the operating field in relation to the position on a clock face, e.g., the location of a specific vessel coursing across the field is from 7 to 2 o'clock.

The instructions given in a previous article (*Journal of Microsurgery* 1:419–427, 1980) on basic focusing of the binocular tube system are also valid for the focusing of the ocular and binocular co-observer tubes. It is also important that the observer set his personal diopter values on the diopter scales and his pupillary distance

on the binocular co-observer tube. Only through these necessary presettings can the "parfocality" of the surgeon and the observer be guaranteed. These preparations are especially important in a situation in which the assistant is responsible for photographic documentation of the procedure. In this case, he should be responsible for supervising the focusing of the entire system. As in all such situations, it is especially recommended that the beginner experiment thoroughly with the focusing relationships in the laboratory before applying them to a clinical situation.

Important Hint. The screw retaining ring on the beam splitter is loosened by turning it clockwise, that is, towards the right when viewing the beam splitter from the side of the accessory. This retaining ring belongs to the beam splitter and is not a part of the accessory. Confusion on this point often leads to a mistake in the proper di-

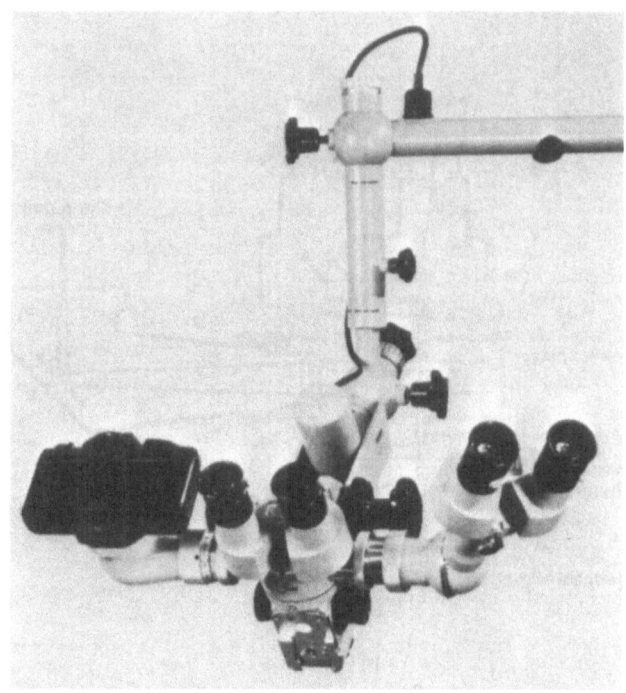

Figure 4. A stereo co-observer tube and photo adapter attached to the beam splitter on an OPMI 1 microscope.

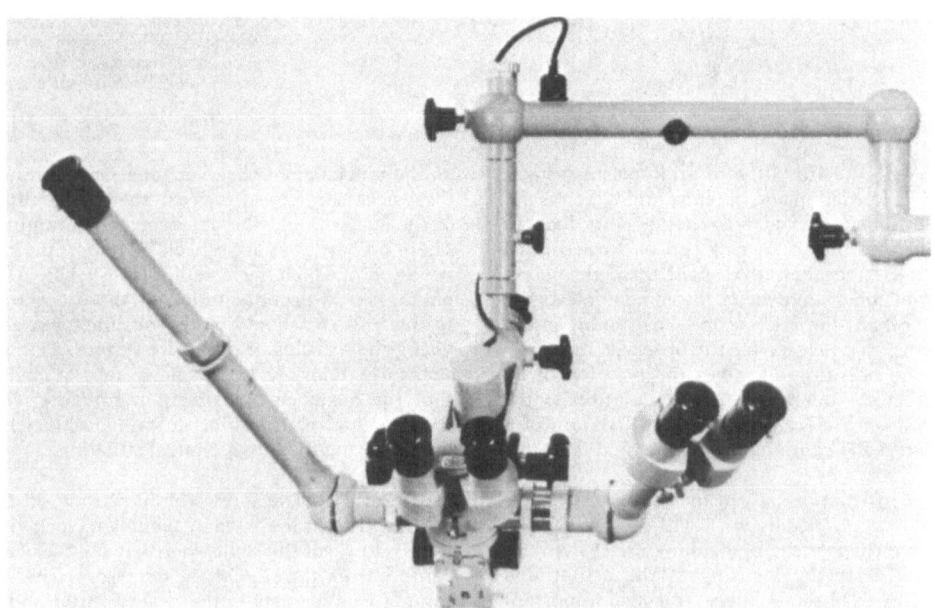

Figure 5. An OPMI 1 microscope with a stereoscopic binocular tube and a long guest observer tube attached to the beam splitter.

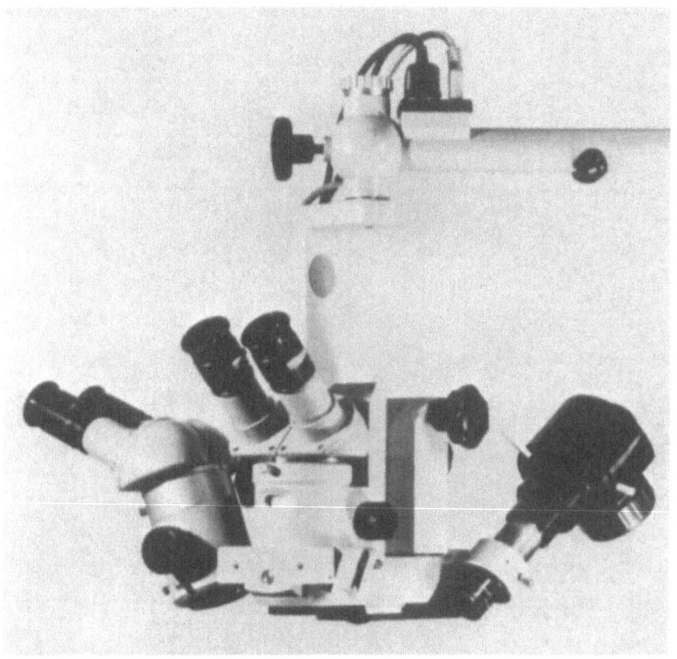

Figure 6. The assistant's microscope for co-observation mounted at a 90° angle to the main microscope.

rection for turning the ring. One should never attempt to loosen this ring forcefully with a wrench or other tool. The ring usually is turned easily in the proper direction by using a rubber cloth for a secure grip and expending a medium amount of force. Some of the newer beam splitters have an arrow engraved on the ring that indicates the proper direction for turning the ring to tighten it over the mount of the accessories. The ring may be loosened by turning it in the opposite direction.

CO-OBSERVATION WITHOUT THE BEAM SPLITTER

In ophthalmic microsurgery, co-observation through the stereo co-observer tube is essential in intraocular work. For operations on the anterior segment of the eye, however, a separate microscope, mounted at a 90° angle on either side of the main microscope, is preferred (Fig. 6). This separate microscope is mounted on a bracket by means of a sliding dovetail and provides an angle of observation of 19°. It is essential that this assistant's microscope (which basically has one fixed magnification of approximately 6×) is carefully aligned so that it is in focus with the

main microscope (parfocality) and its field of view is concentric with the field of view of the main microscope. Adjustment screws in the sliding dovetails allow proper alignment on both sides of the holding bracket. An optional 3-step magnification changer can be attached to the assistant's microscope body to provide magnifications of 4×, 6×, and 10×. The magnification changer is controlled manually like the one on the OPMI 1 series microscopes. For uninhibited use of the "Assistant's Microscope 19°," it is important that before surgery the eyepieces be set at the appropriate diopter values and the pupillary distance be carefully adjusted.

The assistant's microscope can be rotated around its own axis, thereby enabling the assistant to seek out a comfortable position during surgery. It offers full stereo perception similar to that provided by the main instrument and provides the same brightness of image, since light losses resulting from beam splitting are avoided. This kind of assistant's microscope also can be used in other microsurgical disciplines where operations are performed on surface areas and where the assistant can be placed at 90° to the primary surgeon.

237

The methods of documenting microsurgical procedures with 35-mm photography, Super 8 (8-mm) and 16-mm motion pictures, and television are discussed for the Zeiss OPMI 1, OPMI 6-S, and OPMI 7 P/H.

JOURNAL OF MICROSURGERY   2:126–139   1980

THE OPERATING MICROSCOPE. IV. DOCUMENTATION

PETER HOERENZ, Dipl.-Ing.-Phys.

Editor's Note: This is the fourth in a series of five articles by Mr. Hoerenz on the basic principles and handling of the operating microscope. The first article, on optical principles, illumination systems, and support systems, appeared in Journal of Microsurgery *1:364–369, 1980. The second article, on individual parts, handling, assembling, focusing, and balancing, appeared in* Journal of Microsurgery *1:419–427, 1980. The third article, on accessories, appeared in* Journal of Microsurgery *2:22–26, 1980. The fifth article, on care and cleaning, will appear in a future issue.*

The increased application of microsurgery has brought with it an increased interest in methods that allow surgical procedures to be documented. The OPMI series microscopes are designed to allow documentation with a variety of methods:

1. Standard still photography on 35-mm color transparency film with a 35-mm camera back.
2. Stereoscopic still photography on 35-mm color transparency film with two 35-mm camera backs.
3. Stereoscopic still photography on 35-mm color transparency film with the 35-mm half frame method.

From Carl Zeiss, Inc., New York, NY.

Address reprint requests to Mr. Hoerenz at Carl Zeiss, Inc., 444 Fifth Ave., New York, NY 10018.

Received for publication May 27, 1980.

4. Super 8 (8-mm) cinematography on color film with interchangeable film cartridges.
5. Cinematography on 16-mm film using the negative-positive method.
6. Television picture transmission and recording in black and white or color on videotape.
7. Stereoscopic television transmission and recording in color for special use in teaching.

35-mm PHOTOGRAPHY

The OPMI series microscopes can be readily adapted for standard still photography or stereoscopic still photography on either whole or half frames using 35-mm cameras (the first 3 methods listed above). The theoretical and practical discussions below are applicable to all 3 methods.

The Photo Adapter. The Zeiss photo adapter or the Zeiss/Urban Dual Camera Adapter shown in Figure 1 is required for 35-mm photography. The Zeiss photo adapter is equipped with a 220-mm focal length objective, which, like a normal camera objective, has an aperture diaphragm with f-stops of 14, 16, 22, 32, 44, and 64. Figure 2 demonstrates the path of the light rays through the microscope and the photo adapter to the film plane of the camera.

The objective end of the photo adapter is inserted into the side of the beam splitter. Guide slots make it possible to position the photo adapter so that the camera is positioned either above the microscope body or in front of it at a 90° angle (Fig. 3). The retaining ring of the beam splitter should be tightened securely over the

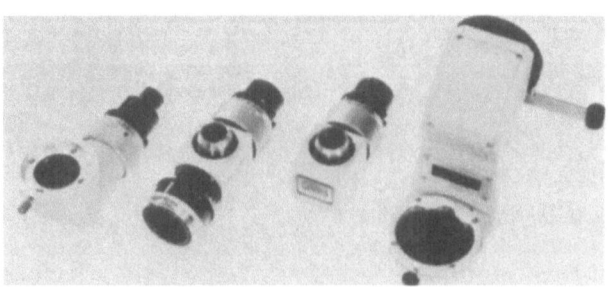

Figure 1. Adapters for the OPMI series microscopes that permit documentation of surgical procedures. (Left to right): The standard Zeiss photo adapter (f = 220 mm); the Zeiss/ Urban Dual Camera Adapter (f = 137/300 mm); the Zeiss cine adapter (f = 74 mm, also available in 137-mm or 107-mm focal lengths); the Urban stereo photo adapter.

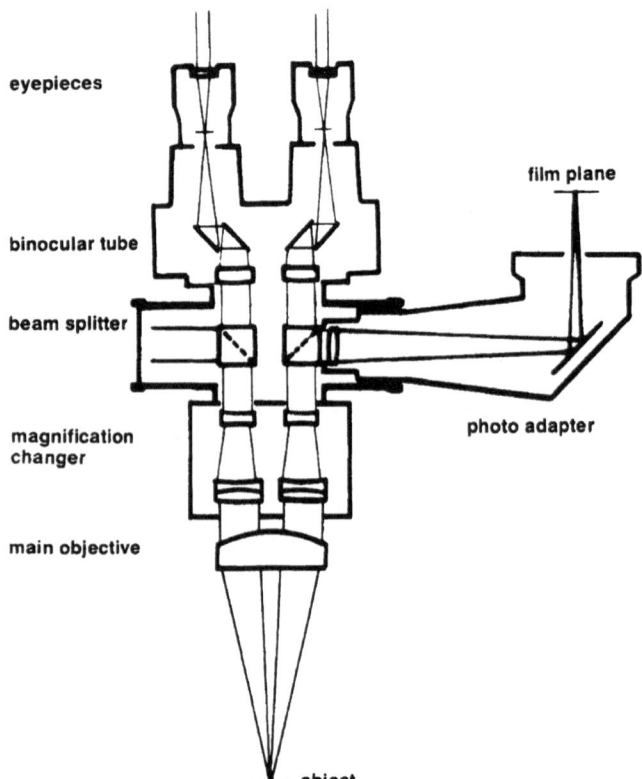

eyepieces

film plane

binocular tube

beam splitter

photo adapter

magnification changer

main objective

object

Figure 2. The path of the light rays in an OPMI microscope with a beam splitter inserted between the magnification changer and the binocular tube system and with a photo adapter attached to the beam splitter.

adapter. The camera end of the photo adapter has a simple dovetail receptacle to which the camera body, minus its own objective, is attached. It can be securely fastened by means of a knurled thumb screw.

There are many camera types that can be used with this photo adapter: for example, the Zeiss-Ikon Contarex, the Zeiss-Ikon Ikarex, the Yashica FR, the Contax RTS, the Contax 139 quartz, all Leica M-series cameras, the Leicaflex, Olympus OM series cameras, the Asahi Pentax, all Nikon F-series cameras, and the Exacta Varex. Zeiss also manufactures a special 35-mm magazine for the photo adapter. A special

240

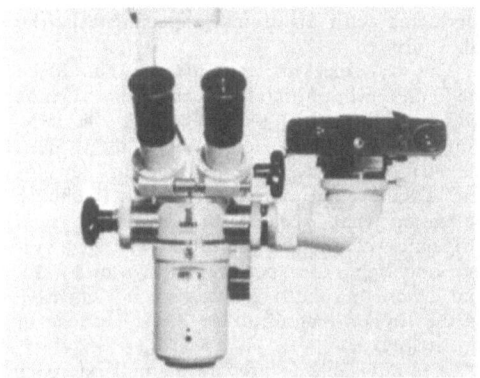 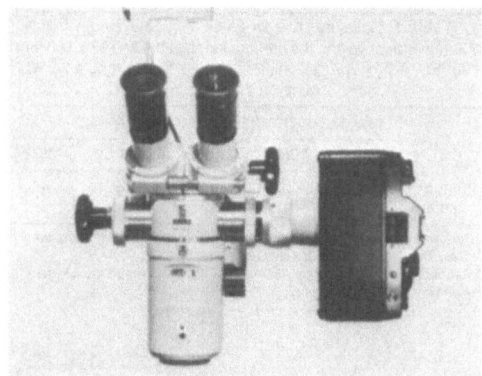

Figure 3. *The two ways of mounting the photo adapter and the camera on the beam splitter. Note the cover over the viewfinder of the camera to prevent false light meter readings.*

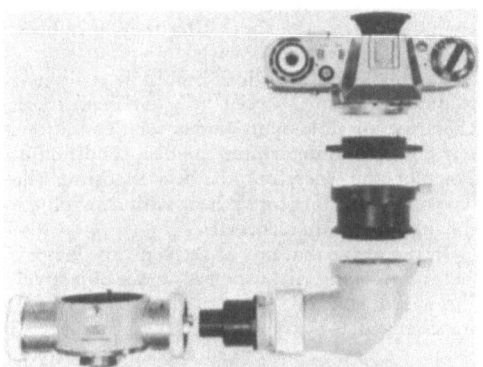

Figure 4. *An exploded view of the parts necessary to attach a 35-mm camera back to the beam splitter. (Top to bottom): Special adapter ring to match the camera back to the photo adapter; optional 2× auxiliary lens for enlarging the image; the photo adapter; the beam splitter.*

adapter ring is available for each of these camera backs that matches them to the dovetail system of the photo adapter as demonstrated in Figure 4.

The camera is attached to the photo adapter once the adapter is installed on the beam splitter in accordance with one of the positions shown in Figure 3. The photo adapter does not have any focusing mechanism. The film plane of the camera is automatically in focus when it is properly mounted on the microscope. When the microscope is focused, the camera is focused. This is called camera parfocality.

In the event that focusing difficulties are encountered, a special ocular is available that contains a cross hair and may be used in the binocular tube as an aid in focusing. If the ocular has been properly focused beforehand, and both the object and the cross hair are in sharp focus, the camera is in focus and the photograph will be at its optimum sharpness.

Proper Exposures. The primary cause of unsatisfactory photographs is negligent focusing. Attention must be paid, however, to other potential causes of blurry photographs, for example, movement of the object or of the microscope. Furthermore, foreground and background blurriness due to insufficient depth of field may be caused by choosing a level of magnification that is too high, or by an aperture setting that is too large. Finally, over- and underexposures may be caused by choosing either the wrong shutter speed or the wrong aperture setting for the available illumination.

Blurs caused by movement can be observed and eliminated by using the cross-hair ocular. The camera shutter should be released only when no relative movement is observed between the cross hair and the object, that is, when the object and microscope are absolutely still. When using a cable release, particular care must be taken that the cable is not pulled or jerked when the shutter is released. This can cause movement of the camera and a ruined photograph.

Blurring caused by insufficient depth of field is more complicated. Image depth will be discussed in greater detail below, and Table 5 gives

Table 1. Exposure table for an OPMI 1 equipped with a 300-mm objective and the camera set at 320 ASA (ASA 160 film for ESP 1 processing), shutter speed 1/15 sec, and a 30-W lamp on overload.[a]

	Magnification changer				
	6(0.4)[b]	10(0.6)	16(1)	25(1.6)	40(2.5)
Aperture setting	44	52	64	52	44

[a]*This table serves only as an example for the preparation of exposure tables. The values shown are only approximate.*
[b]*Numbers in parentheses are the magnification factors on the knobs of the newer OPMI 1 instruments.*

information on the image depth (also known as "depth of field" or erroneously "depth of focus") in relation to the aperture settings of the photo adapter.

It is important to remember that a deviation of half a stop in the aperture setting can lead to noticeable over- or underexposure of the film. This is especially critical when using color films with emulsions in the lower to middle light sensitivity brackets. Incorrect exposure of color film leads to color shift. Therefore, when using a camera that does not have a built-in exposure meter or fully automatic exposure capabilities, it is absolutely necessary to conduct a series of exposure tests beforehand and to prepare an exposure table based on these test results (Table 1). This exposure table should be arranged so that the aperture setting for the photo adapter is given for the particular type of film, for a particular shutter speed (e.g., 1 second), and for a certain level of illumination (e.g., bulb on overload) in connection with the 5 magnification changer positions of the OPMI 1 or certain positions of the zoom system on the OPMI 6-S and 7 P/H.

The test exposure series should be conducted as follows: With the film speed (ASA or DIN rating), shutter speed, and illumination level set and held constant and with the microscope at the highest level of magnification, focus on an object that resembles as closely as possible the actual object to be photographed. Switch to the lowest level of magnification and take 1 photograph at each of the aperture settings: 16, 22, 32, 44, and 64. Then, switch to magnification level 10, or zoom position 0.6, and again take 1 photograph for each aperture setting. Repeat this procedure for each of the remaining magnification levels. This type of exposure test is best

conducted with an animal experiment in the laboratory.

The first series of test exposures should be made on a film of high light sensitivity, such as Kodak Ektachrome 160 (160 ASA, 23 DIN, Tungsten Light Type for artificial light). This makes it possible to use higher aperture settings and to achieve optimum depth of field. (It should be noted that because of certain physical properties of the magnification changer system and light, the aperture settings of 14, 16, and 22 on the photo adapter are not effective at the higher magnification levels because of vignetting.)

It is advisable to prepare a small reference sheet, on which the magnification setting and the aperture setting have been noted, and to photograph it along with the object in the series of test exposures. This will eliminate any errors when evaluating the slides after they have been processed.

The test exposure slides should be evaluated by projection on a screen in a darkened room whenever possible. Only under such conditions is it possible to determine the best rendition of the color and, therefore, the best exposure. The exposure data photographed with the object may also be easily recorded.

In the event that any of the constant factors, such as working distance (i.e., main objective), film speed, shutter speed, or illumination level, are changed for any reason, it is advisable to conduct a new series of test exposures and prepare a new table.

Semiautomatic Cameras. The use of cameras with semi- or fully automatic exposure systems eliminates the need for conducting the series of test exposures described above. Moreover, these types of cameras provide a convenient method for determining the correct exposure factors when changes are made in working distance, film speed, and illumination levels.

Most of the modern semiautomatic single lens reflex camera bodies contain a light metering system that measures the amount of light that comes through the objective (or, in this case, the microscope). This system normally has a needle pointer that must be properly positioned over a mark in the viewfinder. To determine the proper exposure, one proceeds as follows: First, set the film speed of the film being used (e.g., ASA 160) and the shutter speed (e.g., 1 second). Then adjust the aperture of the photo adapter until the needle aligns with the mark in the viewfinder. The camera is then properly adjusted for that particular situation.

Even with semiautomatic cameras, it is advisable to draw up an exposure table because, during the operation, the camera may be covered by a sterile drape and it may be impossible to look into the camera viewfinder and see the exposure meter. To produce an exposure table for a semiautomatic camera, set and fix as constants: the illumination level, the film speed on the camera body, and the shutter speed. Then, focus the microscope over the object at the highest magnification level. Switch the microscope to its lowest magnification level and adjust the aperture of the photo adapter until the light meter needle aligns with the mark in the viewfinder. Make a note of the magnification level and the aperture setting. Then proceed in exactly the same way for all other magnification levels. This method is very quick, and the exposure table can be prepared in a few minutes. In addition, when changes are made in shutter speed, or in the illumination level, the new requisite aperture settings can be determined quickly.

Cameras without light metering systems and semiautomatic cameras both require constant supervision during the operation to ensure that the correct aperture setting is used for the corresponding magnification level. Ideally, a photographer should assist the surgeon.

Fully Automatic Cameras. The new cameras with fully automatic exposure control that have come on the market in the past few years are ideal for use with the operating microscope. These cameras instantly measure and evaluate the light present in the operating field before the shutter is released, and the shutter speed automatically is matched exactly to the available light. If the amount of light reaching the camera changes, whether through changes in the working distance, the illumination level, the magnification level, or the aperture setting, the automatic exposure control will instantly match the shutter speed exactly to the conditions. The only thing that one should monitor when using an automatic camera is the duration of the shutter release noise, based upon which one can estimate the length of the exposure time. Exposure times that far exceed 1 second present a risk of blurring because of possible movement of the object or equipment. Opening the aperture or in-

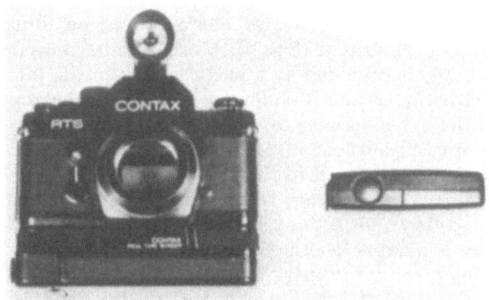

Figure 5. The Contax RTS 35-mm camera with autowinder. Note the infrared sensor shutter release on top. The remote trigger mechanism is on the right.

creasing the illumination level will immediately shorten the shutter speed.

It must be remembered that when using a fully automatic camera, the ocular of the camera viewfinder must be sealed with a cover cap in order to prevent stray light from the operating room illumination from entering the viewfinder and being measured along with the light arriving through the objective of the photo adapter.

Motorized Cameras. The camera systems that have been described up to this point depend upon manual operation of the film advance and shutter release. Such manipulations can disturb the continuity of the operation. Several new motorized camera bodies that can be triggered by a foot or hand switch and that advance the film automatically overcome such difficulties. These cameras receive power from a transformer or an internal battery pack. The transformer for these cameras is either set up on the instrument table or fastened to the microscope column. The power cable and the shutter release cable travel to the motor mechanism over the horizontal arm, and the shutter release switch is plugged into the transformer. The shutter release can be activated by the surgeon or, on his command, by some other member of the surgical team.

Most of the motorized cameras on the market do not have fully automatic exposure systems, so, here again, one must observe the interrelationships between magnification level and aperture setting.

One new camera system that has been introduced recently, the Contax RTS, fulfills all of the requirements of microsurgical photography. This camera not only has a fully automatic exposure system, but it also has a motorized film transport system (Fig. 5). Moreover, its power supply is provided by a battery pack inside the autowinder, and it no longer needs a shutter release cable because the shutter is triggered by a wireless, infrared release system. The infrared receiver is placed in the hot shoe on top of the camera's viewfinder. This receiver can be turned in different directions so that it can be triggered by a hand-held remote triggering device from any point in the operating room. The astounding advantage of the infrared trigger device is that it can function through the sterile drape covering the camera and microscope. It can also be operated by a person standing far away from the microscope and camera. When the button is pressed, the following events take place: an infrared pulse is sent out and is intercepted by the receiver on the camera, the exposure factors are measured by the exposure meter and the exposure mechanism is adjusted, the electronic shutter is triggered, the film frame is advanced, and the shutter is cocked by the autowinder. The camera then is ready for the next photograph. This system allows a series of photographs to be made quickly, one after the other, which is so often necessary for the presentation of consecutive steps in a microsurgical procedure.

Flash Photography. Occasionally, electronic flash photography is preferred over tungsten light photography to avoid any possibility of blurring caused by movement of the object or microscope. In electronic flash photography, daylight type film must be used because the spectrum of the light from the xenon gas discharge in the flash lamp is very similar to natural sunlight.

In many of the older microscope floorstands, a power supply and connector plug were provided for the electronic flash lamp in the base of the microscope stand. These older stands supply the flash with 80 Ws (watt seconds) of flash energy. All newer floorstands have flash power supplies of 160 Ws. The higher flash capacity is always preferable.

The exposure time in flash photography is determined by the duration of the flash discharge; this lies in the range of 1/3,000th of a second. Synchronization between the flash and the open shutter must be achieved. The shutter speed of the camera is therefore set at 1/60th or 1/30th of a second. Many cameras have a special symbol or shutter speed numbers of a different color to

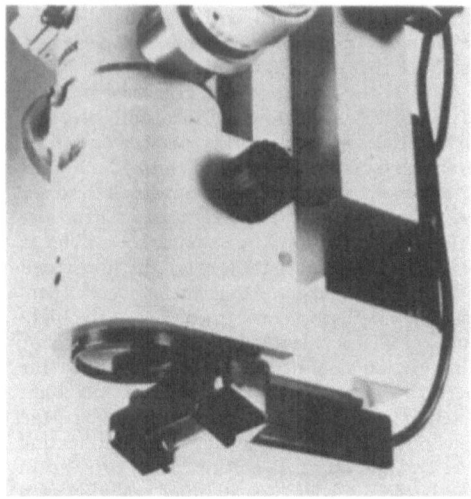

Figure 6. The electronic flash mounted on the dovetail on the lower end of the microscope body. Note that the flash housing should not interfere with the coaxial illumination.

indicate shutter speeds that are synchronized. All shutter speeds slower than the one marked also are synchronized.

The electronic flash is attached to the dovetail on the lower end of the microscope body and is positioned so that it just touches the cone of light produced by the coaxial illumination (Fig. 6). The angle of incidence of the light from the electronic flash is, therefore, somewhat more inclined than the light of the coaxial illumination. It is important to make certain that the upper window of the electronic flash is covered with a metal shield to prevent the flash from being thrown upward into the objective of the microscope.

On the OPMI 7 P/H and 6 P/H, the flash unit is positioned between the 2 fiberoptic illuminators and is held in place by a special flashholder that rotates.

One of the variables in flash photography is the aperture setting of the photo adapter. A series of test exposures should be conducted in the following manner: For every magnification step and every aperture setting, a flash photograph is taken, so that 25 photographs are made in all. Again, a miniature data sheet should be photographed with the object.

The power source for the electronic flash requires at least 10 seconds to fully charge the

Table 2. Magnification factors (M_C) for the OPMI 1, OPMI 6-S, and OPMI 7 P/H magnification changers.

Microscope	Magnification changer dial setting	M_C
OPMI 1	6	0.4
	10	0.6
	16	1.0
	25	1.6
	40	2.5
OPMI 6-S (zoom)	0.5	0.5
	1.0	1.0
	2.0	2.0
OPMI 7 P/H	0.5	0.5
	1.0	1.0
	2.5	2.5

flash capacitors to their maximum load. The flash may be triggered before the maximum load is reached, however, and thus may underexpose the frame. Firing the electronic flash more than 6 times per minute can lead to overheating and damage to the flash unit. Therefore, if a series of photographs is made in a short span of time, the flash unit should be allowed to cool for a few minutes.

Whenever changes are made in the focal length or film speed, or when the optional 2× objective is used, it is recommended that a new series of test exposures be made.

MAGNIFICATION, CAMERA FIELD OF VIEW, AND DEPTH OF FIELD

It is, of course, very important that whatever is viewed in the operating field of the microscope also be photographed. The focal length of 220 mm was chosen in the design of the photo adapter so that the field of view of the camera would approximate the field of view of the microscope in its most commonly equipped form.

Magnification. The calculation of the field of view

of the camera is derived from knowledge of the magnification of the object in the film plane of the camera. The formula for camera magnification (M_{35}) is:

$$M_{35} = (f_p/f_o) \times M_C$$

where f_p = 220 (the focal length of the photo adapter), M_C = the magnification factor, and f_o = the microscope working distance (the focal length of the main objective). The magnification of the object in the film plane of the camera is therefore reduced each time the focal length of the main objective (f_o), that is, the working distance, increases, and is proportionate to the magnification level (M_C) of the magnification changer. The magnification factor (M_C) can be taken from Table 2, and with it the magnification in the film plane of the camera for the usual working distances of 200 mm and 300 mm can be determined (Table 3).

For example, if the magnification changer is set at 16 (M_C = 1), an object 1 cm in size in the operating field will be projected onto the film plane of the camera as 1.1 cm (1.1×), or slightly larger than its real size, with the 200-mm objective, and as 0.7 cm (0.7×), or slightly smaller than its real size, with the 300-mm objective. The comparative values for the visual magnification from Table 4 are 12.5× and 8×, respectively.

Camera Field of View. By comparing the fields of view of the camera and the microscope, it becomes clear that the differences in magnification between the visual and the photographic systems are meaningful. The following formula is helpful for determining the size of the field of view of the camera (F_{35mm}):

$$F_{35\,mm} = (24 \times 36 \text{ mm})/M_{35}$$

It can be seen that the field that the camera "sees" is determined by dividing the film format

Table 3. The size of the field of view of the camera (small side × large side in mm) and the magnification (M_{35}) of an OPMI 1 with the standard photo adapter.

Working distance (f_o) (focal length of main objective)	Magnification changer dial setting									
	6 (0.4)[a]		10 (0.6)		16 (1)		25 (1.6)		40 (2.5)	
	Field of view	Magnification	Field of view	Magnification	Field of view	Magnification	Field of view	Magnification	Field of view	Magnification
200 mm	60 × 90	0.4×	34 × 51	0.7×	22 × 33	1.1×	13 × 20	1.8×	9 × 13	2.7×
300 mm	80 × 120	0.3×	60 × 90	0.4×	34 × 51	0.7×	20 × 30	1.2×	13 × 19	1.9×

[a]*The numbers in parentheses are the magnification factors on the knobs of the newer OPMI 1.*

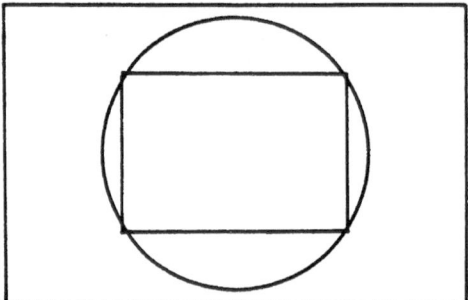

Figure 7. This sketch was traced while looking through both the oculars of the operating microscope and the viewfinder of the camera. The visual field of the microscope is represented by the circle (125-mm binocular tubes and 20 × oculars); the large rectangle represents the field of the 35-mm camera mounted on the photo adapter (f = 220); the small rectangle represents the field of the 35-mm camera with the auxiliary 2× lens attached to the photo adapter.

by the magnification. Returning to the example we used above, with the magnification changer set at 16, we find that rectangular fields are produced that have border lengths of 22 × 33 mm for the 200-mm objective, and 34 × 51 mm for the 300-mm objective (Table 3). For comparative purposes, we determine from Table 4 that the round fields of view of the microscope with these objectives have diameters of 16 and 25 mm, respectively. This means that the visual field of view is totally covered by the field of view of the camera and that all the details that can be seen through the microscope can also be photographed.

Practical hint. With most of the commonly used single lens reflex cameras, it is possible to determine the field of view of the camera directly through the camera viewfinder. It is best to use a piece of graph paper marked in millimeters as an object when doing this. This will enable one to easily determine both the field size and the magnification by counting the millimeters pictured in the viewfinder. For example, when 12 millimeter elements are visible along the short edge of the 35-mm frame, the magnification factor is 2, because this edge is 24 mm. In other words, one divides 24 by the number of millimeters visible along this edge. The total camera field can easily be determined by counting the millimeters visible along both frame edges. While doing this test it is of course possible to also determine the diameter of the microscope field by looking through the oculars. One can also take a pencil and trace both fields on the graph paper while looking through the camera viewfinder and the oculars (Fig. 7). This supplies an immediate document of the available conditions.

Depth of Field. Depth of field in the object viewed is of great importance in microsurgical photography. It is especially important when making photographs for publication, where the levels of the operating field both above and below the detail of interest must be presented in sharp focus. The formula for determining the depth of field (T) for the 35-mm camera is as follows:

$$T_{35} = T'/M_{35}^2$$

where $T' = 2k \times u$ (image depth or depth of focus), and $M_{35} = (f_p/f_o) \times M_C$ (camera magnification). Through transposition we arrive at the following formula:

$$T_{35} = (2k \times u \times f_o^2)/(f_p^2 \times M_C^2)$$

where k = the photo adapter aperture number (14, 16, 22, 32, 44, and 64), u = the maximum allowable diameter of the circle of diffusion

Table 4. The size of the field of view (mm) and the total magnification power of an OPMI 1 equipped with 125-mm binocular tubes and 20× eyepieces.

	Magnification changer dial setting								
	6 (0.4)[a]		10 (0 6)		16 (1)		25 (1.6)		40 (2.5)	
Focal length of the main objective	Field of view	Magnification	Field of view	Magnification	Field of view	Magnification	Field of view	Magnification	Field of view	Magnification
200 mm	40	5×	27	7 5×	16	12 5×	10	20×	6	31×
225 mm	44	4 5×	30	6 5×	18	11×	11	18×	7	28×
250 mm	50	4×	33	6×	20	10×	12 5	16×	8	25×
275 mm	57	3 5×	36	5 5×	22	9×	14	14.5×	9	23×
300 mm	67	3×	40	5×	25	8×	15	13×	10	21×

[a]Numbers in parentheses are the factors on the new OPMI 1 magnification changer knobs.

Table 5. The depth of field (in mm) in relationship to the magnification of the photo adapter with settings of 16, 32, and 64 and working distances of 200 mm and 300 mm.[a]

Working distance (f_o)	Aperture setting	Magnification changer dial setting				
		6 (0.4)	10 (0.6)	16 (1)	25 (1.6)	40 (2.5)
200 mm	16	8.3	3.7	1.3	—	—
	32	16.5	7.3	2.6	1.0	0.4
	64	33.0	14.7	5.3	2.1	0.8
300 mm	16	18.6	8.3	3.7	—	—
	32	37.0	16.5	7.3	2.6	0.9
	64	74.0	33.0	14.7	5.2	1.8

[a]See Table 3 for M_{35} values.

Table 6. The size of the field of view of the camera (small side × large side in mm) and the magnification of an OPMI 1 equipped with the standard photo adapter and the auxiliary 2× lens.

Working distance (f_o) (focal length of main objective)	Magnification changer setting									
	6 (0.4)		10 (0.6)		16 (1)		25 (1.6)		40 (2.5)	
	Field of view	Magnification	Field of view	Magnification	Field of view	Magnification	Field of view	Magnification	Field of view	Magnification
200 mm	30 × 45	0.8×	17 × 25	1.4×	11 × 16	2.2×	6.5 × 10	3.6×	4.5 × 6.5	5.4×
300 mm	40 × 60	0.6×	30 × 45	0.8×	17 × 25	1.4×	10 × 15	2.0×	6.5 × 9.5	3.8×

(agreed upon measurement: 0.05 mm), f_0 = the focal length of the main objective on the microscope, f_p = the focal length of the photo adapter (220 mm, or 440 mm with the 2× auxiliary lens), and M_C = the magnification changer factor (0.4, 0.6, 1, 1.6, and 2.5).

This formula demonstrates that the depth of field is influenced by 2 variables: (*a*) the diameter of the diaphragm (k) of the photo adapter aperture, and (*b*) the magnification. Specifically, the depth of field changes linearly with the aperture number, i.e., it increases as the aperture number (k) increases. On the other hand, the depth of field is unfavorably affected by the degree of magnification, in inverse proportion to it, and, what is more, quadratically, i.e., when the magnification is doubled, the depth of field is reduced 4 times. Again, returning to our example above, we obtain a depth of field of 2.6 mm with the magnification changer set at 16, the photo adapter aperture set at 32, and a working distance of 200 mm. For the working distance of 300 mm, the depth of field is 5.9 mm. When using *f*-stop 64 on the photo adapter, the depth of field is 5.3 mm for the 200-mm objective and 12 mm for the 300-mm objective.

As long as sufficient light is available, it is always advisable to close the aperture of the photo adapter as far as the longest tolerable exposure time permits. It is also always advisable to work with the highest possible illumination in order to reach this goal.

One must always keep in mind the influence that the magnification and the aperture setting have on the depth of field when making photographs for publication. In such cases it makes sense to work with a low camera magnification to ensure that the depth of field includes the entire operating field and to produce the desired image scale for reproduction through subsequent enlargement of the photographs. These relationships are clearly shown in Table 5. The use of magnifications that exceed 1× are especially critical, particularly when aperture settings 44 and 64 are no longer usable because of insufficient light.

Auxiliary 2× objective. In the event that a higher magnification in the film plane of the camera in relation to the visual field is desired, an auxiliary 2× lens is available that fits between the photo adapter and the camera. This lens doubles the

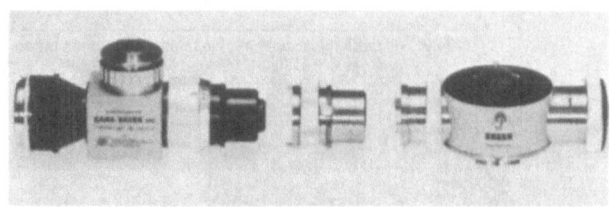

Figure 8. The Dual Camera Adapter manufactured for Zeiss by the Urban Engineering Co. Note the piece in the center for extending the adapter if bulky TV systems are employed.

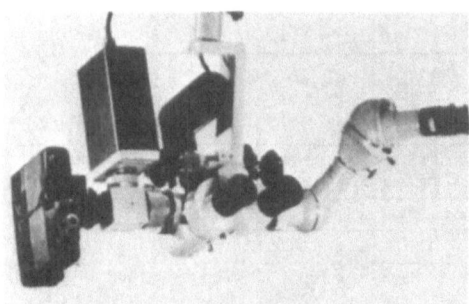

Figure 9. The Dual Camera Adapter mounted on an OPMI 1 with a Contax RTS 35-mm camera and a TV camera.

focal length of the photo adapter to 440 mm and converts the magnifications and fields of the camera to the values given in Table 6.

Again, using the example with the magnification changer set at 16, and comparing the fields of view of the microscope with the fields of view of the camera, it becomes clear that the rectangular camera field now has its corners cut off by the circular microscope field. This size field of view may be preferred when the actual object to be viewed is relatively small in comparison to the total field of view, as is often the case in neurologic and otologic surgery.

THE DUAL CAMERA ADAPTER

A versatile adapter for documentation that has recently been introduced is the Zeiss/Urban Dual Camera Adapter (Fig. 8). This adapter simultaneously accepts a TV or movie camera and a 35-mm camera, using only one opening of the beam splitter (Figs. 9 and 10). This dual capability is especially important to the OPMI 7 P/H in reconstructive surgery and also for the other models in ophthalmic and neurologic microsurgery, where the use of the stereo co-observer tube is mandatory.

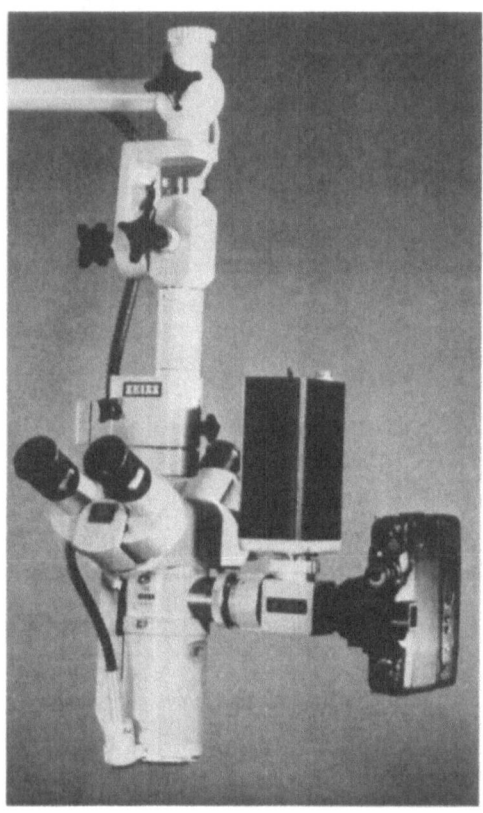

Figure 10. The Dual Camera Adapter mounted on an OPMI 7 P/H for documenting reconstructive surgical procedures.

The Dual Camera Adapter has 2 focal lengths, (a) 137 mm for movie and TV cameras and (b) 300 mm for 35-mm cameras (Table 7), and it contains a beam splitter that divides the incoming light evenly 50/50 between each camera system.

Table 7. Magnifications at the film planes of a 35-mm camera and a 16-mm motion picture camera with the Zeiss/Urban Dual Camera Adapter on the OPMI 1, OPMI 6-S, and OPMI 7 P/H.

Working distance (f_0)	Magnification changer dial setting				
	6 (0.4)	10 (0.6)	16 (1)	25 (1.6)	40 (2.5)
OPMI 1					
35-mm camera					
200 mm	0.6×	0.9×	1.5×	2.4×	3.8×
300 mm	0.4×	0.6×	1.0×	1.6×	2.5×
400 mm	0.3×	0.5×	0.8×	1.2×	1.9×
16-mm camera					
200 mm	0.3×	0.4×	0.6×	1.0×	1.6×
300 mm	0.2×	0.3×	0.5×	0.7×	1.1×
400 mm	0.1×	0.2×	0.3×	0.5×	0.9×

	Magnification changer (zoom)				
	0.5				2.0
OPMI 6-S					
35-mm camera					
150 mm	1.0×				4.0×
200 mm	0.8×				3.0×
300 mm	0.5×				2.0×
16-mm camera					
150 mm	0.5×				1.8×
200 mm	0.3×				1.4×
300 mm	0.2×				0.9×

	Magnification changer (zoom)				
	0.5				2.5
OPMI 7 P/H					
35-mm camera					
200 mm	0.8×				3.8×
225 mm	0.6×				3.0×
16-mm camera					
200 mm	0.4×				1.7×
225 mm	0.3×				1.5×

The advantages of this design are obvious. It is possible to perform 35-mm photography without interrupting the TV system. This means continued TV tape recording as well as uninterrupted observation on the TV screens. The instant readiness of the 35-mm camera relieves the physician or assisting photographer from making manual adjustments on the microscope or adapter system that unavoidably cause the microscope to vibrate. A Yashica bayonet mount for the 35-mm camera permits the fully automatic Contax RTS camera back to be attached without any additional adapter ring. Any TV or movie camera equipped with a standard C-thread lensmount can be attached via the C-thread adapter ring.

Exposure factors for 35-mm photography are the same as for the standard photo adapter.

However, High Speed Ektachrome 160 (160 ASA, Tungsten Light Type) should be used and the ASA scale on the camera should be set at 320. Kodak ESP 1 processing should then be specified when the film is sent to the processor. Regarding exposure factors for movie cameras, no changes are required, except that the diaphragm should be opened one f-stop. Movie cameras with automatic light meters connected to the motorized diaphragm control will function as on the regular single cine adapter.

Regarding TV cameras, the procedure for selecting the appropriate diaphragm setting remains the same. The automatic 35-mm camera is not influenced in the process of determining the proper exposure.

Details regarding the use of the movie and TV cameras will be discussed below.

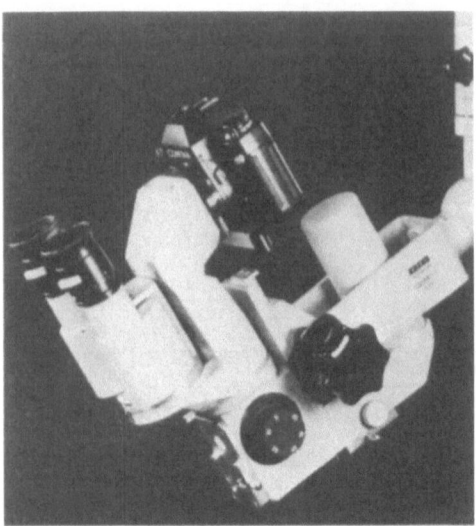

Figure 11. An OPMI 1 equipped with the Zeiss-Urban stereo photo adapter and a Contax automatic camera. Note that the binocular tubes are moved forward approximately 25 mm.

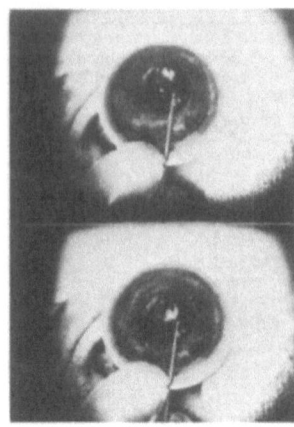

Figure 12. A black and white copy of a stereo color slide taken with the Zeiss/Urban stereo photo adapter.

STEREO PHOTOGRAPHY

The 2 methods available for producing stereoscopic photographs, that is, the full-frame method with 2 cameras and the half-frame method with 1 camera, deliver a perfect 3-dimensional perception of the microstructures in the operating field that is identical to the stereoscopic image viewed through the microscope by the surgeon. This is of special advantage in teaching.

Both methods of stereo photography rest upon the following principle: the light rays in each of the binocular tubes of the microscope produce a slightly different image. These 2 images produce a stereoscopic effect when they are viewed simultaneously through the oculars or when the 2 photographs of the images are viewed in a special viewer.

In the full-frame method, 2 photo adapters are attached to the 2 openings of the beam splitter, and two 35-mm cameras are mounted on the adapters. The two 35-mm cameras must be carefully aligned so that they are parallel to each other, and their apertures must be set at the same f-stop, so that the 2 full-format photographs that are obtained will have the same color values. These 2 photographs are a stereoscopic pair and can be viewed with a special stereo viewer. Stereo projection is also possible. One advantage of this method is that each of the photographs can also be used for monoscopic viewing.

The second method is based on the simultaneous recording of both images on a single 35-mm frame. This involves equipping the microscope with a special stereo photo adapter developed by Urban Engineering (Burbank, CA). This adapter has 2 objectives with focal lengths of 175 mm, and is attached directly to the microscope body in place of the standard beam splitter. The use of this special stereo adapter moves the binocular tube system forward approximately 25 mm; this, however, does not affect the use of the instrument in any way (Fig. 11). Any camera that can be used with the standard photo adapter can be used with the stereo adapter if it is attached with the special adapter ring that ensures horizontal alignment. Cameras with automatic exposure control are best suited. The stereo photo adapter reduces the dimensions of the image from each of the 2 light ray paths to 16 × 24 mm. This permits each image to be recorded on one half of a standard 35-mm frame without mutual interference (Fig. 12).

The method of viewing such a stereo photograph with a stereo viewer is simpler than full-frame stereo viewing. Stereo projection is also possible with a normal projector equipped with a special stereo projection attachment in front of the projector lens. In order to view projected stereo photographs, one needs to wear special polarized eyeglasses.

Table 8. Camera magnifications and camera fields of view (in mm) for Super 8 (8-mm) and 16-mm motion picture cameras mounted on an OPMI 1 with the standard motion picture adapters (f = 74, 107, or 137 mm) at working distances of 200 mm and 300 mm.

	Magnification changer dial setting									
	6 (0.4)		10 (0.6)		16 (1)		25 (1.6)		40 (2.5)	
Working distance (f_a)	Field of view	Magnifica-tion	Field of view	Magnifica-tion	Field of view	Magnifica-tion	Field of view	Magnifica-tion	Field of view	Magnifica-tion
Super 8, 74-mm adapter										
200 mm	42 × 55	0.1×	21 × 28	0.2×	11 × 14	0.4×	7 × 9	0.6×	5 × 6	0.9×
300 mm	46 × 16	0.09×	42 × 55	0.1×	21 × 28	0.2×	11 × 14	0.4×	7 × 9	0.6×
16-mm, 107-mm adapter										
200 mm	38 × 52	0.2×	25 × 34	0.3×	15 × 21	0.5×	8 × 11	0.9×	6 × 9	1.3×
300 mm	75 × 103	0.1×	38 × 52	0.2×	19 × 26	0.4×	13 × 17	0.6×	8 × 11	0.9×
16-mm, 137-mm adapter										
200 mm	25 × 34	0.3×	19 × 26	0.4×	11 × 15	0.7×	7 × 9	1.1×	4 × 6	1.8×
300 mm	38 × 52	0.2×	25 × 34	0.3×	15 × 21	0.5×	10 × 15	0.7×	6 × 9	1.2×

CINEMATOGRAPHY

The production of motion pictures during an operation for use in teaching, discussions, and seminar lectures is also possible on OPMI instruments. Both Super 8 (8-mm) and 16-mm camera systems can be employed. Special adapters, similar to the 35-mm photo adapter, are available that contain their own objectives and are inserted into the standard beam splitter.

For Super 8 motion pictures, a cine adapter with a 74-mm focal length is used; for 16-mm photography, cine adapters with focal lengths of 107 and 137 mm are used. The cine adapters are equipped with an intermediate ring for accommodating movie cameras equipped with the standard C-thread, which permits the direct attachment of these cameras to the cine adapter.

To simplify the setting of the exposure, the cine adapters can be equipped with a fully automatic exposure system, which can be used in connection with the Super 8 and R 16 cameras produced by the Beaulieu Company in France.

The special advantage of the Super 8 system lies in the use of the short objective (f = 74 mm), which means good image brightness and relatively large depth of field. Equally advantageous is the comparatively uncomplicated and fast exchange of film cartridges during an operation. On the other hand, Super 8 movie film cannot be projected onto screens wider than 1.20 m without a definite loss of quality and, therefore, is suitable only for presentation to small audiences. Super 8 is relatively inexpensive, however, which means that films of operations can be produced routinely.

The advantage of the 16-mm film system lies in its high quality when screened for large audiences and in its potential for copy production from color negative material and, thereby, wide distribution. As already noted, the cine adapters with 107- and 137-mm focal lengths are used for 16-mm photography. The 107-mm adapter is preferred in ophthalmology, because its lower magnification permits a wider field to be filmed. The 137-mm Cine Adapter is employed in most other surgical disciplines.

Urban Engineering has developed a special movie camera that can be attached directly to the cine adapter or the Dual Camera Adapter without the use of the intermediate adapter ring. This camera is triggered by a foot pedal and is powered by its own source attached to the microscope column. The correct exposure is provided by a simultaneous increase in the electric current supplied to the incandescent bulb in the microscope. A special characteristic of the Urban camera is its interchangeable film magazines. These magazines are carefully loaded before the operation, and after the film in one magazine is used up, it can be exchanged in seconds without in any way disturbing the continuity of the operation. A warning light on the magazine comes on when the magazine is nearly empty, indicating that only 5 feet of film remain.

To determine the magnification and field of view of the movie camera, we can use the formula given in the section on 35-mm photography. In this case, instead of the photo adapter focal length of 220 mm, we substitute the focal lengths of the cine adapters for Super 8 and 16-mm film, i.e., 74, 107, and 137 mm. For the calculation of the field of view of a movie camera, we must proceed from the size of the film frame, which is 4.2 mm $\times$ 5.5 mm for Super 8, and 7.5 mm $\times$ 10.3 mm for 16-mm film. Table 8 is based upon calculations using these values: f_{cine} = 74 mm, 107 mm, and 137 mm; and working distance = 200 mm or 300 mm.

TELEVISION CAMERAS

In the past few years the electronics industry has made major progress in the miniaturization of TV cameras and in the improvement of color rendition even at low light levels. This means that black and white and color TV cameras weighing as little as 250 g (approximately 1/2 lb) can be permanently installed on the beam splitter of a microscope by means of the 137-mm cine adapter.

Through use of the television camera, the operation may be transmitted to a television screen in the operating room for the orientation of the assisting personnel, or to more distant places, such as the doctor's lounge or the office of the chief surgeon. Audiovisual communication between these locations allows the progress of the operation to be discussed. For teaching institutions, this type of set-up is an absolute necessity. It also makes possible the production of video tapes for teaching.

A large number of color television cameras with excellent color reproduction and resolving power are being offered on the commercial TV market at the moment. It is quite obvious that, like all highly complicated electronic instruments, TV cameras require maintenance, and, therefore, the choice of a system should go to the firm that provides good local service.

The optimum in life-like documentation is seen in color stereo television. This method, up to now, has only been performed on a more or less experimental basis and serves purely the purpose of microsurgical instruction. In the future it will make it possible for numerous observers to experience simultaneously the progress of an operation in color with true 3-dimensional depth perception.

TV cameras to be used with the microscope must be equipped with a standard C-thread mount. They are attached to the cine adapter or the dual camera adapter by means of the C-thread mount adapter ring, which allows them to be locked securely in place. Orientation of the TV camera can be checked on the screen and the camera may be rotated to match the field of view with 12 o'clock on the TV monitor. The diaphragm f-stop on the cine-adapter can be rotated to check for the best color reproduction while the microscope illumination is run on regular load. Of course, the specimen used should closely represent the actual object when adjusting the camera before an operation. A larger f-stop number may be selected if the color reproduction at higher magnifications tends to fade out. The f-stop that is finally selected can be maintained during all procedures, even on the Dual Camera Adapter, since the 35-mm camera automatically adjusts its own exposure.

Methods of cleaning and caring for the Zeiss OPMI
series microscopes are discussed.

JOURNAL OF MICROSURGERY   2:179–182   1981

THE OPERATING MICROSCOPE.
V. MAINTENANCE AND CLEANING

PETER HOERENZ, Dipl.-Ing.-Phys.

*Editor's Note: This is the fifth and last article in a
series by Mr. Hoerenz on the basic principles and
handling of the operating microscope. The first article, on optical principles, illumination systems,
and support systems, appeared in* Journal of Microsurgery *1:364–369, 1980. The second article,
on individual parts, handling, assembling, focusing, and balancing, appeared in* Journal of Microsurgery *1:419–427, 1980. The third article, on
accessories, appeared in* Journal of Microsurgery
*2:22–26, 1980. The fourth article, on documenta-
tion, appeared in* Journal of Microsurgery
2:126–139, 1980.

Although the Zeiss operating microscopes are
designed to give years of trouble-free service,
routine maintenance and cleaning will ensure
optimal performance each time the instrument
is used.

THE OPTICS

Before each use of the microscope, all external
lens surfaces should be inspected and, if need be,
cleaned. The internal glass surfaces also should
be inspected for cleanliness if the binocular tube

From Carl Zeiss, Inc., New York, NY.

Address reprint requests to Mr. Hoerenz at Carl Zeiss, Inc., 444 Fifth Ave.,
New York, NY 10018.

Received for publication June 20, 1980.

0191-3239/0203/0179 $01.25/0

system is changed, if the beam splitter is installed,
or if the oculars are changed.

Not much can be done, of course, to eliminate
mechanical damage, such as scratches in the
lens or chips near the lens flange, that may result
from improper handling or dropping the lens. If
such damage is sustained in the region of the optical light ray paths and illumination ray paths
of an objective lens, the objective will have to be
replaced.

The lens surfaces of the microscope are sus-
ceptible to 3 types of dirt: (*a*) loose deposits such
as dust; (*b*) water-soluble substances such as
spots of blood, irrigating solutions, or water; and
(*c*) substances not soluble in water, such as oil
from eyelashes and fingerprints.

To remove loose particles, especially dust, a
small rubber blowing bulb can be used. This
bulb should be held at an inclined angle approximately 1 cm from the lens surface and
squeezed briskly. This will produce strong blasts
of air that should blow most of the particles
away. The advantage of this method is that it is
not necessary to touch the lens surface in order
to clean it.

Loose particles of dust on the objective also
can be removed with a brush made of badger
hair. This brush must be dipped in a chemical
cleaning solution in order to clean it and remove
any oil. The cleaning solution must be allowed to
evaporate completely before the brush is used,
and the brush should be cleaned frequently.

Very often, after dust has been removed from
a lens, a thin film remains on the surface of the

lens. This film precipitates from the air and can only be removed by wiping the lens. Clean cotton balls are the most suitable material for wiping optical surfaces; linen cloths that are lint-free and have been repeatedly washed also are suitable.

The film on a lens may be removed by breathing carefully onto the surface of the lens to fog it and wiping slowly in a circular fashion from the center of the lens outward to the edge with a clean cotton ball. This procedure should be repeated with new material until the film is gone. In most cases, this type of cleaning is sufficient for all of the lens surfaces except the objective and possibly the eyepieces. The objective should never be cleaned in this manner because the breath may contaminate the lens and the objective cannot be covered by sterile draping in the operating room.

The degree of soiling usually is heavier on the objective and oculars. For example, the objective often becomes soiled during an operation from spattered blood or spots of irrigating solution. It may also become soiled from fingerprints when the instrument is handled after the operation.

A small quantity of cotton applicators, known commercially as "Q-tips," should be used to clean such soiling of the objective or eyepieces. Q-tips are short wooden sticks that have a small portion of cotton wrapped on the ends. (Note: cotton applicators made with *plastic* sticks should not be used, as some of the cleaning solvents tend to dissolve the plastic.)

In order to clean an objective or ocular, one end of a Q-tip should be moistened with distilled water; however, it should not be moistened to the point of being dripping wet. This Q-tip then is used to wipe the lens in a circular motion to remove water-soluble dirt. The surface of the lens then should be wiped with a clean, dry Q-tip. When this has been completed, the dirt that is not soluble in water is removed with a cleaning solvent consisting of 25% denatured alcohol, 10% ether, and 65% acetone. When mixing a stock solution of these highly volatile components, extreme care should be taken. The solvent should be stored in a glass bottle. In applying this cleaning solvent to the optical surface, it is *very* important that the cotton applicator be only lightly moistened with solvent and never dripping wet. Here again, the Q-tip is used to wipe outwardly from the center to the edge of the lens in a circular fashion. This procedure

must be repeated as many times as necessary to render the glass surface absolutely free of streaks.

If it is determined that the inner surface of the objective, which is inside the microscope body, also requires cleaning, the objective should be carefully screwed out of the microscope. The inner surface should be cleaned and the objective reinstalled before the outside surface is cleaned.

Important Reminder. It must be mentioned again that the cleaning fluids should never be used on the objective in such quantities that excess amounts of the solvent flow between the lens and the lens mount. These excess fluids could damage the internal cemented surfaces of the objective. Certain aggressive cleaning substances, such as 100% acetone or pure alcohol, even in small quantities, are powerful enough to destroy the cemented surfaces and therefore should never be used. It also is important that the cleaning substance itself be absolutely clean, and that it contain no foreign material. The cotton applicator should never be dipped into the bottle of stock solution; solvent should be poured into a Petri dish for the cleaning procedure.

CLEANING THE OPERATING MICROSCOPE

The rule of never using an excess amount of cleaning fluid also applies in cleaning the mechanical parts of the microscope. It is, however, permitted and recommended that the external surfaces of the microscope be washed regularly with clean linen cloths that have been dipped in mild soap and water or nonaggressive disinfecting solutions and then wrung out well. The horizontal arm and floor stand may be cleaned in the same manner. As a last step, all parts should be wiped with a dry, lint-free, linen cloth.

Microscopes that are subjected to this maintenance on a regular basis will, over the years, always maintain a factory-new appearance and, above all, will deliver the highest optical performance whenever they are used.

When the surfaces of the microscope are being cleaned, the mechanical functions of the arm joints, the carriage, the casters underneath the base, the base brakes, and the nylon tapes, also should be inspected. It has been mentioned in previous articles that the coupling joints can be greased with petroleum jelly. Should other nonaccessible joints grind or squeak, service by a trained technician is needed.

The up-and-down movement of the carriage should be smooth and rattle-free. Bumpy movement of the carriage indicates that one of the roller-ball bearings has been damaged. Again, service by a technician is needed.

While the carriage is being checked, special attention should be paid to examining the double nylon tape. Should one of the two tapes show any signs of marring, cracking, or other damage, the microscope should be taken out of the operating room *immediately* and a technician should be called.

The three casters underneath the base should roll evenly. A bumpy ride on a smooth floor indicates that the rubber wheels have started to deteriorate and must be replaced; all three casters should be replaced at the same time.

Occasionally, the locking brakes become loose. This condition also should be corrected by a service technician.

CARE OF THE ILLUMINATION EQUIPMENT

Anyone who has ever had to change a burned-out bulb during an operation will know how important it is to inspect the illumination system on a regular basis before surgery.

The following items must be checked on the coaxial and external illumination systems: the 6-V 30-W regular tungsten bulb with centering socket and the 12-V 100-W halogen bulb with centering socket.

The lamp cable, which runs from the lamp holder to the plug receptacle on the horizontal arm, must be free of kinks or breaks. Its 2-pin plug must sit firmly in the receptacle on the horizontal arm and be free of movement. Both contact pins of the plug must be free of corrosion; that is, their metal surfaces should look shiny and should not have any black or brown spots that would indicate contact resistance and sparking in the plug contact. Plugs that contact poorly reduce the amount of current reaching the lamp and hence reduce the amount of light in the operating field. Moreover, corrosion on the pins can build up heat and melt the material, leading to a breakdown in the lighting system.

The lamp cable normally stays cold when the microscope is in use. Should a hot lamp cable be discovered at the end of a long operation, it should be exchanged for a new one through the repair service. A hot cable may indicate that a high electrical current is passing through the cable; this might be caused by a shorted circuit in the lamp housing. In any case, the components of the lamp housing should be examined carefully.

It is recommended that a new bulb be used for operations of long duration (4 or more hours) or whenever a bulb is to be used for a long period on overload. The risk of burning out a bulb during the operation thus will be sharply reduced.

Changing the bulb in the bayonet socket of the lamp house must be done carefully; only a perfectly inserted bulb guarantees shadow-free, even illumination of the operating field. In order to change a bulb, the upper lamp housing is turned approximately 90° in a counter-clockwise direction. It then may be lifted in an upward direction from the microscope illuminator. On microscopes manufactured before 1979, the bulb should be pressed against the bulb housing and turned toward the left; it then will slip out of the bayonet mount. It can be removed by lifting it up and out. On the newer OPMIs, the bulb is sitting in the lower part of the illuminator and can just be lifted out.

A new bulb should not be handled with bare fingers during insertion; rather it should be gripped with a cloth or the carton in which it is packaged. The 3-corner centering plate on the base of the bulb allows it to be inserted in only one way, that is, in the guide grooves of the lamp housing. On the microscopes manufactured before 1979, the pressure of the spring-loaded contacts will be noticeable before the bulb reaches the bayonet grooves. The bulb then should be gently pushed down until it touches the bayonet and turned in a clockwise direction until an obvious click is heard. The correct positioning of the bulb in the socket of the lamp housing should be checked. If a red or blue shadow appears in the field of illumination, the seating of the bulb should be rechecked. On the newer microscope models, the lamp is dropped into the opening in the illuminator and its socket wings are aligned between the locating pins.

Changing the halogen bulb is equally easy. First, the fan housing, which is the upper portion of the halogen illuminator, is lifted off by depressing the two Teflon buttons on the sides of the housing. The socket and connecting pins of the bulb point upward from the lower illuminator part and the bulb is held in place by a spring-loaded clip. The clip is unlocked by turning the white nylon locking button 90°. Then the button and the clip can be raised and the bulb removed. When "dropping" the new bulb into place, the cut-out in the bulb centering socket should be engaged with the tong on the rim of the opening. Finally, the clip is replaced over the bulb socket and turned 90° to lock it. The fan housing is reinstalled by engaging the two guidebars in the holes of the illuminator housing and pushing downward until an audible click indicates full engagement.

Today, fiberoptic illumination systems are being used in great numbers on operating microscopes. In these systems the lamp housing is positioned outside of the sterile microscope drape, and access to the bulb has been simplified by use of a sliding drawer system. This means that a bulb change, together with its drawer, is possible in a few seconds. Therefore, it is not necessary to insert a new bulb before each operation. A spare lamp drawer with a fresh bulb installed in it, however, must always be kept within reach.

The fiberoptic cable of a fiberoptic illumination system should never be bent too sharply; this could lead to fracturing of the thin glass fibers inside the cable. The loss of a large number of such fibers over the years will reduce the illumination level.

Keeping the fiberoptic light cables clean is very easy. Only the polished surfaces at the end of the cable must be kept free of dirt. Here again, cotton applicators can be used for cleaning. When inserting the fiberoptic cable into the lamp housing or into the illumination prism on the microscope, the metal tip of the cable should be pressed in until it is firmly seated against the end stop. The illumination prism of the Vertolux system must be cleaned thoroughly in the same manner as the front objective of the microscope. Here too, cotton applicators and cleaning solutions can be used to clean the surfaces accessible from the outside.

Important Note. The codes of UL 544 (medical and dental equipment) on electrical equipment that is listed by Underwriters Laboratories, Inc. (UL) require that no lay person be able to open and tamper with the electrical power supply if a malfunction occurs. A label on the outside warns: "Not a user-serviceable item." This warning should be taken seriously and no unqualified person should attempt to trouble-shoot such a device. On the other hand, the UL listing assures you that the device has been built in compliance with the strict rules established for equipment that can be used safely in the environment of the operating room. This protects both the user and the patient from possible harm.

B

Patient Information: Laser Surgery

Laser treatment for various gynecologic diseases is a new application of a very important scientific and new therapeutic tool. For the past several years, research and development have made it possible to use the CO_2 laser to treat a wide variety of benign and early malignant diseases of the vulva, vagina, and cervix.

The laser is a beam of infrared light, invisible to the eye, which has the ability to be focused to a minute spot size (1–3 mm). This is similar to focusing sunlight with a magnifying lens to a bright spot. With infrared light from the CO_2 laser so focused, generally by means of an operative microscope, the energy of the laser beam on impact with the cells causes their instantaneous vaporization to a small depth predetermined by the operator. This depth is very shallow and will cause little or no damage to the surrounding cells. Therefore, the healing is very rapid since the remaining cells are healthy and can multiply to heal the area removed. The treatment is generally quick and painless on the cervix and vagina. Most patients are treated in 4–8 min.

The procedure is generally done on an outpatient basis (patients come to the clinic and leave a short time after the procedure). If an anesthetic is required, the treatment will be done in the operating room on an outpatient basis (again allowing patients to leave after the procedure when their recovery from the anesthetic is satisfactory).

C

Discharge Instructions

For the patient who has had laser surgery to the cervix, vagina, vulva, and/or rectum, the following instructions are to be followed very carefully.

C.1. Laser Surgery to Cervix and/or Vagina

If you have had laser surgery of the cervix and/or vagina, you may have a moderate amount of reddish watery discharge during the first 10 days after treatment. A protective sanitary napkin *(not a tampon)* will be necessary. If heavier bright red bleeding occurs, please call your doctor for instructions.

Do not put anything into the vagina (birth canal) for 3 weeks
No douching
No sexual relations (sexual relations can usually be resumed after 3 weeks)
No Tampax or other tampons

You may experience a few cramps somewhat like menstrual cramps. This is to be expected and may require some oral analgesics. If severe, please call your doctor for further instructions.

C.2. Laser Surgery to Vulva and/or Rectum

Do not wear slacks, jeans, or any constricting clothing. A dress is preferable.

Do not wear nylon underpants. Wear *cotton* underpants if you have to go out, otherwise wear no underwear around the house.

Sitz bath: sit in a tub of warm water, without any additions, three times a day for about 10–15 min. Make sure the tub is clean before and after use.

Use a hair dryer to dry the perineal area. *Do not rub* with a towel. When using a hair dryer, put one foot up on a chair and blow the area dry.

Frequently 4–6 weeks are required for the vulva and perineal area to heal. Sexual relations are restricted for this period of time.

Usually one laser treatment is necessary to restore the area treated. The first follow-up visit will be 2 months after treatment.

D

Informed Consent

As laser surgery is now an integral part of otolaryngology, ophthalmology, and gynecology, we believe that a "special or experimental" informed consent is *not* necessary. In fact, the Federal Food and Drug Administration approved this form of surgery for third-party reimbursement under federal insurance programs in 1976. The gynecologist should obtain a routine informed consent that contains all the criteria as set forth for his community. If the instrument is to be used outside of the hospital in a clinical setting, then the individual surgeon may or may not elect to have a *signed* consent. However, in an institutional setting, a signed and witnessed informed consent form should be considered mandatory.

E

Laser Certification

Today, because of medicolegal pressure, the laser surgeon must demonstrate his new capabilities by fulfilling certain prescribed requirements. We have, therefore, set down guidelines that we feel are necessary to qualify a surgeon for CO_2 laser surgery in gynecology.

First, as the CO_2 laser is coupled to the colposcope, the surgeon must be an accomplished colposcopist. Today, as many fine colposcopists have, by virtue of their years of experience, sufficient diagnostic acumen to be considered expert, a definition of who qualifies is best left to the legal community. These surgeons are usually referred to under the grandfather clause, and their skill would stand the test of legal inquiry should the question arise.

However, for surgeons who are younger, the following is suggested. First, a surgeon should submit proof of completion of a basic and advanced course in colposcopy to his credentials committee. Second, he should submit proof of his being a member of the American Society of Colposcopy and Cervical Pathology. Moreover, the successful intra-abdominal microsurgical use of the laser demands that the laser surgeon be a competent microsurgeon, and, when the laser is used in oncology, also an experienced oncologist. In each aspect, basic understanding of the disease process, training in laser surgical techniques and procedures, and familiarity with the laser instrument are mandatory.

The Bureau of Medical Devices of the Food and Drug Administration of the United States Department of Health and Human Services has approved the use of lasers in humans without limiting the applications to disciplines or to types or extent of diseases; voluntary performance standards are in effect. Therefore, at present, it is encumbent upon the providers and users of these medical devices and the institutions in which they are housed, to monitor their applications and to determine their appropriate usage and therapeutic effectiveness.

The Gynecologic Laser Society has prepared the following recommendations for hospital laser programs. Each laser surgeon should obtain appropriate and adequate training in laser surgery. Laser privileges should be issued only to those trained surgeons demonstrating proficiency with the laser instrument. Therefore, one-to-one training with a knowledgeable laser surgeon is suggested. This one-to-one training is believed to be necessary to guide the new surgeon with actual case performance. A minimum of five cases should be completed, or a sufficient number of cases to demonstrate the surgeon's capabilities. The instructor should then give, in writing, a certificate of completion and/or a letter stating that the physician has successfully completed this course. Today, the Gynecologic Laser Society has undertaken this instructional task.

Finally, it is encumbent upon each new laser institution to consider the following minimal criteria before a surgeon is given laser privileges:

1. Certificate of completion of Basic and Advanced Colposcopy Course
2. Certificate of membership in the American Society for Colposcopy and Cervical Pathology
3. Certificate of training under the auspices of the Gynecologic Laser Society

In addition, the following requirements are recommended:

1. Preoperative histologic diagnosis be present in the chart
2. Periodic review by a medical audit committee to evaluate persistence and recurrence rates of precancerous lesions
3. Documentation and careful case follow-up

These requests may seem strenuous, but, in view of our frequent encounters with the legal profession, we feel these precautions should be an adequate demonstration of our continued concern for our patients and for ourselves.

Today, courses sanctioned by the Gynecologic Laser Society are available. Interested physicians and paramedical personnel should write the current president (or his secretary), or:

Joseph H. Bellina, M.D., Ph.D.
Former President and Founder
Gynecologic Laser Society
3439 Kabel Drive, Suite 7
New Orleans, Louisiana 70114

These seminars are structured to include biophysics, instrumentation, and patient care. Most seminars include hands-on training.

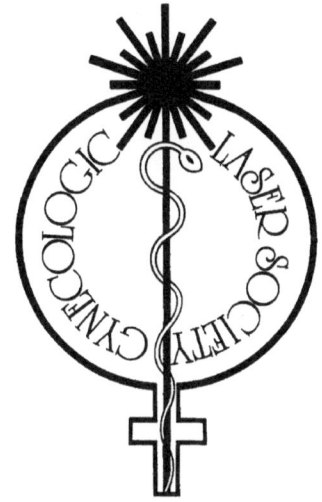

Gynecologic Laser Society emblem.

F

Societies

Listed below are some of the currently active agencies that are using lasers in medicine:

1. Gynecologic Laser Society
   500 Blue Hills Avenue
   Hartford, Connecticut 06112
2. American Society of Laser Medicine and Surgery
   425 Pine Ridge Boulevard
   Suite 203
   Wausau, Wisconsin 54401
3. International Society of Lasers in Surgery and Medicine
   William Aronoff, MD
   Medical Towers Building
   712 North Washington
   Dallas, Texas 75246
4. Italian Society for Laser Surgery and Biomedical Applications
   R. Pariente
   Rome University School of Medicine
   Department of Plastic Surgery
   Policlinico Umberto I
   00161 Rome, Italy
5. Laser Center of Medical Application of the National Research Council
   National Cancer Institute
   Via Venezia 1
   20133 Milan, Italy

Internationally, notably in Japan, Germany, England, and France, new societies that are dedicated to laser medicine have been formed. Soon we expect all countries involved in laser medicine to have their own societies. Each society has annual or biannual meetings. The exact place and time of year vary from country to country. Currently there are more than 1000 surgeons performing laser surgery in all fields of medicine.

The laser is gaining acceptance as a surgical tool by surgeons in all disciplines. As this energy transfer system is explored and tested, its potential application in medicine increases. In gynecology, the laser is being used increasingly and with much success by colposcopists in the management of neoplastic disease of the external genitalia.

Tissue ablation is accomplished both through excision and vaporization procedures. The several advantages of this mode over conventional surgery and cryotherapy include:

1. An unobstructed operating field
2. Cauterization and coagulation of small vascular channels thereby preventing bleeding (which may also aid in preventing metastasis)
3. Minimal damage to adjacent normal tissue and subsequently reduced postoperative sequelae
4. Reduced cost to patients in many instances
5. The lowest recurrence rate (i.e., *highest success rate*) of all standard treatments

Gynecologists employing the molecular gas laser, principally the carbon dioxide laser, have recently formed a professional association, the Gynecologic Laser Society, to serve as a forum for the exchange of information between clinicians and researchers working with the laser. Physicists, laser manufacturers, biomedical engineers, and other interested parties are also invited to participate in the society by becoming associate members and/or by attending the various tutorial seminars and congresses sponsored by the society.

The society is also establishing an international registry of detailed information on etiology, diagnosis, treatment, and outcome, based on patients with gynecologic neoplastic diseases who are treated using the carbon dioxide laser. The society hopes to aid physicians in improving the quality of medical care for their patients by monitoring laser applications and treatment complications, determining the efficacy of this treatment, providing a peer review mechanism, and following up patients. The registry will also serve as a research and teaching data base for continuing education within the society and assistance in preparation of the publications by the members.

G

Publications

Lasers in Surgery and Medicine, published by Alan R. Liss, Inc., New York, is currently the only journal that publishes work exclusively in laser surgery and medicine. The major journals in obstetrics and gynecology lack articles in the fields of gynecologic laser use.

Laser Beam is a newsletter published by the Gynecologic Laser Society that has become a rapid communication system for members of the Society.

Glossary of Laser Terminology

absorption—change of radiant energy to a modified form of energy by inter-action with matter resulting in decrease in power of light passing through a substance.

active medium—the atomic or molecular substance that can provide gain for laser oscillation, often called the laser or lasing medium, or active material.

angstrom (Å)—a unit of length utilized to express wave length or electro-magnetic waves: An angstrom is equal to 10^{-10} m, 10^{-8} cm, 10^{-4} μm, or 10^{-1} nm.

atomic laser—a gas laser in which the medium is of atomic form rather than molecular.

attenuation—the decrease in the radiant flux of an optical beam as it tra-verses an absorbing and/or scattering substance.

axial mode—the mode of frequency of a laser governed primarily by cavity length between the end mirrors, that is, along the cavity length. The mode will have a wavelength which meets the condition that $n\gamma/2 = L$ where γ is the laser wavelength, L is the length between the mirrors, and n is an integer.

beam—a group of light rays that can be parallel, or diverge, or converge.

beam diameter $(1/e^2)$—the diameter of that particular irradiance contour in a laser beam of which the irradiance has fallen to $1/e^2$ (13.5%) of the peak or axial irradiance.

beam divergence—the full angle of the beam spread between diametrically opposed $1/e$ (or $1/e^2$) irradiance points: usually measured in milliradians (1 mrad = 3.4′ of arc).

beam shutter—device used to enclose a laser beam without shutting the laser off.

beam splitter—an optical device which uses controlled reflection to produce two beams from a single incident beam.

beam spot size—the diameter of the laser beam between the $1/e^2$ power points; sometimes used loosely to mean the area of the beam cross section between the $1/e^2$ points.

black body—a body that absorbs all of the incident radiant energy.

bolometer—a radiation detector of thermal type in which absorbed radiation produces a measurable change in the physical property of the sensing element. The change in state is usually that of electrical resistance.

brightness—the power emitted per unit area per unit solid angle ($W/cm^2 \cdot$ sr).

calorie—the quantity of heat required to raise the temperature of 1 g of water by $1\,°C$ (1 cal = 4.184 J).

calorimeter—a device for measuring the total amount of energy absorbed from a source of electromagnetic radiation.

cavity—the device (resonator) that supplies feedback for laser oscillations. The most common form is a laser medium between two reflecting surfaces.

chemical laser—a laser that obtains population inversion directly by a basic chemical reaction.

Class I laser product—any laser, or laser system containing such a laser, that cannot emit laser radiation levels in excess of P_{exempt} or Q_{exempt} for the maximum possible duration inherent in the design of the laser or laser system.

Class II laser product—(1) visible (0.4–0.7 μm) cw laser or laser system which can emit a power exceeding P_{exempt} for the maximum possible duration inherent in the design of the laser or laser system (0.4 μW for emission duration greater than 3×10^4 sec), but not exceeding 1 mW; (2) visible (0.4–0.7 μm) repetitively pulsed laser or laser systems which can emit a power exceeding the appropriate P_{exempt} for the maximum possible duration inherent in the design of the laser or laser system but not P_{exempt} for a 0.25-sec exposure.

Class III laser product—(1) infrared (1.4 μm–1 mm) and ultraviolet (0.2–0.4 μm) laser and laser system which can emit a radiant power in excess of P_{exempt} for the maximum possible duration inherent in the design of the laser or laser system, but cannot emit an average radiant power in excess of 0.5 W for $t_{max} > 0.25$ sec or a radiant exposure of 10 J·cm^{-2} within an exposure time $\leq$ 0.25 sec; (2) visible (0.4–0.7 μm) cw or repetitively pulsed laser or laser system producing a radiant power in excess of P_{exempt} for 0.25-sec exposure (1 mW for a cw laser), but cannot emit an average radiant power greater than 0.5 W; (3) visible and near-infrared (0.4–1.4 μm) single-pulsed lasers which can emit a radiant energy in excess of Q_{exempt}, but which cannot emit a radiant exposure that exceeds 10 J·cm^{-2}; (4) near-infrared (0.7–1.4 μm) cw lasers or single repetitively pulsed lasers which can emit power in excess of P_{exempt} for maximum duration inherent in the design of the laser or laser system, but cannot emit an average power of 0.5 W or greater for periods in excess of 0.25 sec.

Class IV laser product—(1) ultraviolet (0.2–0.4 μm) and infrared (1.4 μm–1 mm) laser and laser systems which emit an average power in excess of 0.5 W for periods greater than 0.25 sec, or a radiant exposure of 10 J·cm^{-2} within an exposure duration of 0.25 sec; (2) visible (0.4–0.7 μm) and near infrared (0.7–1.4 μm) laser and laser systems which emit an average power of 0.5 W or greater for periods greater than 0.25 sec, or a radiant exposure in excess of 10 J·cm^{-2}, or that are required to produce a hazardous diffuse reflection for periods less than 0.25 sec.

coherent light—radiation in which there is a fixed phase relationship between any two points in the electromagnetic field.

collimated beam—a beam of light where the rays are parallel with very small divergence or convergence.

conductivity (thermal)—thermal property of a substance, depending upon the material of which it is made. It is the quantity of heat which flows in unit time through unit area of a layer of the substance of unit thickness with unit difference of temperature between its face [units of (cal·cm)/(cm^2·sec·°C)].

continuous wave (cw)—a laser whose output lasts for a comparatively long uninterrupted time, while the laser is actuated (as compared to a pulsed laser); occasionally, a laser emitting continuously for greater than 0.25 sec.

controlled area—an area where occupancy and activities are controlled and supervised to give protection from optical radiation hazards.

crystal laser—a laser whose active medium is an atomic substance in a crystal, such as ruby.

diffraction-limited—an optical device free of aberrations to a very great extent and limited only by diffraction that unavoidably occurs at the aperture. Diffraction-limited spherical lens in conjunction with a circular aperture will focus a uniform intensity monochromatic light beam to a *spot* (Airy disc) of radius $r = (1.22f\lambda/D)$ where λ equals the wavelength, f equals the focal length of the lens, and D is the lens (or beam) diameter. A laser beam of gaussian intensity variation can be focused to a spot radius of $r = (0.64 f\lambda/D)$ where r is the $1/e^2$ power point.

diffusivity (thermal)—thermal property of a substance depending upon the material of which it is made. It measures the change of temperature which would be produced in unit volume of the substance by the quantity of heat which flows in unit time through unit area of a layer of the substance of unit thickness with unit difference of temperature between its faces (unit of cm^2/sec).

dye laser—a laser for which the medium is an organic dye, usually in solution, with the solution flowing or contained within a cell. Experimental gas dye and solid lasers have been constructed; sometimes called organic dye and tunable dye lasers.

electromagnetic radiation—energy flow formed by vibrating electric and magnetic fields at right angles and lying transverse to the direction of energy. Examples are X rays, ultraviolet light, visible light, infrared radiation, and radio waves, all of which occupy various portions of the electromagnetic spectrum and differ in frequency, wavelength, and energy of a quantum.

electrooptic—describes modulators, Q switches, and other beam control devices that depend on changes in a material's refractive indexes by applying an electrical field. In a Kerr cell, the index variation is proportional to the square of the applied electrical field, with the controlled material generally a liquid. In a pocket cell, the substance is a crystal whose index change varies linearly with the electric field.

emission duration—the temporal duration of a pulse, a series of pulses, or continuous operation, expressed in seconds, during which human access to laser or collateral radiation could be permitted as a result of operation, maintenance, or service of a laser product.

energy(Q)—the capacity for doing work; energy content is commonly used to characterize the output from pulsed lasers, and is generally measured in joules (J).

energy density—the energy per units area expressed in units of joules per square centimeter ($J \cdot cm^{-2}$) (*see* radiant exposure).

error function—a mathematical function defined as:

$$\operatorname{erf}(x) = \frac{2}{\pi} e^{-u^2} \, du$$

exposure—the product of irradiance and the time it lasts.

extinction length—the thickness of the layer of a substance absorbing 90% of the incident radiant energy.

fluorescence—emission of electromagnetic radiation that it is caused by transition from an excited state to the state of molecule or atom. Light emission follows immediately (10^{-6}–10^{-9} sec) the absorption of the exciting radiation. An afterglow of the same or a different wavelength which extend from millisecond to hours or more is called phosphorescence.

focal length—the length between the secondary nodal point of a lens and the primary focal point. For a thin lens, the focal length is the length between the lens and the focal point.

focal point—the focus point toward which light waves converge or from which they diverge or appear to diverge.

gas laser—a laser for which the medium is a gas, of either atomic or molecular form. This laser type is subdivided by medium into atomic (such as helium–neon), molecular (such as carbon dioxide), and ionic (argon, krypton, xenon, and other types such as the metal–vapor helium–cadmium laser). Frequently, "ion" is taken to mean argon or krypton.

gaussian distribution—a frequency distribution curve for a population or collection of variable data, frequently shown as a bell-shaped curve symmetrical about the mean of the data; frequently called normal distribution. A beam having a gaussian irradiance profile is given by an equation of the form $I = I_0 \, e^{-2r^2}/w^2$, where I_0 is the beam centerline irradiance, e is the base of the natural system of logarithms, r is the radius of the contour for irradiance I, and w is the radius of the $1/e^2$ irradiance contour by which beam radius is defined. Both r and w are measured in a plane perpendicular to the beam.

infrared radiation—electromagnetic radiation the wavelengths for which are within the spectrum range of 0.7 μm to 1 mm. This portion of the spectrum is often separated into three bands by wavelength: IR–A (0.7–1.4 μm), or near infrared; IR–B (1.4–3 μm); and IR–C (3 μm–1 mm), or far infrared.

275

integrated radiance—the radiant energy per unit area of a radiating surface per unit solid angle of emission, stated in joules per square centimeter per steradian $(\mathrm{J \cdot cm^{-2} \cdot sr^{-1}})$.

ion laser—a laser for which the active medium is an ionized gas, such as argon or krypton.

ionizing radiation—radiation that can produce ionization; sufficiently energetic charged particles such as alpha and beta rays, and wave-type radiation such as X rays.

irradiance(E)—the radiant power that falls on a surface divided by the area irradiated, expressed in watts per square centimeter $(\mathrm{W \cdot cm^{-2}})$.

joule (J)—a unit of energy; 1 joule = 1 watt for one second $(\mathrm{W \cdot sec})$ or 10^7 ergs, or 0.239 calorie.

joule/cm^2 (J/cm^2)—a unit of radiant exposure utilized when measuring the amount of energy per unit area of surface or per unit area of a laser beam.

Kerr cell—a beam modulator that uses the Kerr effect. The extent of the modulation varies with the square of the applied electric field (*see* electro-optic).

laser—acronym for light amplification (by) stimulated emission (of) radiation. Lasers generate or amplify electromagnetic oscillations at wavelengths from the far infrared (submillimeter) to the ultraviolet. The laser oscillator needs two basic elements: an amplifying medium and a regeneration or feedback mechanism (resonant cavity). The amplifying medium can be any of a variety of substances, such as a gas, semiconductor, dye solution, etc. Feedback is generally created by two mirrors. The distinctive properties of the resulting electromagnetic oscillations include monochromaticity, extremely high intensity, very small bandwidth, very tight beam divergence, and phase coherence.

laser cavity (optical or resonant cavity)—the enclosed volume (resonator) that enables feedback for laser oscillation and light generation. Frequently, the configuration is formed of two reflecting mirrors, separated by the cavity length, L. The lasing medium is positioned between the end mirrors.

laser safety officer—one who is knowledgeable in the evaluation and control of laser hazards and has authority for supervision of the control of laser hazards.

maser—acronym for a device for radio microwave amplification (by the) stimulated emission (of) radiation. In contrast to a laser which emits light, a maser emits microwave radiation.

maximum permissible exposure (MPE)—the radiant exposure to irradiance of laser radiation that, in accordance with present medical knowledge, is not expected to cause detectable corneal or other bodily injury to an individual at any time during his lifetime.

micrometer (μm)—a length equal to 10^{-6} m or 10,000 nm, often termed micron.

microsecond (μsec)—a unit of time equal to 10^{-6} sec.

millisecond (msec)—a unit of time equal to 10^{-3} sec.

monochromaticity—the condition of containing or generating light of only one wavelength from a range of wavelengths present in a beam.

multimode—output or emission at several frequencies simultaneously, usually closely spaced, where each frequency represents a different mode of laser oscillation in the cavity.

nanometer (nm)—a unit of length equal to 10^{-9} m, 10^{-7} cm, 10^{-3} μm, or 10 Å. The nanometer is beginning to replace the angstrom as the principal unit of electromagnetic wavelength.

nanosecond (nsec)—a unit of time equal to 10^{-9} sec.

optical fiber—a long, thin thread of fused silicon or other transparent substance, used to transmit light.

P_{exempt}—that output power (Q_{exempt} that output energy per pulse) of a laser such that no applicable MPE for exposure of the eye may be exceeded, with or without optical instruments.

picosecond (psec)—a unit of time equal to 10^{-12} sec.

photon—the quantum of electromagnetic energy, equal to the product of Planck's constant and the frequency of the radiation.

power (W)—the time rate at which energy is given off, received, or used in some fashion; expressed in watts or in joules per second.

power, average—with a pulsed laser, the pulse energy (joules) times the frequency of the pulse (Hertz), expressed in watts; as compared to the average power of a pulse.

power density—denotes the power per unit area (e.g., $W \cdot cm^{-2}$) contained in a laser beam, or falling on a given target area (*see* irradiance).

Q switch—a device that exhibits a shutter-type effect which prevents laser emission until it is opened. "Q" denotes the quality factor of the laser's resonant cavity. "Active" Q-switching can be accomplished with kerr or pockels cell, a rotating mirror, rotating prism, or acousto-optic devices. "Passive" Q-switching is accomplished using a saturable absorber substance such as a gas or a dye. In a pulsed laser, a Q switch greatly increases pulse power by lessening pulse duration while maintaining the energy constant.

radian—a unit of angular measure equal to the angle subtended at the center of a circle by an arc whose length is equal to the radius of the circle: 1 radian = 57.3°; 2 radians = 360°. One milliradian (10^{-3} radian) subtends an arc whose length is equal to 1 mm at the distance of 1 m.

radiance (L)—the radiant power per unit area of a radiating surface per unit solid angle of emission expressed in watts per square centimeter per steradian ($W \cdot cm^{-2} \cdot sr^{-1}$).

radiant energy (Q)—the energy given off, received, or used in some manner, in the form of radiation, expressed in joules (J).

radiant exposure (H)—the radiant energy irradiating a portion of a surface divided by the area of that portion, in joules per square centimeter ($J \cdot cm^{-2}$).

radiant power (W)—power given off, received, or used in some fashion, in the form of radiation; the time rate of transfer of radiant energy. Expressed in watts (W). Also called radiant flux.

radiant intensity (I)—radiant power of a source in particular direction; ratio of the radiant flux leaving the source transmitted in a portion of the solid angle containing the given direction, and the portion of the solid angle; expressed in watts per steradian ($W \cdot sr^{-1}$).

reflection—the casting back, turning back, or deviation of radiation following its hitting a surface.

semiconductor laser—a laser formed from an active material that is a semiconductor, which can be a diode or homogeneous. Commercial types are usually diodes in which lasing takes place at the junction of n- and p-type semiconductors, typically gallium aluminum arsenide or gallium arsenide. Homogeneous types are composed of undoped semiconductor material and are energized (pumped) by an electron beam.

specific heat—the specific heat of a substance at temperature (t) is defined as dQ/dT where dQ is the quantity of heat necessary to raise the temperature of unit mass of the substance through the small temperature range from t to $t + dt$ (unit of cal/g·°C).

steradian (sr)—the unit of measure for a solid angle. There are four steradians in a sphere.

stimulated emission—emission (radiation) of electromagnetic energy during a transition from a higher-energy state to a lower-energy state in an activated laser medium. The emission is made possible by the presence of a radiation field (stimulating radiation). The stimulated emission is practically the same in every way (frequency, wavelength, momentum, phase, polarization) to the stimulating radiation.

TEM_{00}—the radiation from a laser operating in the fundamental transverse mode. The energy possesses a gaussian (bell-shaped) distribution. All the emitted energy is in one spot, with no side lobes.

transverse modes—laser cavity oscillation modes which give rise to various irradiance distribution in the output beam. These modes are designated TEM_{mn}, where m and n denote the number of nulls in two orthogonal directions within a plane perpendicular to the cavity axis. TEM stands for transverse electromagnetic, since in these modes both the electric and magnetic field vectors are approximately transverse to the cavity axis.

tunable laser—a laser that allows continuous variation of lase emission across a broad wavelength region. A single laser system can be "tuned" to radiate laser light over a continuous spectrum of wavelengths or frequencies.

ultraviolet radiation—electromagnetic radiation that has wavelength from soft X ray to visible, violet light. The spectral region is frequently categorized into three separate bands by wavelength: UV-A (315–400 nm), UV-B (280–315 nm), and UV-C (200–280 nm). Ultraviolet wavelength is shorter than wavelength for visible radiation.

watt (W)—the unit of power or radiant flux; 1 J/sec.

watt/cm²—a term used as a unit of incident power density or irradiance to express the amount of power per unit area of absorbing surface, or per unit area of a cw laser beam.

wavelength (λ)—the distance between two points in a periodic wave which have the same phase.

Index

Abdominal microsurgery, 187, 201, 205, 210
Abdominal surgery, rats, 91, 92
Abnormal colposcopy, 124
Abnormal Pap, 126
Absorption
  CO_2, 32, 34, 83
  coefficient, 33, 44, 84, 88
  definition, 271
  of energy, 257
  of light, 12
  of photons, 27, 99–102, 103, 104, 107
  of water, 74
Adenocarcinoma, 156, 167
Adenosis, 108, 154, 156, 157, 165, 166, 167
Adhesiolysis, 220
American National Standards Institute, 75
Analgesia, 78
Analysis
  of biophysical parameters, 32
  closed form solution, 90
  cytologic, 82
  of heat transfer, 82, 83, 87, 88, 95, 97, 131
  histologic, 83
  plume emission, 97
  SEM, 84–87

Anesthesia
  diathermy, 149–152
  vaporization, 103–105, 111, 113, 116, 127–128, 130, 136, 139–145, 147, 149, 150, 154–156, 165–168, 177, 181, 188, 257
Animal experiments, 6, 23, 24, 102, 212
Aperture, danger labels, 76
Applications, laser, 1, 7, 23, 112, 146, 149, 151, 153, 154, 171, 264, 268
  gynecologic, 111, 115
  liquid laser, 20
Argon laser
  absorption, 33, 81, 84
  applications, 24
  classification, 77
  nonlinear effects, 106
  power output, 106
  thermal action, 102, 104–106

Beam
  absorption, 83, 88
  definitions, 257, 271
  diameter, 102, 105, 106, 108, 130, 137
  focusing, 104–108, 113
  manipulation, 29–30, 54–61, 128, 130, 131, 169, 190, 191–195, 200, 201, 205
  reflection, 72, 81
  splitter, 30, 67, 191

Bioeffects, 81, 111
Biopsy
  colposcopic, 121, 122, 123, 125, 126, 136
  cone, 2, 127, 128, 137
  forceps, 63, 83, 84
  male, 179
  papilloma, 165
  polyp, 156
Bleeding
  cold knife conization, 151
  control of, 132, 137, 169
  postoperative, 141, 147, 151
  reduced, 84, 137, 147, 152, 187
Bowel
  adhesions, 201, 210
  endometriosis, 204, 205
  evacuation of, 75, 211
Bowen's disease, 171, 172
Bureau of Radiologic Health, 76
Burns
  caused by laser, 72, 74
  treatment of, 2

Calculation—power density, 36
Cannula, 130, 199, 207
Capillary hemangioma, 154
Carbon dioxide laser
  absorption, 32–34, 83–84, 88, 102, 104
  advantages, 149, 151, 166, 168, 187
  applications, 1–3, 23, 111–117, 136, 145,
      154, 157, 160–162, 177, 184–186,
      187–204, 207
  beam manipulation, 29, 54, 61, 62, 167,
      173, 184, 188, 190, 191
  bloodless, 84, 114, 181, 204
  cervical applications, 108, 111, 116–166,
      180, 185
  complications, 151, 152, 156, 165
  condyloma acuminatum, 154–162
  conization, 149, 151, 152, 153, 154, 155
  corneal damage, 73, 197
  DES, 185
  excision, 111, 112, 154
  experiments, 82, 91, 102
  gynecologic surgery, 111–117
  hazards, 71–75, 116, 128
  healing, 84, 87, 107, 108, 113, 131, 135,
      142, 143, 147, 152, 155, 157, 168,
      169, 170, 174, 175, 176

Carbon dioxide laser (*cont.*)
  heat transfer analysis, 32, 82–85, 87, 88,
      91, 95
  herpes, 171, 182
  history, 4, 6
  instrumentation, 2, 27, 71, 108, 187, 188,
      190–199
  laser models, 46, 191
  microscope, 166, 169, 187, 190–191,
      193, 195, 196, 198
  vs. other types of treatment, 149–151,
      167
  physics, 3, 6–8, 31
  power density, 36, 37, 39, 84
  prerequisites, 116
  reconstructive surgery, 169–170, 187, 211
  recurrence rates, 135, 179, 181, 182, 183
  regulations, 70–71
  safety, 21–23, 29, 57–59, 70
  scalpel, 61, 111, 128, 135, 165
  TEM, 36, 40
  vaginal applications, 165–167, 170
  vaporization, 103, 111, 116, 165–167,
      170, 172–177
  vulvar applications, 170–178, 257
  wavelength, 3–5, 16, 20, 21, 32, 36, 43,
      44–45, 72, 75, 81, 84, 97, 279
Carcinogenic laser beam, 75
Carcinoma in situ
  definition, 119, 127
  progression, 119–120, 127
  treatment, 82, 165, 167, 171–174, 177
Cavitron, 46
Cavity, optical, 13–14, 16, 19–20, 27, 31,
    37, 59
Cervical applications, 2, 111
Cervical cancer, 117–118, 131
Cervical conization, 149, 151
Cervical, depth of destruction, 104
Cervical discharge instructions, 259
Cervical incompetence, 152, 155
Cervical intraepithelial neoplasia (CIN)
  adolescent sex and, 116
  defined, 115
  diagnosed, 115, 120, 125, 136
  recurrence rate, 115, 129, 135, 143, 144,
      145–148, 149
  treatment, 82, 115, 116, 123–125, 126,
      127, 130, 140, 141, 144–147

Cervical mucus, 128, 135, 154, 156
Cervical treatments, 114, 116, 117, 122, 127, 130, 148, 150–154, 165, 168, 257
Chromopertubation, 202, 203, 209
Cinefluorography, 200
Classification of disease, 124
Coherent, 46, 191
Coitus, 155, 169, 180, 183
Cold knife, 127, 139, 147, 151–154, 167, 178
Collagen, 85, 102, 103, 108, 135
Colpophotographs, 129
Colposcopy, 121, 122, 125, 126, 149, 154, 155, 165, 169, 171, 178
Columnar epithelium, 119, 140, 143
Computer, 20, 90
Conception, 154, 156, 200
Condyloma acuminatum, 99, 165, 168, 171, 179
Cone biopsy, 2, 127, 128, 131, 137, 139, 141
Conservative treatment, 111, 124, 126, 127
Corneal damage, 73, 197
Cornual reimplantation, 188, 202
Cryosurgery, 124–125, 126, 127, 142, 149, 150, 151, 268
Cytology, 82–83, 117–119

Danocrine, 204
Depth of destruction
    calculating, 33, 82
    CIN, 104, 112, 118, 120, 122–125, 131, 135, 139, 146, 150
    persistence, 146
    vaginal, 157
    vulvar, 172
Dermatology, 24
DES (Diethylstilbestrol), 156
Diagnosis, 118, 121, 124, 125–126, 128, 141, 156, 265, 268
Dosimetry, 44
Dysmenorrhea, 152
Dyspareunia, 150, 152, 166–167
Dysplasia
    cervical, 82
    cytology, 167
    recurrence, 126, 166
    and teenage sex, 115–118
    vaporization, 45, 154, 165, 166

Ectocervix, 118, 125, 127
Ectopic pregnancy, 200, 203, 208
Edema, 149, 174–175, 177, 181
Electrocautery, 166
Endometriosis, 190, 195, 204–206
Energy
    absorption, 32, 81
    conductor, 21
    definition, 31
    density, 27, 31, 81, 102
    distribution, 37, 88
    formula, 39
    levels, 3, 8–13, 19–21
    requirements, 106
    shift, 21
    transfer, 1
Enzyme, 20
Epidermoid, 184
Epithelial cells, 82, 85–87, 128, 142, 170, 180
Estrogen, 206
Excision
    margins, 112, 124, 130, 135
    Nd–YAG, 34
    uterine defects, 206
Excitation, 4, 10, 12–14, 16–17, 21, 27
Experiments, 1, 7, 75, 82, 88, 91, 93, 97, 101–102
Extinction length, 33, 90, 275

Failure rate, 150–151, 177
Fallopian tubes, 202, 207–208
Fertility, 116, 152, 154–157
Fiber delivery system, 24
Fimbrioplasty, 188, 201
Fire regulations, 78
Fluoroscopy, 200
Fluorouracil, 168, 178, 181
Follow-up, 117, 127, 142, 143, 145–148, 150, 167, 168, 177
Food and Drug Administration, 76, 263
Future, 70, 76

Gastroenterology, 24
Gaussian curve, 94
Genital tract, 2, 178
Geometry, 107
Granulation tissue, 143, 167, 168, 169
Green's function, 90–91

Gynecologic Laser Society, 264, 268, 269
Gynecologic surgery, 2, 6, 7, 46, 67, 112, 188, 257, 263, 268, 269

Hazards, 71, 116, 128, 273, 276
Healing
  condyloma acuminatum, 168
  cytology, 82, 87–97, 117–120, 155
  intra-abdominal, 187
  time, 11, 111, 148, 149, 150, 168, 173, 175, 257, 260
  vaginal surgery, 165–167
Helium–neon laser, 6, 29–31, 44, 191
Hemangioma, 154, 171
Hemostasis, 137, 143, 148, 187, 206, 207, 210
Herpes, 171, 181, 182
Histology, 82–83, 121, 125, 203, 264
History of lasers, 7, 115, 116
Hydrocortisone, 200
Hysterectomy, 2, 127, 136, 149, 151, 152
Hysterosalpingogram, 155, 199, 200, 206, 208

Incision
  CO_2 laser for, 81, 83, 201, 210
  depth of, 104, 111, 116
  speed of, 36, 44, 84, 111, 113, 136
Infrared light, 4, 25, 44, 74–75, 84, 257, 273, 274, 275
Instrumentation, 2, 27, 71, 197, 265
Intra-abdominal applications, 199, 187–201
Intrauterine applications, 203, 204, 206, 208

Laparoscopy, 155, 199, 205
Laser beam
  ablation, 37, 45, 149, 156
  absorption, 11, 12–13, 33–34, 44, 83
  applications, 1, 71, 112, 127, 136, 188
  argon, 23, 33–35, 102
  burns, 72–74
  carbon dioxide, 35, 39, 75, 81, 83–84, 106, 168, 173, 174
  classification, 23, 33–34
  conization, 115, 121, 127
  danger sign, 76–77
  definition, 276

Laser beam (*cont.*)
  depth of destruction, 34, 39, 45, 82, 146
  heat transfer, 23, 82, 83–85, 88, 95
  hemostasis, 137, 143, 148, 206
  manipulation, 29–30, 54–61, 190–193, 197, 200
  Nd-YAG, 34, 81
  physics, 3, 6–8, 31, 44, 201
  power density, 36–40, 41, 45, 74, 105, 106, 113, 130, 132, 136, 188, 201
  rat experiments, 91, 92
  reflection, 72, 74
  safety, 70–77
  thermal injury, 71–74, 83, 201
  vaporization, 35, 97–98, 103–105, 113, 149, 257
  wavelength, 3–5, 16, 19, 20–21, 23, 32–34, 42–44
Laser irradiation, 23, 98, 102
Laser systems, 20, 21–24, 27, 46, 59, 97
Laser–tissue interaction, 54, 116, 179, 180, 181
Laser treatment
  cervical, 115, 117–128, 135, 141–144, 188
  condyloma acuminatum, 171, 178–181
  vaginal, 156–157, 165–171
  vulvar, 170–172, 173–177
Lesion
  cervical, 2, 117–121, 122–127, 149
  condyloma acuminatum, 154, 165–168
  dysplastic, 45
  malignant, 75, 154
  margins, 124, 137, 143
  recurrence/persistence, 128, 135
  vaginal, 165–168
  vulvar, 170–174, 176–178
Lugol's solution, 66, 128, 131, 166

Maser, 6, 7, 276
Maximum power density, 44–45, 209, 210
Melanoma, 24
Methylprednisolone sodium, 177
Micromanipulator, 7, 62, 131, 136, 190–191, 192–195, 200
Microscope, 2, 6, 23, 29–30, 61, 67, 72, 91, 169–170, 173, 187–193, 197–200, 208, 210, 215–255, 257

Microsurgery
  instrumentation, 29, 61, 75, 187, 190–197
  procedures
    adhesiolysis, 200
    cornual reimplantation, 202
    fimbrioplasty, 201
    linear salpingostomy, 203
    salpingostomy, 201
    septal defects, 206
    tubal reanastomosis, 202
  techniques, 120, 206, 210
Mode
  continuous, pulsed, 7, 59, 147, 272, 273
  cutting, 203
  TEM, 37, 40–44, 70, 81, 90
  zoom, 192
Multicentric, 121, 151, 154

Necrosis, 23, 84, 88, 97, 107–108, 149–150, 201
Neodymium-YAG laser, 6, 7, 21, 23, 25, 33–81
Neoostia, 201, 203
Neoplasia, 112, 113–116, 120–122, 135, 155, 167, 168, 171, 172, 178, 268
Neurodermatitis, 171
Neurosurgery, 23, 25
Nitrogen, 19, 27, 61, 195
N-layer, 88

Oncogenic, 98–99
Oncology, 25
Operating room
  instrumentation, 23, 63, 67, 187–190, 195–197
  personnel, 66, 72
Ophthalmology, 7, 23, 24, 261
Otolaryngology, 24, 261
Ovary, 188, 209

Pain, minimal, 74, 84, 112, 123, 137, 148
Papilloma, 99, 124, 165, 178
Papovavirus tumors, 99
Patient information brochure, 257
Patient preparation, 116, 127, 128
Patient safety, 70, 77
Pelvic infection, 142, 148

Pelvic surgery, 187, 204
Persistent disease, 135, 143, 146, 150, 169
Photon, 3–5, 19, 24, 27, 97, 99, 101–102, 277
Physics, 3, 5–6
Physiology, 187
Postoperative care
  CIN, 116–120, 155
  condyloma acuminatum, 180–181
  herpes, 183
  vaginal, 167, 168
  vulvar, 172–176
Power density
  argon, 106
  basic concepts, 112, 116, 128
  calculation, 36–37, 39, 43–45
  defined, 277
  for procedures, 74, 84, 131–136, 154–156, 166–167, 170, 173–174, 200–210
Precautions, 74, 264
Pregnancy
  cervical incompetence, 152
  condyloma acuminatum in, 178
  ectopic, 200, 203, 208
  high risk, 149
  mucosal, depth in, 121
  rate, 211
  test, 200, 204
Premature labor, 151, 152
Pruritus, 172

Radiation absorption, 33–34, 81
Radiation detection, 272
Radiation, stimulated emission, 1, 3, 5, 6, 20
Reconstructive microsurgery, 187, 203, 204, 211
Recording system, 63, 67, 190, 192, 198
Rectum, 127, 259, 260, 179
Recurrence rate
  cervical disease, 148, 150, 264
  condyloma acuminatum, 178, 180–181
  depth of destruction, 168
  vaginal disease, 175
  vulvar disease, 178
Registry, Gynecologic Laser Society, 267
Regulations, 70, 76–78

Retina, 4, 73
Retractor, 137, 210
Ruby laser, 6, 7, 21, 23–24, 27
Rules of application, 21, 70–71, 131, 136

Safety, 23, 29, 57, 59, 70–72, 75–78
Salpingolysis, 188
Salpingostomy, 188, 201, 203
Scalpel, 61, 111, 128, 132, 183, 195, 206
Scanning electron microscope, 82, 84–85,
    87–88, 97
Scar formation, 88, 142, 148, 167, 170
Silver nitrate, 141, 142, 148
Sitz bath, 176, 260
Sloughing, 149–150, 165, 175
Sperm, 154–156, 169
Squamous epithelium, 82, 83, 85, 119, 124,
    139, 142, 178
Standards, safety, 70–72, 76
Stromal necrosis, 97
Success, 116, 122, 150, 157
Surgical precautions, 72
Surgical procedures, 7, 113, 151, 188, 209,
    212
Succinate, hydrocortisone, 200

TEM
    defined, 279
    modification, 41, 70
    significance, 40–41
    vaporization, 23, 81
Thermal injury, 72, 175
Thymidine, 99
Tissue absorption, 34, 81, 83, 93, 101
Tissue destruction
    depth of, 39, 113, 121, 174–175, 177,
        181
    increased, 174
    preventing, 148
Tissue healing, 83, 87, 97, 107
Tissue, histologic analysis, 82–84
Tissue injury, 72, 74, 150, 167, 170, 200–
    201, 211
Tissue removal, 1–2, 34, 83, 149, 155–156,
    210

Tissue vaporization, 67, 81, 84
Transformation zone, 121, 124, 130, 131,
    145, 150, 152, 180
Transverse vaginal septum, 169
Trypan blue, 98
Tumor, 2, 7, 24, 75, 98, 99, 108, 112, 113,
    153, 154, 166

Ultrasound, 204, 206
Uridine, 99
Urology, 24
Uterine anomalies, 155–156, 206

Vaginal adenosis, 154, 156, 157, 165
Vaginal lesions, 165
Vaginal treatment, 166–169, 175, 179, 210,
    257, 259
Vaporization
    argon, 103–106
    cervical, 97, 127, 131, 154–155, 257
    depth of, 103, 111, 155
    incision, 81
    plume emissions, 75, 97
    results, 101, 172
    vaginal, 165–167, 170
    vulvar, 172–173
Venereal disease, 170
Virus, 99, 182–183
Vulvar applications, 112, 165, 170–176,
    257
Vulvar condyloma acuminatum, 171
Vulvar dystrophy, 167, 172, 174
Vulvectomy, 171, 173, 174, 176

Wavelength
    absorption, 32–35, 74, 97
    argon, 24
    carbon dioxide laser, 44, 72, 84, 103–105
    definition, 279
    of different lasers, 19–20, 21, 23, 33
    principles, 16, 44, 81, 274, 275

X ray, 4–5, 274

Zeiss, 67, 190, 195, 215–255